Geropsychiatric Nursing

❖ *Geropsychiatric Nursing*

SECOND EDITION

Edited by

Mildred O. Hogstel, Ph.D., R.N., C.

Emeritus Professor of Nursing
Harris College of Nursing
Texas Christian University
Fort Worth, Texas

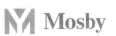 Mosby

St. Louis Baltimore Berlin Boston Carlsbad Chicago London Madrid
Naples New York Philadelphia Sydney Tokyo Toronto

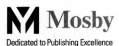
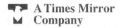

Managing Editor: Jeff Burnham
Associate Developmental Editor: Linda Caldwell
Project Manager: Peg Fagen
Editing and Production: Graphic World Publishing Services

SECOND EDITION

Printed in the United States of America

Composition by Graphic World, Inc.
Printing and Binding by R. R. Donnelley

Mosby–Year Book, Inc.
11830 Westline Industrial Drive
St. Louis, Missouri 63146

Library of Congress Cataloging-in-Publication Data

Geropsychiatric nursing/edited by Mildred O. Hogstel.—2nd ed.
    p.   cm.
    Includes bibliographical references and index.
    ISBN 0-8016-7811-0
    1. Aged—Mental health. 2. Aged—Care. 3. Geriatric psychiatry.
  4. Geriatric nursing. I. Hogstel, Mildred O.
    [DNLM: 1. Geriatric Nursing. 2. Psychiatric Nursing. 3. Mental
Disorders—in old age—Nurses' instruction. WY 152 G37778 1995]
RC451.4.A5G485 1995
610.73′65—dc20
DNLM/DLC
for Library of Congress   94-22935
                                         CIP

95   96   97   98   99   /   9   8   7   6   5   4   3   2   1

*In loving memory of
my parents, brother, and grandparents*

❖ *Contributors*

Marta Askew Browning, M.S.N., R.N.
Assistant Professor of Nursing
Department of Nursing
Temple University College of Allied Health Professions
Philadelphia, Pennsylvania

Kathleen C. Buckwalter, Ph.D., R.N., F.A.A.N.
Professor and Associate Director
University of Iowa College of Nursing
Iowa City, Iowa

Janis M. Campbell, Ph.D., R.N.
Associate Professor of Nursing
The University of Akron College of Nursing
Akron, Ohio

Gail Hamilton, Ph.D., R.N.
Associate Professor of Nursing
Temple University College of Allied Health Professions
Philadelphia, Pennsylvania

Mary S. Harper, Ph.D., R.N., F.A.A.N.
Coordinator, Long Term Care Programs
Mental Disorders of Aging Research Branch
U.S. Department of Health and Human Services
National Institute of Mental Health
Rockville, Maryland

Mildred O. Hogstel, Ph.D., R.N., C.
Emeritus Professor of Nursing
Harris College of Nursing
Texas Christian University
Fort Worth, Texas

Maisie Schmidt Kashka, Ph.D., R.N.
Associate Professor
College of Nursing
Texas Women's University
Denton, Texas

Anne Langston Lind, M.S., R.N.
Assistant Professor
Harris College of Nursing
Texas Christian University
Fort Worth, Texas

Edward A. Luke, Jr., D.O.
Fort Worth Family Institute
Geriatric Services
Fort Worth, Texas

M. Kathryn Nichols, M.S.N., R.N., C.S.
Emeritus Associate Professor of Nursing
Harris College of Nursing
Texas Christian University
Fort Worth, Texas

Brenda Riley, D.S.N., R.N.
Associate Professor
Troy State University
Troy, Alabama

Jacqueline M. Stolley, M.A., R.N., C.
Research Associate and Doctoral Student
University of Iowa College of Nursing
Iowa City, Iowa

Sandra Helene Tweed, Ph.D., R.N., C.A.R.N.
Assistant Professor
School of Nursing
State University of New York at Buffalo
Buffalo, New York

Joan Wagner, M.S.N., M.A., R.N., C.
Vice President, Nursing Systems
Geriatric Medical Care
Knoxville, Tennessee

Kay Weiler, M.A., J.D., R.N.
Assistant Professor
University of Iowa College of Nursing
Iowa City, Iowa

❖ *Reviewers*

Geri Richards Hall, M.A., R.N., C.S.
Gerontology Clinical Nursing Specialist II
Department of Nursing
The University of Iowa
Iowa City, Iowa

Barbara Kupchak, Ph.D., R.N., C.
Assistant Professor of Nursing
West Virginia University
Morgantown, West Virginia

Judith R. Lentz, M.S.N., M.A., R.N.
Doctoral Candidate, Rice University
Houston, Texas
Adjunct Instructor, School of Nursing
St. Louis University
St. Louis, Missouri

❖ *Preface*

Caring for the specific mental health problems and needs of older adults is now recognized as a subspecialty in the field of gerontological nursing. Still, the large majority of older people who have mental health problems are not being identified, evaluated, or treated. This is especially true for those older people who are residing in nursing homes and those who are isolated in their homes in the community. Too often, confusion, disorientation, depression, paranoid behavior, and other mental and emotional problems of older people have been blamed on "just getting old," both by older people themselves and by health care professionals. Therefore, many older people have not been diagnosed and treated for their mental health problems, thus decreasing the quality, and sometimes the length, of their lives.

The purpose of this book is to help nurses and others who care for and about older people to become more aware of the special mental health problems and care of older adults.

This book is intended for practicing nurses in psychiatric nursing, gerontological nursing, community health nursing, and medical-surgical nursing, as well as nurses who work in hospitals, nursing homes, home health care agencies, adult day care centers, outpatient clinics, day surgery centers, and retirement centers. Social workers, recreational therapists, and activity directors who work with older adults will also find much helpful information in the book. This book will also be useful for nursing students enrolled in courses in each of the above clinical fields, because they all care for older people with possible mental and emotional problems.

Chapter 1 presents an overview of geropsychiatric nursing by a nurse who started working with mentally ill older patients in the 1940s. She discusses the development of the field up to the current time and lists some challenging research ideas. Chapter 2 reminds the reader that one of the primary goals of nursing is to help maintain and promote mental health in all older people. Chapter 3 discusses the human and physical resources and standards now available and those needed for the future in geriatric psychiatry and geropsychiatric nursing. The need for a total assessment—physical, functional, social, emotional, environmental, and mental—is presented in Chapter 4. Clinical applications and precautions needed in using the most important psychotropic drugs with older adults are summarized by a geriatric psychiatrist in Chapter 5.

Chapters 6 through 9 are devoted to the most common mental health problems found in the older population: depression; cognitive disorders, particularly Alzheimer's disease; schizophrenia, especially paranoid behavior and paraphrenia; and substance-related disorders, with emphasis on alcohol abuse and polypharmacy. Each of these chapters has a sample nursing care plan for the major problems discussed.

Chapter 10, new in this edition, presents a recent trend: that of inpatient geropsychiatric nursing in a general hospital, where the *physical* and *mental health* problems and needs of older persons can be assessed and treated on an interdisciplinary basis.

Chapter 11 focuses on the varied mental health problems of older adults in nursing homes and provides many specific practical nursing interventions useful when caring for those residents with behavioral and mental problems. Chapter 12 concentrates on the care of mentally ill older people in the home, with special emphasis on the problems and needs of family caregivers. Chapter 13 discusses a variety of community resources available to help older people maintain or regain their mental health. A new section in this chapter addresses legal issues important for older persons and their families to consider when cognitive changes affect the older person's ability to make choices and decisions.

The Appendixes are quite extensive, and include assessment guides and tools; psychiatric diagnoses most common in older adults as adapted from the 1994 *Diagnostic and Statistical Manual of Mental Disorders,* fourth edition, American Psychiatric Association; guidelines to reduce environmental stimuli in patients with Alzheimer's disease; and a list of additional geropsychiatric resources such as agencies, organizations, and publications.

I wish to express my thanks to each of the contributing authors who gave of their time and expertise to help make this second edition possible. I also appreciate the assistance of typists Susan Moore and Esther Ochoa and the many small but important ways Terry Sheridan helped.

Nurses and others who work with and care for older adults in any setting have a responsibility and unique challenge to identify, assess, assist, and refer clients with mental and behavioral problems to appropriate services and facilities for treatment and care so that they may have the opportunity to live life to the fullest for as long as possible.

Mildred O. Hogstel

❖ Contents

❖ Detailed Contents

## Chapter 1

❖ *An Overview of Mental Health and Older Adults*

Mary S. Harper

The older adult population is increasing and will continue to increase significantly in the United States. In the United States 5700 people celebrated their 65th birthday each day in 1992, which means that about 2.1 million people are added to the older population each year. This age group numbered 32.3 million in 1992. They represent 12.7% of the United States population. From 2010 to 2030, the older population will grow 73% while the population under age 65 decreases almost 3%. By the year 2040 there may be more people aged 65 or older than persons under 20 years of age. The fastest growing age groups are those 85 years old, the poor, and minority elders.

Minority populations are projected to constitute 25% of the older population in 2030, up from 13% in 1990. Between 1990 and 2040 the Caucasian population aged 65 and older is projected to increase by 93%, compared with 328% for minorities. At present there are 3.3 million persons 85 years of age—26 times as many as in 1900. There were 6.9 million aged 80 and older in 1990, and this population will grow to more than 25 million by 2050 (1 in 12 will be 80). The centenarian groups more than doubled during the 1980s. In 1990 100-year-olds numbered 35,808 (*A Profile*, 1993; U.S. Bureau of the Census, 1992).

Today in the United States, for the first time the average family has more parents than children at home. It is not uncommon for people aged 60 and over to be caring for parents aged 80 to 100 or more. The stress of the "36-hour day" leads them to develop emotional problems, disturbances of the immune system, and increased dependency on alcohol and psychotropic drugs (Lebowitz & Light, 1992; American Association of Colleges of Nursing, 1993). Although older people represent 13% of the U.S. population, they account for over 30% of the health care expenditures and use over half of the acute and chronic hospital beds in the nation (Miller & Kelman, 1992).

❖ *Definitions of Health and Mental Illness*

Health for older people can be defined as the ability to live and function effectively in society and to exercise self-reliance and autonomy to the maximum extent feasible, but not necessarily total freedom from disease. Mental illness can occur at any time when a cluster of behavioral signs and symptoms come together and disrupt the individual's ability to function effectively in a family, home, or community.

❖ *Profile of the Mental Health of Older Adults*

Psychopathology increases with age. Older adults have disproportionately more psychiatric disorders, behavioral stress, and adjustment problems than younger adults at a time when their quality of life should be the best. The incidence of suicide and functional disorders, for example, depression and paranoid states, increases with age. Organic brain diseases increase after age 60 and the suicide rate is four times higher for the older Caucasian man than it is for younger adults (Osgood & Brant, 1991; Riley, 1994; Wasylenki, 1982).

Depression occurs in 10% to 15% of individuals over the age of 65 and 10% to 20% of the population over age 60 (Branconnier, 1980; Ruegg, Zisook, & Swerdlow, 1988). Also, the prevalence of depression in medically ill older people is 20% to 35% (Ruegg, Zisook, & Swerdlow, 1988).

In a survey and screening of patients admitted to a large surgical unit at an academic medical center, the researchers found that 60% of those admitted to the hospital had diagnosable psychiatric disorders. From a review of the records, 2% to 10% of the patients admitted had been diagnosed with common psychiatric disorders (Strain, 1977). The most common diagnosis was delirium. With more than 200,000 hip fractures occurring annually in the United States, it seems appropriate to staff such a surgical ward with a geropsychiatric clinical nurse specialist.

There are 16,000 Medicare-Medicaid eligible nursing homes in the United States with 1.6 million older people. In one survey it was reported that 843,000 residents have a mental, social, behavioral, or emotional disorder, but only 2% have contact with a mental health professional. It was estimated that 51% have dementia, 4% schizophrenia, and 11% other mental disorders. With this number of mentally ill older people, the nursing home should be the primary provider of mental health services for this group (Burns, et al., 1993; Harper, 1986). In 1990 the Department of Veterans Affairs, in a study of its nursing homes, revealed that 72% of all residents had a primary or associated psychiatric diagnosis (Kelly & Urquhart, 1993).

In a study of 9,000 noninstitutionalized older persons, Regier et al. (1984) did not find a statistically significant number of psychiatric problems such as schizophrenia, panic disorders, personality disorders, or substance abuse; however, they did find that 14% of the subjects were cognitively impaired, with depression and dementia of the Alzheimer's type.

❖ *Factors Affecting the Mental Health of the Older Population*

Nocturnal sleep tends to change with age. Older people do not sleep with the same efficiency as young adults. Some 30% to 50% of older people have chronic sleep disturbance, which commonly results in the use of sleeping medications, reduced quality of life, and increased morbidity and mortality. Consequently, the combination of altered sleep, sleep pathologies, and pharmacology in aging results in higher risk of drug-induced insomnia and excessive daytime sleepiness (Webb, 1989).

There are 11 million people with diabetes in the United States, and 38% are over 65 years of age. The most common atypical finding of diabetes mellitus in older adults is an alteration in mentation (confusion, delirium, dementia, depression, cognitive impairment, and memory impairment, particularly in non–insulin dependent diabetes mellitus [NIDDM]). Many symptoms associated with both hyperglycemia and hypoglycemia have been found to be more closely related to depressive mood than to the level of glycemic control (Lustman, Clouse, & Carney, 1988; Tun, Nathan, & Perlmuter, 1990).

For millions of older people, the greatest threats to health and well-being are not cancer and heart disease but anxiety, stress, loneliness, social isolation, depression, fear of abandonment, abuse, and poverty. In 1992, 29% of noninstitutionalized persons aged 65 and older assessed their health as fair to poor, compared with 7% for persons under age 65. There was little difference between the sexes, but African-American older people were much more likely to rate their health as fair or poor (44%) than were older Caucasians (28%).

Some older people say that their health is good or fair although they have four or five diagnosable conditions. Older people generally have an enormous pool of tolerated illnesses and/or psychopathology at any one time that has been denied, ignored, underreported, or not diagnosed or treated. One of the problems frequently observed with African-American elders is their delay in seeking care and treatment. The health care system relies on the patient to initiate care, and that is precisely what older people do not do. This problem makes undetected decline likely among many frail older people.

These are some of the unique problems relating to the mental health of older adults:

◆ Multiple pathologies (comorbidity)
◆ Atypical or nonspecific presentation of illness
◆ Delay in reporting problems

◆ Underreporting of symptoms
◆ Polypharmacy

Another factor predisposing older individuals to decline because of late detection of illness is the clustering of diseases in this age group. Surveys of community-dwelling older people have found on average nearly five important disabilities per person, and surveys of those in institutions have found more than double this figure. Some of the most common problems that coexist in older people include the following:

◆ Substance abuse and mental illness
◆ Diabetes and depression
◆ Selected cancers and depression
◆ Sleep disturbances and substance abuse
◆ Hypertension and diabetes
◆ Myocardial infarct and diabetes
◆ Dementia and depression

In a medical outcome study of 9,386 people, 844 (9.4%) had diabetes mellitus. Of these diabetic patients 33% were depressed, 56.9% also had hypertension, 36% had arthritis, and 10.3% had congestive heart failure. It is a challenge to treat and coordinate the complex array of physical, psychological, economic, and social problems of an older person with diabetes (Froom, 1990). A nurse practitioner in New York described her nurse-managed diabetic clinic as a depression clinic because over 50% of the diabetic patients were also clinically depressed.

Older people often present their illness atypically. Many who have fecal impaction will be confused or delirious; myocardial infarction commonly presents as shortness of breath without the typical chest pain; and hypothyroidism may present as apathy and cachexia. Pneumonia may present as anorexia and acute confusional state with normal pulse, no elevation of temperature, and no rise in white blood cell count. Transient ischemic attacks may present as acute confusional state or falls. Urinary tract infections may present as an acute confusional state with absence of pyrexia and no rise in white blood cell count, incontinence, or general slowness (Gambert, 1990).

It is important, therefore, for the geropsychiatric nurse to remember that virtually any disease with a classic complex of symptoms or signs in old age frequently shows few or none of the characteristic findings. The classic presentation is often replaced by one or more nonspecific symptoms. The most common are refusal to eat or drink, falling, incontinence, dizziness, acute confusion, weight loss, disturbance of gait, restlessness, agitation, insomnia, and failure to thrive.

Because of the comorbidity, atypical presentation of illness, delay in reporting and underreporting symptoms, and polypharmacy of older persons in addition to psychopathology, the specially trained geropsychiatric nurse is essential.

❖ *Major Mental Health Problems*

The major mental health problems of older persons reported by providers and researchers Liptzin (1986), Ouslander (1982), Harper (1987), Gurland (1982), and Matteson and McConnell (1988) include the following:

- ◆ Delirium
- ◆ Dementia
- ◆ Depression
- ◆ Agitation
- ◆ Emotional problems associated with poor physical health
- ◆ Crying spells
- ◆ Irritability
- ◆ Pacing
- ◆ Wandering
- ◆ Assaultiveness
- ◆ Expressions of feelings of unworthiness, hopelessness
- ◆ Diminished memory, orientation, and judgment
- ◆ Apathy
- ◆ Withdrawal
- ◆ Suicidal impulses and/or attempts
- ◆ Loneliness/lonesomeness
- ◆ Paranoid delusions
- ◆ Demanding behavior
- ◆ Anxiety disorders
- ◆ Alcohol abuse
- ◆ Impaired concentration
- ◆ Short attention span
- ◆ Tendencies to hoard personal items, including feces
- ◆ Stress incontinence
- ◆ Disorientation

Emotional reactions to hospitalization or entry into a long-term care facility are significant in all age groups but may be more intense in older adults. Anxiety, depression, agitation, and disorientation are emotional reactions that can result from fears of hospitalization, diagnostic testing, the outcome of diagnostic testing and treatment, or hospital routine. Admission to a hospital often signals impending death, and this fear is heightened with the daily routines of the hospital such as blood drawing, specimen collecting, and attitudes of staff providers and occasionally the family. The hospital can induce feelings of helplessness, role loss, status loss, dependency, and isolation. Meaningful relationships may be jeopardized by limited visiting hours. This deprivation emphasizes an alienation process inherent in hospitalization. Older patients who are left alone for periods of time often complain of ill-defined malaise that can progress quickly to confusion (Matteson & McConnell, 1988).

❖ *Mental Health Care by Nonpsychiatric Physicians*

Primary care physicians are the primary providers of mental health services to older adults. According to Schurman and Mitchell (1985), nonpsychiatric physicians (NPP) provided over 7.8 million mental illness visits for patients age 65 or over between 1979 and 1981 and provided 80% of the ambulatory mental health care. NPPs are responsible for four out of six office visits by older patients who require mental health services. Access to the private psychiatrist for older adults did not change measurably between 1974 and 1981. Only 6% of the users of community mental health centers (CMHC) are older clients. This rate has not changed significantly in the past 10 years (Flemming, Buchanan, Santos, & Richards, 1984; Schurman & Mitchell, 1985).

Although older people may be present in a multiagency program or facility that offers primary health care, psychiatric services, podiatry, visual screening, cancer detection, or ecological care in the same setting, older adults frequently will not use the CMHC. Instead they visit a nonmental health professional for mental health services.

In many instances the CMHC may not have staff members who are specialized or interested in mental health services for older clients. Lack of funds and the stigma often associated with mental illness are other reasons that older adults seek NPP care. This situation presents a challenge for the geropsychiatric nurse.

❖ *Geropsychiatric Nursing*

Historical Evolution

Gerontological nursing was formalized as a specialty in 1966, although the need for a gerontological nursing specialty was identified as early as 1900. Between 1900 and 1950 widowed and retired nurses cared for the aged in board-and-care homes (McConnell, 1988). The first gerontological nursing textbook was published in 1950 (Newton, 1950). Like many nursing texts of that era, the material was long on aphorism and short on scientific rationale. During this period nursing research was concerned with chronic disease, and the older population began to grow (Mack, 1952).

A search of the literature on nursing, gerontological nursing, and psychiatric nursing revealed that Dorothy Schwartz was the first nurse to publish a book concerned with psychosocial needs of older ambulatory patients (Schwartz, Henley, & Zeitz, 1964). These nursing activities, the increased political action generated to establish governmental health insurance for the older population (Medicare), the establishment of a Center of Mental Health and Aging within the National Institute of Mental Health in 1975 and the American Nurses' Association first meeting of a conference group on Geriatric Nursing Practice set the stage for the establishment of geropsychiatric nursing as a specialty.

Geropsychiatric nursing became a specialty after 1970. Schwartz's book emphasized the psychosocial aspects of the care of the aged. Her book was very useful to nurses in psychiatric veterans' hospitals that had many back wards. A back ward included mentally impaired patients whose ages ranged from 50 to 100 years. Little more than custodial care was provided in these wards with 70 to 100 patients. Few of the nursing assistants knew anything about the patients except their names, even though the patients had been there for 10 to 15 years. There was very little employment turnover of nurse assistants. Most of the nurse assistants had some training, but little of their training included psychiatric nursing. Most of the training was disease and procedure oriented. On each ward there were nurse assistants, an on-call social worker, and an on-call physician who also covered other wards. Eventually the development of individual patient care plans and study of the participant-observation recordings for psychodynamics of behavior improved the quality of care of the aged mentally ill.

National Perspective

The interest in geropsychiatric nursing is slowly increasing, with a number of nurses providing strong leadership in this field. An invitational national conference on geropsychiatric nursing, "Bringing Advances in Practice and Research to Education," was held in November 1993 for the purpose of sharing (Abraham, Buckwalter, Harper, & Hight, 1994). Several leaders in the field made presentations on the status of geropsychiatric nursing, including suggested curriculum content and clinical experiences for the preparation of advanced practice nurses. Other presentations focused on the needs for research in geropsychiatric nursing and essentials of prevention in mental health and aging. There were 22 participants, and evaluation comments included suggestions for a follow-up conference. Details of this conference and its content appeared in the April 1994 issue of the *Journal of Psychosocial Nursing* (Special Issue, 1994), with the entire issue devoted to articles on geropsychiatric nursing.

Teaching Caregivers

The geropsychiatric nurse must teach, monitor, and supervise caregivers (nurse aides, licensed practical nurses [LPNs], members of the patients' families, and significant others). In long-term care (LTC) 80% of the noninstitutional care is given by members of the family (spouse, daughter, daughter-in-law), and 13% of the caregivers are men, who often need special kinds of help.

Eighty percent of the care in LTC institutions is provided by the nurse aide, LPN, or other nonprofessional caregiver. There are about 7 million caregivers between the ages of 45 and 60 (American Association of Retired Persons, 1993). These caregivers need instructions in meeting the mental health needs of older people. Bruce and McNamara (1992) found that 21.8% of their 2,553 noninstitutional elders were cognitively impaired, 2.3% had depression, 3.9% had dysthymia, and 2.2% had anxiety disorders.

Many family caregivers undergo stress in the performance of the task. Zarit (1987) has concluded that family members who provide care to ill relatives undergo emotional, physical, and social strain and suffer higher rates of depression, perceived burden, social isolation, family discord, and physical ill health. Zarit (1987) developed a scale to measure family member burden in caregiving. Ferris (1993) demonstrated the effectiveness of psychosocial education in reducing stress and depression in the caregiver in addition to delaying for 2 months admission of the care recipient to a nursing home.

Rabins, Filling, Eastham, and Zabora (1990) compared the emotional adaptation of caring for an Alzheimer's patient with caring for a cancer patient. With psychosocial support, both caregiver groups showed a decline in anxiety and negative mood. Morycz, Malloy, Bozich, and Martz (1987) found that African-American caregivers were under less strain when caring for elders with Alzheimer's disease and were less likely to institutionalize family members with late-life organic brain disorders than were Caucasian caregivers. The African-American caregivers were slightly younger, had less formal education, and less income. Montgomery (1993) indicated several studies revealing that many people are not stressed or burdened by caregiving. An excellent resource for caregivers is the Family Caregiver Alliance (Appendix G). This organization has literature and videotapes, and it sponsors conferences for providers and members of the family.

Since the primary providers of long-term care are members of the family, nurse aides, LPNs, and the registered nurse in selected situations, it is imperative that a geropsychiatric nurse be available to provide information, help, and supervision as indicated.

Ethical Aspects

Many dilemmas arise with advances in the delivery of health care. When should aggressive or heroic treatment be pursued? Who should receive the transplant or dialysis or other limited resources? Is it right to stop all medical treatment or withhold or withdraw food and water from patients in the last stage of Alzheimer's disease? What are the circumstances under which such actions might be considered morally permissible? Should chemical and physical restraints be used? When should resuscitation be performed?

Patients' Rights

Equally important and even more pervasive are the day-to-day ethical concerns such as the following patients' rights:

- Right to refuse treatment or medication
- Right to refuse psychosurgery and electroconvulsive therapy
- Right to informed consent
- Right to privacy
- Right to receive mail unopened

- Right to see family and visitors
- Right to treatment services that take place in the least restrictive setting to maximize independent functioning
- Right to religious expressions
- Right to prompt medical care and treatment
- Right to be free from dangerous procedures
- Right to freedom from excessive or unnecessary use of restraints, seclusion, medication abuse, or neglect; specifically, medication should not be used as punishment or for staff convenience or as a substitute for other programs (Keglovits, 1983, pp. 801-811).

Effective implementation of patients' rights frequently depends on awareness, support, and advocacy by the geropsychiatric nurse. It is imperative that the nurse know the laws for mandatory reporting in such areas as elder abuse, ethical practices, suicide attempts, theft from the patient, informed consent, freedom of information, confidentiality of information, and privacy laws.

Contemporary forensic considerations important to humanistic geropsychiatric nursing practice include involuntary admissions, criteria for the right to treatment, civil rights of the patient, nurse-patient relationship, decision-making capacity or incapacity, withdrawal or withholding of food, do not resuscitate (DNR) orders, transfer of a patient that places his or her health in jeopardy, rationing of health services and treatments such as organ transplants or renal dialysis, denial of admission because of method of payment (Medicaid vs. private pay), chemical and physical restraints, and unlawful retention of a voluntary patient.

Legal does not mean *ethical*. In fact, many laws demand less than ethical behavior. If a geropsychiatric nurse is suspicious that a resident has in his or her possession over-the-counter or prescription drugs and is saving pills for a suicide attempt, does the nurse have the right to search the resident and his or her room? The constitution protects all citizens from unreasonable search and seizure. People do not lose that protection when they are admitted to a nursing home. Some searches lead to lawsuits on the grounds of deprivation of constitutional rights (Ethics Grand Rounds, 1989).

Ethics and politics interfere and overlap for nursing administrators, educators, researchers, and practitioners. Ethics is about *right* and *good* actions and politics is concerned with *power* and *manipulations*. Ethics is concerned with individuals and society (Aroskar, 1987). Politics can also refer to relations between leaders and nonleaders in social groups and various governmental and nongovernmental activities. Health care is largely governed by political forces such as reimbursement (Medicare, Medicaid) and politics is increasingly concerned with the allocation of resources such as money, health care, and facilities. Therefore, a geropsychiatric nurse must be aware of ethical issues and use political forces and advocacy to improve quality of care.

Life-sustaining treatment is defined as "any medical intervention, technology, procedure, or medication that is administered to a patient in order to forestall the moment of death, whether or not the treatment is intended to affect the underlying life threatening disease(s) or biological processes" (Hastings Center, 1987, p. 57). According to a report from the Office of Technology Assessment (1986), the total utilization of life-sustaining technologies ranges from a few thousand persons (in the case of mechanical ventilation, 750,000) to 1.4 million persons in the case of nutritional support. The use among the older population ranges from 2200 for ventilation to 680,000 for nutritional support.

The geropsychiatric nurse must be concerned about safety, appropriate use, policies for use, withdrawal and withholding of treatment, informed consent for the use of the life-sustaining treatment, and the fears of the patient and family.

The five life-sustaining technologies studied by the Office of Technology Assessment (1986) included dialysis, resuscitation, long-term mechanical ventilation, enteral (tube) nutritional support, and parenteral (intravenous) nutritional support.

One study reported that only 70% of the nursing facilities studied have written policies and procedures regarding ethical decision making including life and death decisions. Conversely, 75% of the facilities indicated that they do not have an ethics committee to provide assistance in dealing with ethical issues. Eighty-nine percent of the existing ethics committees included a nurse. A physician, administrator, social worker, resident, and family members were included in the membership of the ethics committee less than half the time. An attorney or clergyman was included in about one quarter of the committees. One third of the nursing homes studied reported having no residents with living wills (written expression or statement by the patient expressing his or her wishes about the use of life support machines, mechanisms, and procedures in case of serious illness) (Maturity News Service, 1987; American Health Care Association, 1988). One physician stated that "doctors and family tend to override a living will if there is a conflict between the patient's wishes and the family's desires" (Kelly, 1988, p. 9).

The number of right-to-die cases is rising as medical science discovers new methods of extending life. Sophisticated technology including respirators, feeding machines, and surgical techniques save thousands of lives every year but also create moral, medical, ethical, nursing, and legal dilemmas.

The President's Commission report (1983) focused on ethical, medical, and legal issues in treatment decisions. This report made important recommendations for treatment decisions that involve vulnerable patient groups such as those who lack decision-making capacity, those with permanent loss of consciousness, and hospitalized patients in need of resuscitation. The commission clarified that the term *withholding* refers to *not starting* treatment, whereas the term *withdrawing* refers to *stopping* treatment after it has been started. The geropsychiatric nurse must be aware that greater moral justification may be required for withholding treatment, because such a decision is made without knowledge of positive effects of treatment. The President's Commission report (1983) argued that life-sustaining treatments are expendable if they are useless or if the burden of the treatment exceeds its benefits. Geropsychiatric nurses are urged to obtain a copy of the American Nurses'

Association (ANA) guidelines on withdrawing and withholding food and fluids prepared by the ANA Committee on Ethics.

The term *capacity* refers to the patient's functional ability to make informed health care decisions according to personal values, instead of *competence* and *incompetence,* which are legal terms applied to patients as a result of a judicial proceeding. A patient may be declared legally incompetent but still have decision-making capacity (Fry, 1988).

There are many ethical and moral decisions that the geropsychiatric nurse must face. However, the nurse must use such basic guidelines as these:

- ◆ Providing for the safeguard of the patient's rights to privacy, dignity, and protection
- ◆ Balancing the needs of the individual with those of society
- ◆ Serving as an advocate for the patient
- ◆ Respecting the patient and family at all times
- ◆ Participating actively in ethics and other policy committees
- ◆ Becoming familiar with the Patient's Bill of Rights (American Hospital Association, 1973)

The active concerns of the geropsychiatric nurse with the older patient will include discussions about the following:

- ◆ Access to treatment
- ◆ Rationing of treatment and care
- ◆ Death and suicide
- ◆ Competency
- ◆ Decision-making capacity
- ◆ Disclosure of health care resources and services

Quality of Life

The quality of life for older adults is greatly influenced by their previous lifestyle, culture, education, health care beliefs, education, family strengths, and integration into the community.

The overall goal of the more than 1 million employees in long-term care facilities is to improve the quality of life of older persons, maximize their functional independence and capacities, and promote health. More of this philosophy must be included in the education of registered nurses, licensed practical nurses, and nurse aides. The Institute of Medicine (1986) clearly defined the importance of quality of life as "intimately related to the quality of care, but encompassing a resident's sense of well-being, level of satisfaction with life, and feeling of self-worth and self-esteem" (p. 371).

Quality of life for older adults is greatly enhanced by their involvement in planning, sponsoring, and evaluating programs and services in institutional, outpatient, and community settings.

Traditionally, long-term care planning and policy-making groups have depended on interaction among a variety of groups: providers and related organizations, long-term care nurses, legislators, consumer advocacy groups, organized labor groups, residents, families, ombudsmen, religious groups, corporate and business coalitions, research individuals and groups, and regulatory agencies.

The various resident councils in nursing homes raise important issues. The nursing home leadership must offer an opportunity for collaboration among the leadership of the council, the nursing home, and the ombudsman (DiCenso, 1988).

A study conducted by the National Citizen's Coalition for Nursing Home Reform asked nursing home residents across the country to rate the importance of various quality of life issues. The outcomes of the study resulted in several quality of life guidelines (Karen, 1988).

Guidelines for quality of life protocols:

- Environment
- Activities
- Facility philosophy
- Privacy
- Choice and informed decision making
- Interactions
- Personal, social, and spiritual life
- Security

Other factors that contribute to the quality of life (Holder & Frank, 1988):

- Maintenance of the best possible physical condition with discomfort and pain minimized; movement of body; exercise; action; continued functioning at maximum potential
- Self-determination, personal control, involvement in group efforts and group decision making, participation in civic affairs, kindness, cheerfulness, laughter from and with others
- Good listening, empathy, sympathy, and supportive, positive, constructive attitudes of individuals one lives with or who are always nearby
- Attractive, clean, comfortable surroundings
- Positive presentation of one's self in one's own lifestyle
- Positive relationship with staff, family, and peers

One of the residents in a nursing home remarked, "Our physical weakness and mental fatigue, limited vision, hearing, and mobility have robbed us of much of our independence and often lowered our self-esteem, but we need the opportunity to make more of our decisions" (Wyckoff, 1988, p. 26). A good geropsychiatric nurse should actively participate in resident councils, have scheduled individual conferences with residents and/or members of the family, and announce staff and programmatic changes in the resident council's newsletter. Visits by surveyors and inspectors should also be announced.

Challenges for the Future

Mental illness in older people is associated with increased family stress, lengthened recovery periods from acute and chronic illness, multiple hospitalizations, multiple providers often without network communications, social isolation, and increased health care cost, which impose unnecessary suffering, reduced functioning and diminished quality of life. At the same time, a variety of factors including age, bias on the part of providers, consumer stigma against psychiatric treatment, insurance stigma causing inadequate coverage, lack of provider training in geropsychiatric nursing and geropsychiatry, and negative reimbursement incentives have combined to render mentally ill older persons vastly underserved by the current mental health system in both the private and public sectors.

Geropsychiatric nursing as a specialty is needed because, as concluded by Lipowski (1967, 1975) and Hale (1986), 30% to 60% of inpatients and 50% to 80% of outpatients suffer from psychiatric disorders of sufficient magnitude to cause problems for the primary health care provider. Hale (1986) also found in a literature review that between 20% and 50% of both psychiatric and medical patients had significant concomitant physical and psychiatric illnesses.

Because of the graying of the population, the high prevalence of comorbidity (physical and mental illnesses), and the lack of properly educated health care providers, it is imperative that the roles of the geropsychiatric nurse be expanded. Those roles include the following:

- ◆ Preventing iatrogenesis
- ◆ Maintaining or restoring function within a framework encompassing the physical, psychological, social, and economic needs of older adults
- ◆ Increasing self-care abilities and functions
- ◆ Modifying the environment to eliminate physical and psychological barriers to desired autonomy
- ◆ Maintaining and furthering the quality of life
- ◆ Providing equal or greater attention to preserving functional capacity, including rehabilitation

Older people have both physical and cognitive impairment, so they require a different kind of support. Generally, the cognitively impaired require more assistive devices, standby supervision, and teaching of self-care activities. The physically ill require more assistance with the activities of daily living, doing for them the things that they cannot do or are unwilling to do for themselves. Therefore, other important roles of the geropsychiatric nurse are assessment, implementation, and evaluation. Comprehensive assessment should include the following:

- ◆ Physical functioning
- ◆ Enabling services and family and community support
- ◆ Need for specific medical and rehabilitation therapies
- ◆ Mental and emotional functioning

- Environment conducive to empowerment
- Potential for productive or personally rewarding life
- Cognitive, behavioral, and emotional status
- Effects of race, ethnicity, culture, and religion on the treatment outcomes
- Early detection of dementia, delirium, and depression
- Impact on family functions and family resources

The geropsychiatric nurse must be prepared to function in both institutional and community settings. Rovner et al. (1990) reported a prevalence of 80% psychiatric disorders among 454 consecutive new nursing home admissions. The most common disorder was dementia (67.4%), and 40% of the demented patients had additional psychiatric syndromes such as delusions and depression. These patients constituted a distinct subgroup that predicted frequent use of restraints and neuroleptics and the greatest consumption of nursing time. Ten percent of the new admissions had a diagnosis of affective disorders. Therefore, the need for a nurse prepared in the care of older persons with mental disorders is essential in a nursing home setting.

Research Needs

Research by geropsychiatric nurses is slowly increasing. However, organized efforts and funding have been devoted to preparation of research faculties, development of geropsychiatric nursing curricula, and educating nurses who care for older clients in settings such as home health care agencies and adult day care centers. Nurses who work on surgical, medical, oncology, and orthopedic units also need to learn more about older patients with behavioral, emotional, social, and mental disorders.

One of the greatest challenges to the geropsychiatric nurse is the provision of mental health services in the home and in community-based programs. Ninety-five percent of the older population live in the community; yet most nursing research, education and training focuses on institutional settings. Research is desperately needed in the areas of studying the mental health needs of older people who live at home and the most cost-effective techniques for delivery of mental health services in the home. The family provides 80% of the services to older people in noninstitutional settings. What is the role of the nurse in assuring the delivery of quality care by family members?

The following topics are suggested for research in geropsychiatric nursing:

1. Development of assessment instruments to measure change and/or progress in the behavioral, emotional, and mental disorders of older adults in various settings (in-home, adult day care, and institutions). Establishment of norms for the 65-year-old and over, 85-year-old and over, and 100-year-old and over groups. Establishment of validity and reliability for these tests.
2. Development of assessment instruments that can be administered by members of the family, nurse aides, and nonpsychologist health providers.
3. Development of assessment instruments that are appropriate for measuring behavior in various levels or phases of illness, for example, Reisberg's seven stages of Alzheimer's disease (Reisberg, Ferris, DeLeon, & Crook, 1982). It is

essential that nurses become knowledgeable about characteristics of behavior for phases of disorders and develop nursing care plans for the unique needs at each phase. It is cost effective to provide care according to the phase of illness. Such a plan may prevent premature dependency.

4. Study of the quality of care delivered by the family, licensed practical nurses, nurse aides, and registered nurses to improve the quality of care.
5. Study of the impact of long-term care legislation on the quality of care; for example, the Omnibus Budget Reconciliation Act of 1987, which requires mental as well as physical evaluation of all nursing home residents, as well as a plan for active treatment if needed (The 100th Congress, 1988, p. 12).
6. Development of strategies for the prevention of fragmentation and the promotion of continuity of care within a facility and between facilities and home.
7. Identification and analysis of some of the precipitating and predisposing factors associated with excessive disability of the old-old (85 to 100 years) and patients with Alzheimer's disease.
8. Study of the nature, consequences, and interaction of stress associated with caregiving on individual family caregivers who are 65 years of age and older.
9. Identification of the behavioral, social, emotional, and mental health needs of homebound older adults between the ages of 85 and 100.
10. Identification of the functions, roles, and barriers in geropsychiatric nursing in an acute care hospital setting (e.g., orthopedic, medical oncology, and surgical units).
11. Study of the incidence and prevalence of falls, confusion, and polypharmacy (for example, older patients who take more than 10 prescribed medications).
12. Study of the mental health needs of the older population living alone in rural areas.
13. Critical analysis of instruments and theories used in geropsychiatric nursing, with recommendations for improving the quality of nursing research.
14. Study of the outcomes of various methods used to teach behavioral management to nurse aides and members of the family of mentally retarded older persons.
15. Analysis of the relationship between depression of the caregiver and the severity and/or stage of Alzheimer's disease.

Another area where nursing research is needed is self-care. For example:

1. What is the profile of an older adult who can safely provide quality self-care?
2. What procedures are most suitable for self-care? What is the impact of memory decline on an older person's ability to provide self-care?
3. What are the barriers to self-care for the very old living at home?
4. From an ethical and legal framework, is withholding fluids or withdrawing of fluids an assisted suicide? To what extent are nurses guided by a patient's living will?
5. What are appropriate nursing alternatives to physical and chemical restraints?

Geropsychiatric nurses should be cautious about what they read and select as instruments to measure anxiety, hostility, and depression in older adults. Many instruments commonly used in geropsychiatric nursing research have never been validated in older populations. The nurse is in a unique position to develop reliable and valid instruments for this group. Older people tend to deny or somaticize feelings of depression, anxiety, and tension, either because of social desirability factors such as looking good to others and projecting an image of self-reliance or a lack of self-awareness as to what they are really experiencing. It is hard to sort out the contributions of physiological factors to the reported affective distress. Sleep disturbances, which often accompany depression, may be particularly difficult to evaluate. It is not easy to distinguish apathy, fatigue, and motor retardation from emotional withdrawal for assessing either depression or anxiety disorders. Nurses are in a unique position to assist in sorting out the physiological contributions to depression and anxiety through nursing research.

Nursing research in long-term care facilities is very scarce and often very deficient in research design (e.g., absence of theoretical framework, data analysis, operational definitions) (Haight, 1989).

Nurses must become involved in (1) valuation, policy, pricing, and cost of nursing care; (2) ethical implications of nursing care; (3) quality of care; (4) care of older people in noninstitutional settings; (5) impact of the prospective payment system (DRGs) on the quality, location, and cost of geropsychiatric nursing; (6) rehabilitation; (7) caregiver's stress; (8) techniques and practices for promoting and maintaining functional capabilities and independent functioning, and (9) outcomes for care in institutions *and* the community and home.

Public Policy

Public policy and the politics of aging greatly influence health care in the United States. It is important that geropsychiatric nurses at every level know the legislation directing long-term care and collaborate in shaping and developing it. Public policy determines the length of stay in a health care facility, the type of treatment, the type of provider, the reimbursement pay or denial, the type of patient who can be admitted to a given institution, the location of the facility, tax credit or incentive for health services, and the use of life support. In some instances, health policies are made with health professionals and policymakers, and in other instances health policy may be made without the endorsement or collaboration of health professionals.

Geropsychiatric nurses must read the *Federal Register* and become a part of the lawmaking that governs their practice. The deadline for the comment period is published in the *Federal Register*. Nurses must recognize that the initiatives in health policy will come increasingly from the federal government. Recent changes in long-term care regulations are governed primarily by political platforms and fiscal necessities. The total Medicare-Medicaid budget for 1987 was $118 billion, (Davis, 1988, p. 6) and the need is increasing every year.

Geropsychiatric nurses should especially become involved in the health care debate and encourage the passage of responsible cost-effective legislation that will increase the quantity and quality of mental health care for older adults in institutional and noninstitutional settings.

❖ Summary

More emphasis must be placed on geropsychiatric nursing because almost half of the adult population will be over 65 years of age within the next 40 years and more than half of the 2 million older persons in long-term care facilities have behavioral, social, emotional, or mental disorders. There are more than 8 million episodes (admissions, transfer, consultation, and discharges) in the acute health care facilities that involve persons over 65 years of age. A high percentage of older patients are admitted to acute care hospitals for emotional and mental problems or because they become depressed or confused during their treatment or after surgery (Campbell, 1986; Gurland, 1982; Liptzin, 1986; Bootzin & Shadish, 1986).

There is a national prevalence of 18% to 25% of mental illness among older adults. Psychopathology increases with age (Liptzin, 1986); therefore, more geropsychiatric nurses are needed than ever before. Much more research is needed in this area (Harper & Lebowitz, 1986).

Geropsychiatric nursing is a blend of knowledge, practices, and skills from medical and surgical nursing, psychiatric nursing, gerontological nursing, and community health nursing. Geropsychiatric nurses serve in a variety of roles; counselor, consultant, case manager, advocate, direct care provider, therapist, policy maker, policy analyst, researcher, administrator, and home health care team leader. For the most part, geropsychiatric nurses have focused on institutional care. There must be more focus on in-home and community-based programs for mentally ill older adults. Ninety-five percent of the older population live in noninstitutional settings, and 6 million of them have one or more limitations in activities of daily living. They are underserved by the mental health system, although they have a high prevalence of mental disorders.

❖ References

Abraham, I. L., Buckwalter, K. C., Harper, M. S., & Hight, V. A. (1994). Geropsychiatric nursing: Bringing advances in practice and research to education. (Editorial). *Journal of Psychosocial Nursing, 32*(4), p. 5.

American Association of Colleges of Nursing. (1993, June 25). *Memorandum: Advanced Practice Nursing.* Washington, DC: AACN.

American Association of Retired Persons. (1993). *Newsletter for Volunteers.* May-June, 1993, p. 8.

American Health Care Association. (1988). Management, ethics, opinions, providers. *Long Term Care Professionals, 14*(10), 28-33.

American Hospital Association. (1973). *A patient's bill of rights.* Chicago: Author.

Aroskar, M. (1987). The interface of ethics and policies in nursing. *Nursing Outlook, 35*(6), 268-272.

Bootzin, R. R., & Shadish, W. R. (1986). Assessment and treatment in nursing homes: Implications for research. In M. S. Harper & B. D. Lebowitz (Eds.), *Mental illness in nursing homes: Agenda for research* (pp. 95-109). Washington, DC: DHHS Publication No. (ADM) 86-1459.

Branconnier, R. J., Cole, J. O., & Shazvinian, S. (1990). Treating the depressed elderly: The comparative behavioral pharmacology of Mianserian and amitriptyline. In E. Costa & E. Recogni (Eds.), *Typical and atypical antidepressants: Clinical practice* (pp. 183-190). New York: Raven Press.

Bruce, M. L., & McNamara, R. (1992). Psychiatric status among the homebound elderly: An epidemiologic perspective. *Journal of the American Geriatrics Society, 40*(6), 561-566.

Burns, B. J., Wagner, H. R., Taube, J. E., Magaziner, J., Permutt, T., & Landerman, L. R. (1993). Mental health service use by the elderly in nursing homes. *American Journal of Public Health, 83*(3), 331-337.

Campbell, E. G. (1986). After the fall: Confusion. *American Journal of Nursing, 86*(2), 151-154

Davis, C. (1988). Home care and its financial support: Future directions and present policies—impact on care. In *Home Health Care: Issues, Trends and Strategies* (pp. 3-18). Rockville, MD: Health Resources and Services Administration, Division of Nursing.

DiCenso, R. D. (1988). How residents can keep regulators on track. *Provider: For Long Term Care Professionals, 14*(12), 18-20.

Ethics Grand Rounds. (1989). Should you protect a patient from himself? *Nursing 89, 19*(1), 67-69.

Ferris, S. (1993, October 22). Caregiver intervention project: Preliminary cost savings estimates. Personal communication on progress report.

Flemming, A., Buchanan, J. G., Santos, J. F., & Richards, L. D. (1984). *Mental health services for the elderly: Report of a survey of community mental health centers*. Washington, DC: The Action Committee to Implement the Mental Health Recommendations of the 1981 White House Conference on Aging.

Froom, J. (1990). Diabetes mellitus in the elderly. *Clinics in Geriatric Medicine, 6*(4), 150

Fry, S. T. (1988). Outlook on ethics. *Nursing Outlook, 36*(3), 122-150.

Gambert, S. R. (1990). Atypical presentation of diabetes mellitus in the elderly. *Clinics in Geriatric Medicine, 6*(4), 721-729.

Gurland, B. J. (1982). Epidemiology of psychopathology in old age: Some implications for clinical services. *Psychiatric Clinics of North America, 5*(1), 11-26.

Haight, B. K. (1989). Nursing research in long term care facilities (1984-1988). *Nursing Health Care, 10*(3), 147-150.

Hale, R. E. (1986). The diagnosis and treatment of psychiatric disorders in medically ill patients. *Military Medicine, 151*(11), 587-589.

Harper, M. S. (1986). Introduction. In M. S. Harper & B. Lebowitz (Eds.), *Mental illness in nursing homes: Agenda for research* (pp. 1-6). Washington, DC: DHHS Publication No. (ADM) 86-1459.

Harper, M. S. (1987). Mental health and aging. *Aging Network News, 3*(12), 1, 10, 14.

Harper, M. S., & Lebowitz, B. D. (Eds.), (1986). *Mental illness in nursing homes: Agenda for research*. Washington, DC: DHHS Publication No. (ADM) 86-1459.

Hastings Center. (1987). *Guidelines on the termination of life sustaining treatment and the care of the dying*. Bloomington, IN: Indiana University Press.

Holder, E. L., & Frank, B. (1988). Residents speak out on what makes quality. *Provider of Long Term Care Professionals, 14*(12), 28-29.

Institute of Medicine, Committee on Nursing Home Regulation. (1986). *Improving the quality of care in nursing homes* (p. 371). Washington, DC: National Academy Press.

Karen, M. J. (1988). Quality assurance in New York State: Resident-centered protocols the basis. *Provider: For Long Term Care Professionals, 24*(12), 21-22.

Keglovits, J. (1983). Legal considerations in psychiatric nursing practice. In H. S. Wilson & C. R. Kneisl (Eds.), *Psychiatric nursing* (pp. 787-815). Menlo Park, CA: Addison-Wesley.

Kelly, M. (1988). Age-old dilemmas. In *Health Sciences* (pp. 7-10). Minneapolis: University of Minnesota.

Kelly, J., & Urquhart, A. (1993). *A report on caring for the mentally ill nursing home patient: Introduction and care planning.* Washington, DC: U.S. Department of Veterans Affairs.

Lebowitz, B., & Light, E. (1992). Caregiver stress. In T. T. Yoshikawa, E. L. Cobbs, & K. Brummel-Smith (Eds.), *Ambulatory geriatric care* (pp. 47-54). St. Louis, MO: Mosby.

Lipowski, Z. J. (1967). Review of consultation psychiatry and psychosomatic medicine: 2. Clinical aspects. *Psychosomatic Medicine, 19* 113-201.

Lipowski, Z. J. (1975). Psychiatry of somatic diseases: Epidemiology pathogenesis classification. *Comprehensive Psychiatry, 16* 105-124.

Liptzin, B. (1986). Major mental disorders/problems in nursing homes: Implications for research and public policy. In M. S. Harper & B. D. Lebowitz (Eds.), *Mental illness in nursing homes: Agenda for research* (pp. 41-55). Washington, DC: DHHS Publication No. (ADM) 86-1459.

Lustman, P. J., Clouse, R. E., & Carney, R. M. (1988). Depression and the reporting of diabetes symptoms. *International Journal of Psychiatric Medicine, 18*(4), 295-303.

Mack, M. (1952). Personal adjustment of chronically ill people under home care. *Nursing Research, 1,* 9-30.

Matteson, M. A., & McConnell, E. S. (1988). Gerontological nursing in acute care settings. In M. A. Matteson & E. S. McConnell (Eds.), *Gerontological nursing* (pp. 721-761). Philadelphia: Saunders.

Maturity News Service. (1987). *Does one have the right to die?* New York: New York Times Syndication Sales Corp.

McConnell, E. S. (1988). Outlook for gerontological nursing as a specialty. In M. A. Matteson & E. S. McConnell (Eds.), *Gerontological nursing* (pp. 123-136). Philadelphia: Saunders.

Miller, L. S., & Kelman, D. S. (1992). Estimates of the loss of individual productivity from alcohol and drug abuse, and mental illness. In R. G. Frank & W. G. Manning (Eds.), *Economics and mental health* (pp. 91-129). Baltimore: The Johns Hopkins University Press.

Montgomery, R. J. V. (1993). Seven markers for caregiver research. *Aging Today, 14*(6), 9.

Morycz, R.K., Malloy, J., Bozich, M. & Martz, P. (1987) Racial differences in family burden: Clinical implications for social work. *Journal of Gerontological Social Work 10,* 133-142.

Newsletter for Volunteers. (1993, May-June). American Association of Retired Person, p. 8.

Newton, K. (1950). *Geriatric nursing.* St. Louis: Mosby.

Office of Technology Assessment. (1986, June). *Life-sustaining technologies and the elderly.* Washington, DC: Author.

The 100th Congress and mental health. (1988). Alexandria, VA: The National Mental Health Association.

Osgood, N. J., & Brant, B. A. (1991). Suicide among the elderly in institutional and community settings. In M. S. Harper (Ed.), *Management and care of the elderly* (pp. 37-71). Newbury Park, California: Sage.

Ouslander, J. G. (1982). Illness and psychopathology in the elderly. *Psychiatric Clinics of North America, 5*(1), 145-158.

President's Commission for the Study of Ethical Problems in Medicine and Biomedical and Behavioral Research. *Deciding to forgo life-sustaining treatment: A report on the ethical, medical, and legal issues in treatment decisions.* (1983). Washington, DC: U.S. Government Printing Office.

A profile of older Americans. (1993). Washington, DC: American Association of Retired Persons.

Rabins, P. V., Fitting, M. D., Eastham, J., & Zabora, J. (1990). Emotional adaptation over time in care-givers for chronically ill elderly people. *Age and Ageing, 19*(2), 185-190.

Regier, D. A., Myers, J. K., Kramer, M., Robin, L. M., Blaser, D. G., Hough, R. L., Eaton, W. W., & Lucke, B. Z. (1984). The NIMH epidemiologic catchment area programs, historical context, major objectives and study population characteristics. *Archives of General Psychiatry, 41,* 934-944.

Reisberg, B., Ferris, S. H., DeLeon, M. J., & Crook, T. (1982). The global deterioration scale for assessment of primary degenerative dementia. *The American Journal of Psychiatry, 139*(9), 1136-1139.

Riley, B. B. (1994). Mental disorders. In M. O. Hogstel (Ed.), *Nursing care of the older adult.* 3rd ed. (pp. 204-233). New York: Delmar.

Rovner, B. W., German, P. S., Broadhead, J., Morriss, R. K., Brant, L. J., Blaustein, J., & Folstein, M. F. (1990). The diagnoses in nursing homes. *International Psychogeriatrics, 2*(1), 13-24.

Ruegg, R. G., Zisook, S., & Swerdlow, N. R. (1988). Depression in the aged: An overview. *Psychiatric Clinics of North America, 11*(1), 83-97.

Schurman, R., & Mitchell, J. B. (1985, June). *Nonpsychiatrist physicians: Mental health care for the aged, final report.* Washington, DC: National Institute of Mental Health.

Schwartz, D., Henley, B., & Zeitz, L. (1964). *The elderly ambulatory patient: Nursing and psychosocial needs.* New York: Macmillan.

Special Issue: Geropsychiatric Nursing. (1994). *Journal of Psychosocial Nursing, 32*(4).

Strain, J. J. (1977). Mental disorders in surgical services. *American Journal of Psychiatry, 22*(8), 1044-1049.

Tun, P. A., Nathan, D. M., & Perlmuter, L. C. (1990). Cognitive and affective disorders in elderly diabetics. *Clinics in Geriatric Medicine, 6*(4), 731-746.

United States Bureau of the Census Current Population Reports, Special Studies. (1992). *Sixty-five plus in America* (pp. 23-178). Washington, DC: U.S. Government Printing Office.

Wasylenki, D. (1982). The psychogeriatric problem. *Canada's Mental Health, 30*(3), 16-19.

Webb, W. B. (1989). Age-related changes in sleep. *Clinics in Geriatric Medicine, 5*(2), 275-287.

Wyckoff, B. (1988). A resident's thoughts on quality of life. *Provider: For Long Term Care Professionals, 14*(2), 26.

Zarit, S. H. (1987). The burdens of caregivers. In A. C. Kalicki (Ed.), *Confronting Alzheimer's disease* (pp. 68-76). Owings Mills, MD: Rynd Communications.

Chapter 2

❖ *Promotion of Mental Health in Older Adults*

Gail P. Hamilton

"Mental health refers to an individual's ability to negotiate the daily challenges and social interactions of life, without experiencing undue emotional or behavioral incapacity." (*Healthy People 2000*, 1991, p. 60). Health care professionals as well as the informed population at large value health promotion and recognize its importance. Although health promotional activities are frequently equated with physical health, the physical, psychological, social, and spiritual aspects of the human condition are interwoven. All are interdependent and must be considered as a unit.

When a person progresses from middle to later life, roles, abilities, insights, perspectives, and attitudes are in a state of transition. This chapter discusses many of the issues that become important during this stage of living. The gerontological nurse can educate and encourage older people to confront the challenges and use available resources to enhance their quality of life. The nurse, providing holistic care, will use helping strategies to assist the client in achieving optimal mental health. Successful client outcomes will result in the older client achieving optimal independence, maximum participation in decision making, positive feelings of self-worth, and full involvement in productive and self-fulfilling activities.

Emphasis upon abilities rather than disabilities will help the older client transcend physical, social, and psychological losses. When lifestyle changes are necessary, the nurse assumes an educational role and teaches useful environmental strategies. Individual responsibility is stressed. The focus of supportive care is on strengths rather than weaknesses. An upbeat, positive attitude in combination with short-term achievable goals and daily pleasures offers encouragement and hope to a person or family who may feel overwhelmed with problems and frustrations. The nurse and the older adult form a partnership. The client uses available attributes and strengths; the nurse offers support and management strategies. The interdisciplinary team will provide services outside nursing. Often it is the nurse who recognizes the necessity of referral and coordinates the team effort.

❖ Successful Aging

In a review article summarizing the literature related to personal adjustment to aging, Coleman (1992) discusses subjective indicators of successful aging. The concepts of perceived control and adaptation have been recently added to the more traditional measurements of life satisfaction, morale, and self-esteem. Using the available research literature, George (1990) and George and Clipp (1991) made the following conclusions regarding subjective well-being: (1) The majority of older persons (about 85%) are satisfied with their lives. (2) Levels of life satisfaction tend to be stable over time. (3) Life satisfaction is strongly related to objective measurements, including health, socioeconomic status, friends, and family relationships. George and Clipp (1991) suggest that a comprehensive dimension of subjective well-being includes an assessment of self and an assessment of the meaning of life.

❖ Social Theories of Aging

A successful social and psychological adjustment in old age is an object of interest and research for gerontologists. Encouraging positive lifestyle practices necessitates a comprehensive knowledge base about successful aging. Scientific studies of aging 4 and 5 decades ago coalesced into major theories. These include the theories of disengagement, activity, and continuity.

The disengagement and activity theories, taking opposing views, dominated the social gerontological literature in the 1960s and continue to be cited. The continuity theory followed. These theories attempt to predict and explain the social interactions and role involvements that contribute to a successful life adjustment of a person in old age. No theory has advanced to the point that accurate generalizations can be made about an individual's behavior. To the contrary, older adults are extremely diverse, and the concept of successful aging varies according to the individual. However, formulation of these theories has revealed areas that need further study, has raised particular questions that have not been fully answered, and has served as a framework to organize knowledge.

Disengagement Theory

Disengagement theory postulates that "aging is an inevitable mutual withdrawal or disengagement, resulting in decreased interaction between the aging person and others in the social systems he belongs to" (Cummings & Henry, 1961, p. 13). Gerontologists have criticized the disengagement theory, saying that it insulates the general population from the loneliness of older people. Some say this theory reflects the bias of an industrial society.

Larson, Zuzanek, and Mannell (1985) studied the quantity and quality of time spent alone by healthy, affluent older persons. They found that living situation and marital status were the two strongest predictors of solitude. Although all subjects spent a considerable time alone despite access to family and friends, men and unmarried persons spent more time in solitude. Generally speaking, the absence of another person was not considered a negative. Married persons felt particularly positive about aloneness and enjoyed this time for personal absorption in a chosen activity.

When dealing with a person who chooses a disengaged lifestyle, the nurse is confronted by a dilemma. Is it best to accept the disengagement theory and allow this person the chosen aloneness? Is this person depressed? What intervention, if any, will serve the best interests of the older person? Society generally does not approve of an inactive lifestyle. Nonetheless, disengaged persons are often invisible, and the easiest solution may, indeed, be none at all. Decisions should be made jointly, with suggestions from both the older person and the nurse. In choosing a plan and intervention, the nurse must be sensitive to the belief system of self and society and avoid expediency, which can interfere with decision making.

Some older persons prefer social inactivity. When isolation reflects similar choices from the past, aloneness may indeed be appropriate. Conversely, disengagement in the face of a past lifestyle of sociability and active participation signals an incongruency. With such an assessment the nurse, in cooperation with the family and the older person, can explore other explanations and develop a therapeutic plan. A baseline personality profile is very useful in evaluating present behavior.

Activity Theory

Some older persons disengage voluntarily, and others choose to remain active throughout life. As individuals differ, so do their chosen lifestyles. Proponents of the activity theory accentuate research findings that correlate activity with higher life satisfaction (Havighurst, 1968).

In the 1950s many social gerontologists accepted the principles of activity theory. However, when the disengagement theory became well known in the 1960s, the activity theory was offered as a separate view. This theory suggests that older people enjoy and need activity and social interaction to achieve contentment and a sense of well-being. The principles of activity are harmonious with the American lifestyle and adherence to the work ethic. People intuitively believe that persons who are retired from the workplace can find many other useful roles in society. People differ, however, and physical, economic, social, intellectual, and emotional needs and abilities vary considerably. Persons who have had numerous interests and opportunities in earlier life tend to satisfy the personality qualifications necessary for successful adaptations to a new, fulfilling lifestyle. In contrast, there are many who do not choose to participate in active new social roles. For some, a hobby or sport does not fill the void left by retirement from a fulfilling role in the workplace.

Neugarten, Havighurst, & Tobin (1968) found a diversity of social role activity and life satisfaction among older persons. Some people showed high social activity and life satisfaction. Others exhibited low-low, low-high, or high-low activity and life satisfaction. The majority of the older persons studied were competent and well functioning, with high levels of life satisfaction. They were said to have *integrated personalities*. Their activity differed from high to disengaged. Another category, those with *defended personalities*, maintained acceptable levels of life satisfaction when they maintained tight controls over their impulse life. Their levels of social engagement also varied. Other persons, said to have *passive-dependent* and *unintegrated personalities*, had medium to low life satisfaction and exhibited low or medium levels of activity. This study points out the differences among individuals and the complexities in formulating a theory of aging.

Continuity Theory

Personality characteristics are formed early and continue across a lifetime. According to Atchley (1994), changes in life circumstances are assimilated by the individual without loss of old perspectives. Individual traits evolve and change with life circumstances. The new merges with the old. Continuity (Atchley, 1989) is an adaptive strategy that allows change to be integrated harmoniously through existing internal and external structures. Internal continuity requires memory and is determined by past personality, preferences, and workings of the inner character. Thus the person's abilities to adapt to changes, make decisions, and respond predictably are interconnected and built upon the past. Inner continuity leads to a sense of solid identity and self-esteem. When the physical and social environments are recalled and persist into the present, they can provide a sense of external continuity. Although change is inevitable, a familiar framework can facilitate the person's adjustment.

Applications to Nursing

The nurse can use these theories to help the older person achieve personal fulfillment. The research has shown some contradictions but has consistently indicated that persons are not all the same and therefore cannot be expected to respond to old age predictably. It is important for the nurse to learn as much as possible about the past life of the individual, specifically hobbies, social activities, moral and spiritual values, and work. How the person responded throughout life to losses, disappointments, crises, and successes will be invaluable information. Older persons who have always been joiners are good candidates for planned social activities or for continued work roles. Others, who have been introspective throughout life, will be happier if they continue with similar patterns. Social events may best be limited to family affairs or inclusion of selected close friends. If a hobby relates to past interests, encouragement is valuable. It is important to retain continuity, or connection to the past. Old habits, values, and interests are integral to a person's present life. The nurse can best facilitate adaptation and life fulfillment if the present reflects the past.

❖ Developmental Tasks in Later Life

Erikson (1963) described the eight stages of human life, which begin with infancy and progress to old age. Each stage presents new challenges for the individual. The final task, the challenge of old age, is called ego integrity versus despair. This stage of life represents the culmination of all life events for the older person, a psychological reflection on the self. Successful progression through these stages and a satisfactory achievement of tasks results in a positive feeling about oneself and a personal sense of self-worth and satisfaction (integrity). When tasks are confronted but are resolved incompletely or not at all, the person is left with feelings of dissatisfaction and inadequacy (despair). A person with ego integrity feels satisfied and fulfilled and accepts the inevitability of death. Despair, the negative resolution, is a sense of incompleteness in meeting life's challenges. The despair results because time has run out and the person will not be able to make things right. This frustration will cause the older person to fear death. A sense of meaninglessness and uselessness pervades.

Erikson's reformulated theory (Erikson, Erikson, & Kivnick, 1986) challenges the older adult to renew, review, and rework the eight psychosocial themes. To establish integrity, the individual can draw sustenance from the past but also should remain vitally involved in the present. Throughout life the older person has developed internal and external resources. Inner strengths take on a greater importance when they must compensate for loss of physical abilities in old age. In recognizing one's life strengths and weaknesses, an elder can plan life events in a way that will maximize positive mental health (Kivnik, 1993).

Havighurst lists a series of social and personal tasks that occur over a lifetime. Contentment and happiness result; otherwise social disapproval, unhappiness, and difficulty with later tasks follow. Tasks of later maturity include adjusting to decreases in physical strength and health, retirement, reduced income, and death of a spouse. Social tasks include establishing affiliation with one's age group, adopting and adapting to social roles in a flexible way, and establishing satisfactory physical living arrangements (Havighurst, 1972). To achieve successful later life adjustment, the following adaptations are recommended for the older person: (1) maintenance of feelings of self-worth, (2) resolution of old conflicts, (3) adjustment to loss of power roles, (4) adjustment to the deaths of significant others, (5) adaptation to environmental changes, and (6) maintenance of an optimal level of wellness (Hamilton, 1992).

❖ Self-Esteem

Self-concept is the cognitive component of a person's self-perception. The *ideal self* is subjective and specifies the person's conception of desirable self-characteristics. In comparing the self-concept with the ideal self the person achieves *self-esteem.*

Negative or positive self-esteem is a judgment that reflects the person's self-opinion (Atchely, 1994; George, 1990). In later life many occurrences and situations threaten a positive self-concept. Ageism exemplifies this. Research has shown that many negative stereotypes, such as lowered attributes of competence, activity, intelligence, attractiveness, and health, as well as increased levels of dependency, illness, nonproductivity, and inflexibility, are attributed to older persons (Levin, 1988). Stereotypes contribute to the negative feelings and devaluation by American society of our aging population. Ageism is evident among all age groups, including older people, many of whom devalue themselves and their peers.

Continuity of self provides the older person with defense against erosion of self-esteem. Because the present self is inevitably woven with the past, memories of past competence, success, and achievement support a positive self-image. Atchley (1994, p. 143) asserts that about 80% of older persons use psychological defenses to maintain their self-esteem. This leaves a remaining 20% with a lowered self-esteem.

The heterogeneity of the older population makes it impossible to attribute a reduced self-image to a single specific cause. Self-image alterations may result from a perceived loss of control and competence within the physical environment, a change in physical status, or a change in the social or economic environment (Bensink, Godbey, Marshall, & Yarandi, 1992; Frey, Kelbley, Durham, & James, 1992; Thomas, 1988).

The nurse is able to intervene on several levels to enhance the client's self-esteem and feelings of personal worth. These interventions include (1) encouraging ventilation of feelings, (2) acknowledging and accepting the feelings expressed, (3) accepting client behaviors, (4) assisting clients to understand and accept their own feelings, (5) identifying problems cooperatively with the client, (6) setting realistic goals cooperatively, (7) teaching and counseling as needed, (8) supporting abilities and encouraging independence, (9) focusing on client strengths, (10) suggesting the use of self-help or reminiscence groups to increase positive feelings about past accomplishments, (11) assisting clients to develop new interests, (12) reinforcing positively all new skills as they are developed, and (13) using environmental manipulation to enhance the abilities of the older person (Penn, 1988; Pfister-Minogue, 1993).

Losses are legitimate and personally unsettling and should be recognized as such. The older person who is grieving may benefit from talking about fears, sadness, and other feelings. Active listening can nurture trust and signifies the nurse's interest and concern for personal losses. When the problem has been verbalized, the nurse and older person can then cooperatively solve the problem. It is essential that the older person participate in all elements of the plan of care. Together the nurse and client can identify strengths and set goals. This cooperative effort has been found useful to enhance positive feelings in the older person.

The value of interventions by the nurse cannot be overemphasized. Outside influences affect self-esteem. Measures that affirm the individual's worth can be simple but vital to a positive quality of life for older persons.

❖ *Life Planning*

A comfortable and secure old age is a commonly voiced desire of older persons. There are certainly many differences in persons' perceptions of what constitutes comfort and security. Three important factors include adequate finances, good health, and relationships with family and friends. Independence is usually a high priority of the older person. Some choose to live in a protected environment such as a continuing care or retirement community rather than incur the risk of dependence upon children. Others choose to live alone despite financial, health, and social instabilities accompanied by voiced worries of the adult children. Many relate that they are not afraid to die but that they are afraid of the long illness and dependency that may precede death. Although most persons are not preoccupied by this worry, some express it as a significant issue.

The financial burden of long-term illness is difficult for all but the wealthiest. Women, minorities, and those who live alone are 70% of noninstitutionalized older persons. These persons are at highest risk for poverty (U.S. Senate Special Committee on Aging, 1991, p. 54). Many of them have very little disposable income and therefore are unable to spend money for leisure activities. Statistically, income level and perception of one's health status are directly correlated (U.S. Senate Special Committee on Aging, 1991). Persons who have a limited income tend not to seek preventive health care. Physical health, life satisfaction, and peace of mind can be affected adversely.

Preretirement Planning

The nurse who is aware of the negative implications of financial insecurities can urge families to seek preretirement counseling. In middle age a couple can anticipate retirement income by means of a pension plan, investments, and savings. Most companies have a benefits counselor who can calculate the employee's assets at the time of retirement. Clients often do not appreciate the financial vulnerability of retirement unless it is emphasized. Experts recommend that a specific plan should be drawn up 5 years prior to retirement with implementation of the plan beginning 2 years ahead (Hardy, 1989). Planning ahead may relieve future problems. Because life expectancy for women is about 7 years more than for men (U.S. Senate Special Committee on Aging, 1991), provisions should safeguard the woman's financial security in the event of her husband's death. Pension benefits and Social Security benefits should be evaluated with this in mind.

Financial considerations are only part of preretirement planning. In connection with income and pension considerations should be included estate planning with attention to wills, trusts, and life insurance; health management; housing; social relationships; leisure time; developmental changes of aging; and use of community resources (Hardy, 1989).

If an existing program is available, the nurse can encourage the potential retiree to attend. If not, it may be feasible to set one up. In that case the nurse should work as a member of the multidisciplinary team to prepare the curriculum and presentations. Specific content information can be provided by a guest expert in a lecture with questions and answers. Other methods of presentation include group discussion and active participation, study materials, individual counseling, and encounter sessions. These methods or combinations of them have been used successfully. Neuhs (1991) has developed a Retirement Self-Efficacy Scale that is useful for identifying high-risk individuals before and after retirement. Retirement concerns can be recognized and the nurse can provide individual counseling where indicated.

Programs can be presented in numerous settings. Many businesses incorporate preretirement programs into the organizational structure to smooth the transition from employment to retirement. Continuing education courses may be included in collegiate curricula. The information is useful also for the person who is already retired. Classes may be offered through community programs in churches and schools. For the person who is motivated to do independent study, many books and workbooks are available. Although this information is designed to prepare the person for retirement, new retirees may also wish to attend.

Retirement

Labor force participation of men and women declines steadily in the older age groups. In 1989 among persons 70 years and older, only 10.9% of men and 4.6% of women were in the labor force (U.S. Special Committee on Aging, 1991). Retirement from work can present a significant adjustment challenge for the older population financially, socially, and emotionally. Work provides both a structured activity within a regular time frame and a sense of purpose and daily meaning. Energy is channeled into intellectual, creative, and/or physical tasks that offer a sense of satisfaction when they are completed. The worker, regardless of the work role, functions within a social structure. Social interactions occur; friendships and acquaintances often extend beyond the workplace. The financial reward, originally the motivating force behind the chosen occupation, is only one facet of the work benefits. Persons assume an identity from their choice of career. This determines how others view them and often affects how persons view themselves. Fewer social interactions and role change may cause the retiree to feel useless, bored, and lonely.

Despite these problems, persons are retiring earlier. In 1989 only 54.8% of men and 35.5% of women aged 60 to 64 were in the labor force. People retire for many reasons, including declining health, financial support from Social Security and pensions, the retirement of a spouse, and the opportunity to participate in leisure and volunteer pursuits. In addition, with the economic shift to service industries in the United States there is an increased emphasis on retirement options (Ruhm, 1989; U.S. Special Committee on Aging, 1991).

Research suggests that persons who have a high commitment to the work role place little value on leisure time. Such people are relatively unlikely to view retirement favorably. People who are most likely to succeed in retirement are those who are actively involved in service organizations and have a positive outlook toward leisure activities (Hooker and Ventis, 1984). The routine that is necessary for work can frustrate leisure activities. Time and energy are finite, and there may not be enough of them for the worker's personal and social interests. A retiree will have ample time to pursue hobbies, creative activities, interact with family, and help others in volunteer pursuits.

As retirement has become an expected transition in American life, so adjustment to retirement has become easier. Using data from the Normative Aging Study, Bosse, Aldwin, Levenson, and Workman-Daniels (1991) found that only 30% of the male participants found retirement to be stressful. Major predictors for a stressful retirement were poor health and financial difficulties. Research indicates that a stable social situation, personal control, secure finances, and realistic expectations contribute to a positive adaptation (Atchley, 1994; Daly & Futrell, 1989; Vinick & Ekerdt, 1989).

The decision to retire may be a matter of personal choice or necessity. About two thirds of retirees age 65 and older report that they stopped working by choice. Others were forced to retire because of unemployment or health problems. Persons who have little or no financial reserve, including personal savings, home ownership, and pensions, tend to stay at work longer. About one fourth of older people have resources and incomes below or barely above the poverty level. Those at greatest risk are the oldest old, those not living in families, and minority women living alone (U.S. Senate Special Committee on Aging, 1991, p. 38-53).

Governmental assistance programs are available to these vulnerable older persons. In housing, for example, rent reductions through public housing developments or rent subsidies on a federal, state, or local level are available for some. Thirty percent of the federal budget is set aside for programs benefiting older people. Included are Social Security and Supplemental Security Income (54%), Medicare (26%), Medicaid (6%), and other programs providing assorted social, energy, and housing benefits (14%) (U.S. Senate Special Committee on Aging, 1991, pp. 197, 238-239).

Partial Retirement

The adjustment to retirement may be facilitated by a gradual rather than abrupt relinquishment of work. It seems reasonable that a shift to part-time work can ease retirement trauma. Many new retirees change from career jobs to part-time jobs. These seem to provide a transition to full retirement.

More than 25% of new retirees between the ages of 58 and 73 assume a new job role. A government study found that 22% of older women and 24% of older men continued to be employed for up to 2 years after receiving their first Social Security retirement benefits (U.S. Special Committee on Aging, 1991, p. 90). These positions are often characterized by a change in employer from that of the preretirement job, a switch in both industry and occupation, a decrease in the wage rate, and a decrease in annual earnings (Parnes, 1989; Quinn & Burkhauser, 1990;

Ruhm, 1989). Questions remain unanswered about partial retirement. Why do workers not continue in their career jobs on a part-time basis? Is this because of Social Security incentives? Why do such workers take on new jobs? (Ruhm, 1989). In 1986, 48% of the men and 61% of the women over age 65 held part-time jobs (U.S. Senate Special Committee on Aging, 1991).

Use of Leisure Time

The state of retirement as an accepted lifestyle in combination with an expanded life expectancy allows older people to spend a substantial portion of their lives in activities outside the labor force (U.S. Special Committee on Aging, 1991, p.86). Research suggests that retired people use leisure time as they did prior to retirement. Favorite activities include television, visiting, reading, home maintenance, and hobbies. After retirement, only a few people adopt new hobbies. There is continuity throughout the life course, and recreational interests are no exception (Kunkel, 1989).

❖ Late-Life Learning

Late-life learning has come of age. The myth that depicts our older generation as unable to learn has been exploded. Indeed, older people not only can learn, they want to learn, and many participate in varied educational experiences. A class or informal learning experience will enrich the older person with new information and also provide a social opportunity. Instructional topics abound. Learning opportunities include a variety of subjects that range from hobbies, science, arts, and health promotion to career enhancement and work skills. Older persons are very much interested in learning about health promotion and quality of life issues. Nurses can capitalize on this motivation and offer health information classes. Examples of popular topics include commonly occurring illnesses, with symptoms, medications, and management; nutritional advice; home safety; cancer detection measures; skin care; and selecting a physician.

Age-related physiological changes may be barriers to learning if not addressed. Teaching will be more meaningful for the participants if the nurse uses the following classroom strategies: (1) Develop a list of topics with suggestions from the participants. (2) Select a quiet room away from distractions. (3) Develop short-term outcomes in cooperation with the learners. (4) Encourage the use of glasses and hearing aids. (5) Provide glare-free lighting. (6) Furnish refreshments whenever possible. (7) Pace learning tasks according to group stamina. (8) Limit the length of the class period. (9) Encourage participation from the group. (10) Give positive reinforcement for successful learning (Weinrich, Boyd, and Nussbaum, 1989; Hamilton, 1992).

Various teaching aids make classes more interesting and understandable and their benefits longer-lasting. Pamphlets and other reading materials can be studied at home and shared with significant others. Language used on all visual aids should be uncomplicated and straightforward. This allows for educational deficits in participants (Weinrich & Boyd, 1992). Only 51% of those who are 65 years and older are high school graduates (U.S. Senate Special Committee on Aging, 1991, p.193). Overheads and posters should have distinctly visible high-contrast lettering that is large enough to be seen at a distance. White lettering on a dark background is best for posters (Weinrich & Boyd, 1992).

Some educational programs based in high schools, community colleges, universities, or community centers train retirees who want to develop new careers or expand their knowledge. Some university programs waive tuition or reduce rates for older persons. Many offer support services in reading, writing, public speaking, counseling, and placement. Depending upon the needs and goals of the older participants, a variety of paths can be followed. In 1988, 140,000 people over the age of 55 were enrolled in college or high school courses (U.S. Senate Special Committee on Aging, 1991). Some students earn a degree and pursue a new career. Others find full- or part-time work with the help of the placement services. Some choose to volunteer their skills.

Enrichment Education

Informal and often nontraditional enrichment programs reflect the educational demands of the older generations (Fagelson, 1990). Many older people are enrolled in noncredit part-time courses taken for personal fulfillment or to enhance career expertise (Fagelson, 1990). In 1984, 2.7 million persons over age 55 were taking one or more such courses (U.S. Senate Special Committee on Aging, 1991). Elderhostel is one such initiative that has been flourishing since 1976 and has registered thousands of persons over age 60 (or over age 50 when accompanying someone over 60). This self-supporting program uses college campuses throughout the world for short-term (usually 1 week) residency. Participants pay a tuition charge that will meet program costs. A vast choice of courses meets varied interests; subsidized travel and ongoing satisfaction to learners have contributed to its success (Elderhostel, 1993; Verschueren, 1993).

The National Council on Aging offers the Discovery Program, which has also been very successful offering enrichment learning. Many thousands of persons have attended this subsidized program at low cost. Less affluent and underserved older people have been the primary beneficiaries.

Desirable outgrowths of older adult education go beyond the explicit purposes of the programs. These include intergenerational bonding, reductions in dependency, increased autonomy, and self-help. Successful activities provide an opportunity for older adults to achieve abundance of life.

❖ Volunteerism

The search for purpose and constructive use of leisure time that motivates older people to attend classes and learning sessions also impels them to volunteer their services to a cause perceived as worthwhile. It is not uncommon for an older person to adopt an elder's role in society, providing guidance, support, and counseling to a younger and more innocent generation. Moreover, this role has been formalized through specific programs. Local voluntary organizations recognize a community need and informally gather resources to meet it. There are also formal federally sponsored projects that rely on the older generations for manpower.

A telephone survey of people 60 years and older in 962 interviews revealed that more than 41% of the respondents performed some form of volunteer work in the past year. Those aged 65 to 74 had the highest rate, about 45%. Usually more than one day a week was volunteered. Reasons given for volunteering include moral responsibility (52%), a social obligation (33%), a way of finding companionship (25%), and a way to alleviate feelings of guilt (5%). Those with a college education were more likely to volunteer (66%) than those who had a high school education (37.5%) (Marriott Seniors Volunteerism Study, 1991).

ACTION, a federal volunteer agency, sponsors three programs that use only people over 60 years as volunteers: Senior Companion Program, Retired Senior Volunteer Program (RSVP), and Foster Grandparents. When the Foster Grandparents program began in 1965, older people volunteered their services to benefit handicapped and ill children. These programs have expanded, and now 23,300 older people offer support services totaling 21 million hours that address a myriad of social problems of the younger generations. Services are well organized, creative, and effective. For example, older volunteers are model parents for children at risk as a result of family crises such as abuse, neglect, abandonment, and absence of parents. They work individually with such children and provide love, support, and necessary caring tasks (ACTION, 1992). Senior Companions offers personal assistance and peer support to low-income, homebound, and chronically ill older people. These volunteers are required to perform 20 hours of service each week. Along with comfort and support, they provide household services on a one-to-one basis. Volunteers for Foster Grandparents and Senior Companions receive a small hourly stipend, one free meal, and transportation costs. They must meet standards of low income to qualify as volunteers for these programs.

RSVP is ACTION's largest program, with more than 400,000 volunteers. Public and private organizations sponsor local RSVP activities cooperatively with ACTION. RSVP volunteers provide services in defined projects ranging from first aid to tutoring. They serve with no compensation.

Senior adults can volunteer their services in many programs for and with all ages. In schools they can serve as teacher aides, tutors, demonstrators, and guest speakers. Retired professionals provide their services free of charge to needy older people. Through these and many other programs older volunteers give time, energy, and knowledge that benefit and support troubled individuals. Many volunteer services are provided informally to friends and neighbors. These, in combination with services and care channeled through church-sponsored and community agencies, are not necessarily calculated as volunteer hours. If every American over the age of 65 were to give one hour a week to a volunteer activity, an annual total of 1.5 billion hours would be donated (Kerschner & Butler, 1988).

Although many people embrace the voluntary experience with enthusiasm, a substantial number discontinue services after a short time. Attrition can be minimized if predictors for successful candidates are identified. A survey of 151 senior volunteers revealed four role characteristics associated with role satisfaction and retention. The first, role recognition, demonstrates the importance of positive feedback from peers, supervisor, clients, and the organization. The second, role-set interaction, illustrates the need for contact with other volunteers and paid staff. The third, role congruence, establishes the importance of agreement between expectations and the actual job experience. And the fourth, service activity pattern, signifies the value of past involvement in community experience (Stevens, 1991).

Volunteers are rewarded by knowing that they are truly needed. The personal involvement is beneficial to both the giver and the recipient, and time spent is worthwhile. Goals are set and achieved. Loneliness is replaced by concern for someone with a profound need. Social interactions occur and new friends are made. Thoughts are turned outward and focus on others instead of oneself. Not everyone wants to be a volunteer; however, those who choose to become involved derive intrinsic satisfactions and simultaneously furnish services that would otherwise be unavailable.

❖ *Leisure*

Implicit in the theories of successful adjustment to old age is the chosen lifestyle that accompanies newfound leisure time. Use of free time varies according to the desires of the retired person and constraints that include finances, health, and social milieu, community opportunities, and abilities of the older person (Cutler & Hendricks, 1990). Beyond choices that include work, volunteerism, and educational pursuits, some older persons want to devote their free time to activities separate from a work orientation. These may be creative, challenging, and/or expressive.

Usually there is a continuity with the past, and the older person will select something that is congruent with earlier living. Creative and artistic pursuits provide a satisfying, stimulating outlet. Music, painting, and writing are but a few modes of creative expression available for the older person to enjoy actively or passively. The fine arts, including music, drama, literature, and museums also can enhance the quality of life. When the weather permits, nature itself can contribute to the esthetic pleasure of the older adult. All five senses can receive stimulation during a nature hike or when gardening (Catlin, Milliorn & Milliorn, 1992).

In research involving leisure activities of 30 community-residing African-American women, four themes were verbalized: loneliness; church, worship, and duty; affiliative activities; and solitary activities (Chin-Sang & Allen, 1991). Activities varied from active and vigorous behaviors to artistic and creative activities such as playing a musical instrument and performing handwork. All the participants read the Bible and newspapers, watched television, and listened to the radio.

A review of studies by Cutler and Hendricks (1990) notes that time spent on physically active leisure activities decreases with increasing age. However, moderate-intensity and low-intensity patterns of activities do not decrease with aging. Evidence supporting continuity and stability across the lifespan is very strong. A high level of leisure participation in youth is associated with high levels of participation in maturity (p. 174). Gender differences occur, with men more interested in outdoor recreational sports such as hunting, fishing, travel, and spectator sports. Conversely, women tend to enjoy home-based and cultural activities. Well-being seems to be associated with active involvement in leisure activities (Cutler & Hendricks, 1990).

To enhance maximum leisure in later years, the nurse can make the following suggestions to middle-aged adults and young-older persons: (1) Make leisure a daily high-priority activity. (2) Do not neglect leisure activity for any period of time; additional free time may become problematic if patterns of leisure are not already present. (3) Continue to cultivate new leisure interests. (4) Be adaptable with personal and social changes (Leitner & Leitner, 1989, p. 277).

❖ *Social Relationships*

Social relationships enable the older person to enjoy life more fully. Family and friends provide the older person with a sense of security, identity, and self-worth. In addition to furnishing essential psychosocial support, the social network also is the major provider of instrumental aid. In times of illnesses and other personal crises, the older person's social network may indeed be the deciding variable that determines place of residence, living conditions, and physical care.

Marriage

The later-life family has launched its children and shed its child-rearing responsibilities. Nevertheless, the family point of reference rests with the husband-wife dyad. Within their marriage and relationship, they can expect to encounter new life events associated with developmental changes of later life. Interdependency and interactions of the generations within this family network furnish the older couple with a vital support system (Brubaker, 1990).

The couple relationship has weathered many years; with increased life expectancy they can anticipate many more years together. Researchers have investigated the character of long-standing marriages. What special attributes may have contributed to the longevity of this relationship? Does marital satisfaction ebb and wane over the lifespan? These and many other questions have been investigated, and some findings have been contradictory.

Much research has addressed the relationship between health, life satisfaction, and the social support system of older persons (Condie, 1989; Vinick & Ekerdt, 1989; Willits and Crider, 1988). Persons living alone are less satisfied with their lives and worry more about money and health (Kasper, 1988). Research supports the conclusion that married older persons have higher levels of morale, life satisfaction, mental and physical health, economic resources, and social support (Bengston, Rosenthal, and Burton, 1990). Life satisfaction can easily be affected by many variables, depending on the circumstances of the individual. Health is a major determinant, outranking the number of friends, marital status, and income (Willits & Crider, 1988). However, the positive effect of social relationships on health cannot be overlooked (Huss, Buckwalter, & Stolley, 1988).

Quality and quantity are two dimensions of relationships that must be considered. Quantity addresses the numbers of persons and frequency of contacts. Quality considers the perception of support by the older person as well as intimacy and scope. Atchley (1994) discusses marital satisfaction using the describers of intimacy, sexual intimacy, interdependence, and belonging. Intimacy encompasses trust, affection, and regard. Interdependence involves the sharing of housework, income, and other resources. Belonging is an identification of the person with the dyad. It includes a sharing of values and perspectives. Intimacy can be social, emotional, and/or physical; any and all are important. Touching, clinging, stroking, sexual expression, confiding, and reassurance contribute to preservation and maintenance of affiliative bonds.

Confiding relationships, one form of intimacy, have been found to have a major positive influence on well-being. Such a trust relationship must include mutual sharing of feelings and personal problems. When it is present in old age, there are associated lower levels of loneliness and higher levels of self-esteem and mental and physical health (Kendig, Coles, Pittelkow, & Wilson, 1988; Huss et al., 1988). Most older people have confidants and a few intimate relationships even when they do not have close family members. The range of individual interactions varies considerably. Often the wife assumes a major supportive role within the marital dyad. Although men in retirement have shared activities and interests with other friends, the wife continues to be named as closest friend and confidant. However, married women sometimes use family, specifically a daughter, and friends for socioemotional support instead of their spouses (Anderson & McCulloch, 1993; Atchley, 1994; Reisman, 1988).

Research (Kendig et al., 1988) indicates that older people are most likely to confide in a spouse, second in a child, followed by a sibling or friend. Father-son and mother-daughter liaisons are often important. In parent-child relationships, the daughter is often a confidant for the mother (Anderson & McCulloch, 1993).

A successful marriage enhances life satisfaction for older persons. Contentment with marriage is the strongest predictor of life satisfaction for women. For men, only good health is a more important predictor. Most marriages of older people are stable. Rarity of divorces is a phenomenon often associated with a lifestyle from an era past. Although research findings are contradictory, it is generally agreed that marital satisfaction is higher in later life than in middle life (Atchley, 1994; Condie, 1989).

Over a lifetime a couple has developed a cooperative and comfortable interaction. Values and perspectives become similar through mutual life experiences. The family unit offers a sense of belonging and unity. With retirement comes added leisure time. Although strains are sometimes associated with new role adjustments (Preston & Dellasega, 1990), a sharing of housework, income, and household tasks also leads to added interdependence. Some research studies indicate that retirement of the husband with a wife who continues to work can have a significantly negative effect upon the marital satisfaction of the woman. The researchers suggest that a husband's unwillingness to accept household responsibilities may explain this phenomenon (Lee and Sheehan, 1989).

Couples with grown children often find themselves in the role of grandparent. They provide such functions as historian, family arbitrator, mentor, emergency helper, surrogate parent, and value shaper. When couples find themselves providing surrogate parenting to their grandchildren, strains often occur. Parenting grandchildren is rewarding, but this added responsibility will cause the couple to lose privacy and the freedom they gained when they retired. They will have less time to pursue hobbies, socializing, and interacting with each other. The burdens of child care may drain them physically and emotionally (Atchley, 1994).

Many happy and positive marriages end in later life with the death of one partner. After the painful period of recovery from such a loss, some widows and widowers decide to remarry. Due to the sex differentials on life expectancy, there are more marriageable women than there are men. Furthermore, society norms dictate that women marry men older than themselves. Thus the marriage rates of older men are eight times those of older women (U.S. Special Committee on Aging, 1991). New partners are often old friends who have also been widowed, neighbors, or members of the same church. Although financial security or need for a helper or nurse may be the motivator, companionship is given as the major reason for remarriage. With age and life experience to help overcome potential conflict, most older remarriages are successful. Interestingly, research indicates that remarried men tend to be more satisfied in their marriages than remarried women (Bowers & Bahr, 1989). Five variables that seem to contribute to remarriage success are (1) the older persons have known one another well, (2) friends and family approve, (3) the individuals have adapted to role changes of later life, (4) the couple does not live in either person's previous home, and (5) the couple has sufficient income (Atchley, 1994; Travis, 1987).

Sexuality

Unfortunately, prevailing ageism in American society has fostered an insensitivity to the intimacy and relationship needs of older persons. Sexuality of older persons in particular is viewed negatively. Sexual activity of older persons has received recent attention, but prevailing myths and attitudes are difficult to change. Sexually active older persons are often judged to be practicing aberrant behavior. Sexual practice is often denied or ignored by society at large, and concerns by older adults remain unspoken and unanswered.

The reproductive physiology of older persons indeed changes drastically. It takes longer to achieve an erection and orgasm, and hormonal alterations may present physical gynecological changes that cause painful and difficult coitus. Also, chronic illness, lack of physical and psychic energy, side effects of medications, lack of social sanctioning, disinterest and boredom, preoccupation, and fear of failure may deter any attempts. However, some of these barriers can be overcome with appropriate counseling and hormone replacement. Many older couples continue sexual relationships well into old age (Comfort & Dial, 1991; McCracken, 1988).

Although sexuality is equated with intercourse, other sexual expressions of holding, touching, and closeness may afford satisfaction and fulfillment to older adults. Nurses can listen, suggest, and facilitate a positive, healthy sexual outlook. To achieve this role, nurses must first deal with their own beliefs and attitudes. Sexual intimacy and loving play a necessary and desirable role in life, regardless of age.

Friendships

Friends validate the existence of a person. Old friends were voluntarily selected and have stood the test of many years. As they age, these friends get sick, die, move away, or have no means of transportation. It is often difficult for long-standing friends to see one another and reinforce their relationship. Nevertheless, friendship networks offer companionship, emotional, and service support to many older people. They are particularly important to people who have little or no family support (Jerome, 1991).

Women are more likely than men to have stable, intimate, and supportive friendships (Connidis & Davies, 1992). There is a positive relationship between friendship and psychological well-being. Friendships offer several advantages over family relationships: age differences are minimal, the relationship is voluntary, and social involvement with others is frequent (Adams, 1989). Friends can offer comfort and support when the death of a loved person occur. Social activities and keeping busy with friends and family are useful coping strategies for the grieving widow and widower. Friends do not always share a past. Older persons, particularly in the absence of family, may develop new friendships in later life (Mullins & Mushel, 1992).

A person enters a nursing home when the social support system is unable to care adequately for him or her. Research shows that institutionalization is more likely if a person lives alone and has a mental or physical incapacity (Steinbach, 1992). Nurses have many opportunities to develop friendships with older persons. Sometimes they become confidants to older persons. Close ties with the staff are significantly related to the life satisfaction, health, and mental functioning of the older person (Huss et al., 1988). In providing holistic care, the nurse uses contact time with residents therapeutically and effectively.

Nursing Home Communication

Physically impaired elders need others within their environment to provide socioemotional support. Substantive interactions among the residents is often minimal. Research has affirmed constrictive norms among residents of nursing homes. These serve to inhibit communication and limit intimacy. Kaakinen (1992) calls it a "forlorn silence." During her research in eight nursing homes, she found many norms and taboos among the residents regarding behavior and interactions. Some of the most commonly held self-regulatory statements were (1) ignore those perceived to be "senile," (2) talk only with those who are willing to talk, (3) don't talk to those who are hearing-impaired, and (4) use silence to regulate talking behaviors (Kaakinen, 1992, p. 261). She found that the residents comply with these taboos. Because they insulate themselves from others, they place themselves at high risk for isolation.

The nurse can use this information to plan counteracting interventions. It may be necessary to segregate confused residents. For those who are cognitively intact, (1) place talkative persons in rooms with other talkative persons; (2) encourage activities designed to stimulate conversation; (3) change the large-group format of the residents' council to small group task forces; (4) establish small discussion groups; (5) offer memorial services for those who died (this may encourage verbalization about cumulative losses); (6) increase residents' contacts with talking people coming into the home (volunteer programs); (7) develop recreational activities that enhance interactions (reminiscence, current events, Bible study, etc.); (8) rearrange the environment to promote communication (placement of chairs and wheelchairs facing one another, small conversation corners, etc.); (9) install adaptive equipment for the hearing-impaired; (10) decrease environmental noise in the dining room (Kaakinen, 1992).

❖ *Religion*

Throughout history religion has been a source of support for older persons (Koenig, 1993). Only families and the federal government provide more instrumental assistance (Blazer, 1991). Through voluntary services initiated and provided by the church, many community-based persons achieve maximum independence. Church members are often directly involved in providing physical and emotional care. The care is often provided by persons who themselves are past 65 years of age. Indirectly through the use of the church building, churches sponsor activities for older persons including recreational and nutritional programs. Some churches sponsor and administer institutional care.

Many older persons attach great importance to religion. In a telephone survey, 96% of those 65 or older agreed with the statement, "There is a God who watches over you and answers your prayers" (Koenig, 1993). Older persons who are actively involved and committed to religious activities have a signifgicantly higher morale (Koenig, Kvale, & Ferrel, 1988). Engagement is often participative through church services and church-related activity. The older person also may take quiet time to reflect on values and beliefs and to pray and read religious material. Prayer and Bible reading are reported to be helpful to many newly bereaved widowed people (Nelson, 1990). In a survey of older persons to determine coping strategies, religious coping behaviors were named most frequently. These behaviors include placing faith and trust in God, prayer, and obtaining help and strength from God to handle the situation (Koenig, 1993; Koenig, George, & Siegler, 1988).

Holistic nursing must incorporate the spiritual aspects of a person into care. This aspect is sometimes avoided or forgotten. It is important for the nurse to acknowledge this spiritual dimension of the patient and facilitate religious expression and growth. An assessment through questions and observations helps to outline the person's religious affiliation and needs. Appropriate referrals, sharing, and active listening all will help to support spirituality of the older person (Forbis, 1988; Hamner, 1990; Nelson, 1990).

❖ *Companion Animals*

Pets can enhance the quality of life of older people. Intuitively and anecdotally, society recognizes the value of a friendly animal for an older person living alone. With a rising awareness of the need for social support, many encourage the use of companion animals (Boldt, 1992; Harris & Gellin, 1990; Miller & Lago, 1990). Pets fill a void in the lives of older persons. However, pets do not replace people. Self-reported morale is higher for women living alone with a pet than for those living without one. Nevertheless, living with people raises the morale higher than living with a pet (Goldmeier, 1986).

Pet therapy is the application of the bond between humans and companion animals. Pets are friendly companions that distract and divert attention from losses. People like to stroke and hug their pets. They talk to them and may tell them about their problems. Pets need daily care and provide regular purpose to a life that may otherwise be aimless. The animal may facilitate social engagement by providing a focus for conversation (Cusack, 1988; Weisberg & Pack, 1991).

Many qualitative reports and some quantitative studies have documented the varied benefits to older people of the companion animal–human bond. Animals have been used successfully in nursing homes and in hospitals. Such programs must be carefully planned and implemented with cooperation from administration and staff. A design for evaluation should be incorporated (Rosenkoetter & Bowes, 1991; Schantz, 1990; Weisberg & Pack, 1991).

❖ *Personal Space*

The internal environment of a human being is clearly defined by the physical body. Surrounding the body is a poorly defined area with a boundary that separates it from the external environment. This zone is known as personal space. It goes with the individual and may be compressed or expanded according to circumstances. For example, on a crowded bus there is little personal space beyond the body. However, in a library, the personal space is inclined to expand. The external environment begins where the personal space ends. In the external environment, people have an innate need for privacy, a personal haven (territory) set apart that belongs exclusively to them. This territory varies in size according to the culture, situation, and personal status of the person. It has clearly delineated boundaries that leave no doubts about ownership (Roberts, 1980).

Relocation

The territory of an older person is more commonly known as a house or an apartment. It signifies independence, autonomy, home, and privacy and offers a societal role to its inhabitant. Most older people want to remain in their own homes and maintain their independence. Many are willing to jeopardize their safety, their economic stability, and their optimal health to do so. They may endure a great deal of discomfort, inconvenience, and loneliness before relinquishing this independence. When an old person leaves home to live elsewhere, there are inevitable regrets and a sense of loss.

Cherished possessions often must be left behind when a person moves. However, whenever possible the older person should be encouraged to move items that support memories, serve a useful function, and facilitate role continuance (Mikhail, 1992; Thomasma, 1990). The nurse should be sensitive to the person's need for personal space, privacy, and autonomy in the new living quarters. For a positive adjustment the definition of a new territory must be completed to the older person's satisfaction. When possible the nurse should encourage discussions on the meaning of possessions. The nurse can provide education and information about the new community, point out community resources, help with problem solving, attend to emotional issues, encourage use of familiar coping strategies, and make needed referrals for counseling (Brooke, 1989b; Mikhail, 1992).

Relocation is a traumatic and difficult event for all older persons. However, several factors specifically affect adjustment to relocation. These can serve as predictors of the attitudes of the resident. Mikhail (1992) discusses three of these: voluntary admission, involuntary admission, and family dynamics.

If the elder is unable to manage self-care and has no other way to meet daily needs, placement may be necessary. In this situation the older person controls the admission process and may even be familiar with the setting. With careful preadmission planning, which ideally includes an introductory visit and meeting some staff and residents, some familiarization will occur prior to admission. Predictably, the transition will be less traumatic (Brooke, 1989a, Mikhail, 1992; Reinardy, 1992).

Conversely, the older person may have not been included in the decision-making process. Press of time, sudden dependency, prior hospitalization, or insensitive family judgments may have precipitated a hasty nursing home admission without the necessary emotional preparation. The older person may feel hurt, angry, abandoned, depressed, or any combination of negative emotions (Brooke, 1989a; Mikhail, 1992; Reinardy, 1992).

The family should be supportive to the older person, particularly during this time of anxiety. However, if guilt, family conflict, or some other personal issue is paramount, the family members can become part of the problem. Their conflict may be evident to the older person as well as to the nursing home staff, interfering with a smooth adaptation (Mikhail, 1992).

Based upon her research, Brooke (1989a) suggests that there are four phases in the process of relocation adjustment. The first, *disorganization,* is characterized by such negative feelings as loss, abandonment and anxiety. Secondly, *reorganization* occurs. During this stage, the older person is trying to assign meaning to this new experience. It is a time when feelings and self-confidence are particularly evident. In the third phase, *relationship building,* the person is establishing ties with the people around him or her. When losses and feelings have been adequately resolved, the *stabilization* stage occurs. Although they may prefer their past circumstances, they have adapted and come to terms with their new home.

❖ *Autonomy*

The nursing home environment requires a radical life adjustment by the older adult. Staffing economics dictate a routine that robs the residents of autonomous choices. Baths, meals, activities, and visiting are scheduled for staff convenience. However, certain measures within the environment can restore some control to the older adult. Residents can be encouraged to arrange personal items and furniture in their room. They can decide what to wear and be given options where opportunities present themselves. Activities should be offered, and the residents should have autonomy in their choice of activities. Residents can be requested to share their special talents but should not be coerced to participate. The nurse recognizes and reinforces achievement of accomplishments such as daily exercises, artwork, task completion, and group activity (Cox, Kaeser, Montgomery, & Marion, 1991; Penn, 1988).

Increased autonomy implies increased responsibility. Within their physical and mental capabilities, residents can be encouraged and even expected to participate in certain ongoing activities. These obligations should be negotiated and monitored skillfully and fairly by the nurse or other professional. Such duties as basic self-care, mail delivery, making announcements, tending pets, gardening, repairing clothes, greeting visitors, minor maintenance, and helping other residents are examples of regular chores that residents can do. Participation in responsible activities fosters empowerment, dignity, and a sense of community (Jameton, 1988). Such activities are commonly performed by residents in continuing care and retirement communities. However, nursing home residents are rarely given such obligations, although they might benefit from encouragement by the nursing staff.

Other less conventional methods can increase self-esteem and autonomy. One 550-bed nursing home organized a political and social action group that they call Seniors for Justice (SFJ). This group began as a discussion group with topics generated by the recreational therapist. The success of SFJ became evident when the residents brought their own topics to this forum and adopted a democratic process of discussion and vote. From this beginning has evolved social action. Members have become involved with such questions as gun control, the plight of the homeless, and a nursing home recycling program.

The SFJ group's work has become known outside of the nursing home and has elicited responses from the community at large. They now receive letters, pro and con, and have hosted elected officials. Other outcomes of their work include a recycling program within their facility and a contribution of a small sum of money and a vanload of food to a homeless shelter. Members of the SFJ have seen positive changes directly resulting from their efforts. They feel empowered and effective (Hubbard, Werner, Cohen-Mansfield, & Shusterman, 1992).

❖ *Environmental Supports*

Because of possible decremental changes in the sensory organs and decreases in mobility caused by chronic illness, the milieu of the older person often becomes restricted. The person may be receiving only partial messages or none at all from an environment that appears to the caregiver to offer a variety of stimuli. A person relates to the environment only to the degree that it has relevance for him or her. The nurse can help older persons establish a more significant communication with their surroundings. The environment must supply meaningful stimuli. A cluttered, object-filled area may provide needed tactile experiences as well as remembrances of the past. When there are few close friends and relatives, the need for cherished and consequential inanimate objects is greater. Surfaces of floors, walls, and furniture should offer interesting and varied textures. Smells and sounds can be varied. The environment should be inviting and important to the older person.

Lawton (1986) formulated the environmental docility hypothesis, which states that the reduced competency of an individual, whether caused by personal disability or deprived status, renders that person's behavior more susceptible to immediate environmental situations. This hypothesis implies that a favorable environment will enhance desirable behavioral change and increase competence. Small changes in the environment for the less competent person may produce substantial changes in the adaptiveness of behavior and may support independence and autonomy.

Homes that will allow the older person to age in place are now being designed and built. Exterior steps are eliminated; levels within the home can be negotiated without stairways. Doors and corridors will accommodate a wheelchair. Counters and sinks can be adjusted up and down. Bathroom walls are designed to hold grab bars (Noakes, 1988; Sit, 1992). Many environmental supports exist to help the individual. The nurse can be aware that technical innovations may be all that is necessary to provide safety and well-being to the community-based older person. The developmental trends include (1) increased interest in mobility, (2) expansion of agility aids, (3) wider use of sensory enhancements, (4) identification of products as memory aids or devices to improve mental function, (5) application of new materials and construction, and (6) use of creative methods for introducing the general public to technology (Hiatt, 1986). Most devices are available through medical or hospital supply stores and catalogs.

❖ *Humor*

Sometimes a situation seems so serious that laughter is out of the question. Yet this may be an appropriate moment for the participants to step away and focus upon the elements of humor. The role of humor in the care of older persons is not well recognized as a therapeutic modality. However, it can be very useful in geronto-logical care. It is valuable for stress management, building relationships, as a coping mechanism, as a tool to promote physical and psychological healing, and as a communication technique (Davidhizar & Schearer, 1992).

Humor may help to defuse an awkward situation and facilitate communication when one is trying to develop a sense of trust or introducing a difficult or uncomfortable issue. For example, an outgoing and personable older gentleman was diagnosed as having cancer of the larynx. After a laryngectomy and radical neck surgery, friends were understandably hesitant to visit him at home. Despite his emotional turmoil and discomfort, he managed to crack jokes using pencil and paper and inject humor into this sad situation. Visitors were put at ease and all were more comfortable. They marveled at his sense of humor and complimented him on his ability to laugh in the face of adversity. He gained in self-esteem, and family and friends enjoyed their visits and repeated them.

Humor can also be a valuable tool within the institutional setting. The hospital hierarchy dictates patient and staff expectations; the patient is dependent and assumes a sick person's role, while the staff is in charge and assumes an active role. Embarrassing and awkward episodes develop that would be incongruous in other settings. A well-timed and appropriate comment on such an occasion reduces tension and allows the patient to see the caregiver's empathy and awareness of his or her discomfort.

Some people have a natural and inborn sense of humor. They provoke laughter. Others are not so gifted. If humor is forced, poorly timed, or inappropriate, it is not perceived as humorous. Humor with sexual, ethnic, racial, or religious overtones should be avoided. Patients who are already stressed and highly anxious may be very sensitive to a joke that they perceive as making light of their problem. A better approach may be to allow patients to laugh at themselves or for the caregivers to deprecate themselves or a situation rather than target the patient. Laughter *with* a person rather than *at* a person is a caution that should be heeded.

A newly bereaved widow had undergone at least 6 difficult months at the side of her dying husband. She was exhausted and emotionally drained when he died. According to his wishes, she had his remains cremated. A memorial service and burial were scheduled in his hometown many miles away. She had to carry his ashes onto the plane in a small suitcase. This highly charged drama was defused with mirth and her need to laugh in the face of grief. Her description of the trip regaled her listeners. If this topic had been addressed by anyone else, it would have been met with dismay and hostility. In another situation this discussion would have been taboo. Yet mourners were given permission to laugh. The burden of grief was temporarily lifted and everyone felt a little better.

The gerontological nurse can encourage the use of laughter. However, confused and depressed persons are less than ideal candidates. Rather, humor must be individualized to the situation and the person. A joke may be funniest if it is general rather than specific to the older person's immediate concern. A silly movie starring the Three Stooges or the Marx Brothers may stimulate old memories as well as laughter.

One nursing home has been highly successful in developing original and humorous musical dramas for residents, staff, and family. The players are the families of the nursing home residents. Through this medium they poke fun at the staff and common nursing home events. In a clever, entertaining way they can ventilate their emotions, and at the same time they show their appreciation to the staff (Weisberg & Haberman, 1992). Through humor the nurse can encourage a lighter approach to problems. It is better to laugh and not take ourselves so seriously (Simon, 1988; Sullivan & Deane, 1988; Ruxton, 1988).

❖ *Physical, Social, and Psychological Health Maintenance*

Physical Health

Losses of physical health have some direct effects on the quality of life for older people. Chronic illness accompanies old age. During this century, problems of chronic disease increased while those of acute disease decreased. Hospital admissions are often for acute exacerbations of chronic conditions. Over 80% of people 65 and older have at least one chronic condition; multiple conditions are common. The older the person, the greater are the disabilities and activity limitations. Illness presents special problems for persons living alone. In 1989, 30.5% of the noninstitutionalized group over 65 lived alone (U.S. Senate Special Committee on Aging, 1991, p. 187). If community resources and/or adult children are unable to provide care, these persons are at high risk for institutionalization. This in itself can have a disquieting effect on the older person who is dealing with daily problems of self-maintenance.

Many of the chronic health problems of later life, for example osteoporosis, coronary artery disease, glaucoma, malignancies, and malnutrition, are slow to develop and difficult to treat. Some of these conditions are life-threatening; they all jeopardize quality of life. Primary prevention measures taken prior to the onset of any illness may actually prevent the health problem. Secondary promotion efforts begun early in the disease process can delay or possibly reverse the progression of disease. Tertiary preventive care may help the older person to maintain function and independence as long as possible. The gerontological nurse, assuming the role of health educator and advocate, can make a very important contribution to the positive health of older individuals.

Urinary incontinence, a very common problem for older adults, is socially disruptive and upsetting. Thomas and Morse (1991) surveyed 60 community-based persons to elicit their descriptions of incontinence. Many persons who endure incontinence report that it interferes with everyday activities and is difficult to control. Some report embarrassment and worry about odor or leakage. The various strategies used, often self-devised, are often uncomfortable; commercial products are expensive and bulky. A majority had sought medical advice and received numerous recommendations. A few had spoken with a nurse, but some did not realize that nurses dealt with incontinence issues.

Nursing interventions are valuable in the management of incontinence. Yet too often the nurse fails to assess or discuss it. Through counseling and health suggestions the client can receive emotional support and practical ideas regarding the use of easily manipulated clothing, adequate fluid intake, regular toileting, and pelvic floor muscle exercises. This gives the older person a sense of control. Even if there is little or no success with the incontinence problem, the nurse's interest and concern will reduce some feelings of isolation.

Falls are another source of psychological pain. Loss of balance as a result of medications, weakness, dizziness, hypertension, sensory decrements, environment, or neurological disease can result in a fall. The possibility of an incapacitating injury can destroy feelings of well-being. The nurse may use the interdisciplinary team (physician, occupational therapist, physical therapist) to provide suggestions for treatment and prevention. The concern of others may uplift feelings of self-worth. Interventions may reduce the risks of falling.

Everyday pleasures fundamental to quality of life for all persons are sometimes diminished in old age because of physical problems. Restricted eyesight interferes with reading; losses of taste and smell rob the person of food enjoyment. For persons who enjoy concerts, plays, and shows, hearing losses can be devastating. The nurse can suggest pertinent interventions and help the person with adaptations. Appropriate choices made according to the needs and desires of the older person will provide feelings of control and enhance the quality of life. If sensory deficits of eyesight and hearing develop, the sense of touch becomes more important. Communication is enhanced if the nurse takes advantage of opportunities to touch and be touched by older persons.

Nutrition

Dining provides a source of pleasure to many older persons. Whether in a restaurant or at home, social engagement traditionally takes place around the dinner table. Because of its potential as a regular and positive life event for all ages, a shared, regular mealtime should be encouraged. In combination with a well-balanced diet, both physical and emotional needs are supported.

Older persons often equate good nutrition with good health. Although caloric needs are reduced in older people, the body's needs for basic nutrients remain the same as younger adults' needs. Proteins and complex carbohydrates are vital, as are essential minerals, vitamins, fiber, and calories. Fat adds satiety and flavor, but its use should be limited because fatty foods are high in calories and contribute to atherosclerosis. Excessive salting should be discouraged, especially in the presence of hypertension or diseases predisposing to edema. Food flavors can be enhanced by lemon and spices. The nurse can reinforce and encourage positive dietary practices.

Foods should contain vital nutrients with a minimum of empty calories. Healthful living practices are reinforcing. In the absence of illness, older persons who maintain an optimal weight and eat a well-balanced diet will feel more energetic and motivated to participate in daily activities. This in turn provides a positive outlook and a healthy appetite, so the cycle of wellness continues.

Certain environmental and situational stresses interfere with dietary practices. Health problems including sensory deficits, dental and digestive impairments, disability, immobility, and depression all negatively affect food intake (Schlenker, 1993). Lack of money, inadequate housing, inability to cook, and apathy may also interfere with eating pleasures. The older person living alone may feel discouraged about cooking for one. The nurse can suggest that the full recipe be prepared and the excess be frozen for future meals. Perhaps it is the association between eating and socialization that intensifies lack of appetite and indifference toward food when the single older person has no dinner companion. This can be remedied by inviting a neighbor to dinner. Some older persons have been known to allow their pet to sit at the dinner table. Eating near a window, watching television, and reading all make mealtime more interesting for the solitary eater. Senior centers provide a hot, nutritious meal free or for a low cost for those who are mobile.

Wellness Clinics

Health promotion activities are supported on a federal level by the Administration on Aging, by state and area agencies on aging, and by many privately supported nonprofit organizations such as the National Council on Aging and the American Association of Retired Persons. Throughout the country versatile and creative programs educate and inspire older adults to take responsibility for health maintenance. These wellness programs teach good health practices and involve older people in health promotion activities, often in small groups. Health screening, chronic illness management, referral services, and life enrichment activities are some of the services available. Many clinics and programs are nurse managed and are closely allied with the local multipurpose senior centers (Igou, Hawkins, Johnson, & Utley, 1989; Pelican, Barbieri, & Blair, 1990; Utley, Hawkins, Igou, & Johnson, 1988; Wilson, Patterson, & Alford, 1989).

In the past 2 decades, researchers have demonstrated the value of physical activity in maintaining physical fitness and slowing the aging process. Loss of strength, flexibility, and endurance in muscles and joints become particularly evident when the person reaches the seventh decade. Although exercise cannot be expected to keep an old person young, it helps to retard degenerative processes attributable to disuse and inactivity. Certainly a program of exercise can heighten the quality of life by enhancing functional abilities and independence (Carter, Williams, & Macera, 1993; Schilke, 1991).

Fitness Programs

Exercise programs are physiologically beneficial for persons of all ages. The improvements that result when a regular fitness program is initiated are greater and more perceptible in inverse proportion to the fitness level. When fitness levels are low, greater improvement is achieved. Good physical health is only one result of a regular exercise program. When a person feels better physically, psychological well-being follows. Older people who are immobile often experience poor self-esteem, depression, insomnia, social isolation, loneliness, and feelings of inadequacy and helplessness. Regular exercise and physical fitness can change such feelings. It can enhance a person's independence and result in a better self-image. Sleeping habits, appetite, mental concentration, and energy levels may increase; constipation, apathy, and psychosomatic complaints diminish (Exercise, 1991; Gillett et al., 1993).

Improved mobility enhances opportunities for socialization. Exercise programs are often most successful within a group setting. The local YMCA, community centers, senior citizen centers, high schools, and community colleges may have such programs for older persons. Participants offer encouragement to one another, and the fitness program becomes fun, a time for joking and camaraderie. Older persons who are grieving can find others with similar or worse problems; this helps to lessen feelings of isolation and vulnerability (Gueldner & Spradley, 1988; Moore, 1989).

Persons who enjoy walking outdoors may need to devise creative alternatives for days of inclement weather. A shopping mall has regulated temperature and is an ideal place on a rainy, cold, or hot day. Videotapes of exercise programs provide reinforcing music and encouragement for those who want to stay at home. However, a change of environment and social opportunities are the optimal choices.

It is important for the nurse and older person to work cooperatively to set reasonable short-term goals that encourage the attainment of fitness. Goals themselves are important for older persons. Goals may provide a sense of purpose and order for those whose existence is aimless and boring. The exercise program may become the most important activity in such a person's life. Measurable physical changes will give persons satisfaction and pleasure that are attributable to their own personal effort and encourage them to take pride in their accomplishments and strive to achieve even greater changes. In combination with new friends, these outcomes may produce a higher quality of life.

Senior Centers

Senior centers are the community service agencies most widely used by older adults. More than 10,000 senior centers in the United States serve approximately 25% of the older population. State and local legislation has actively supported the development of multipurpose senior centers and has encouraged their presence in areas accessible to all older citizens. These centers have recreational, educational, and service components. Most centers provide transportation. They offer information and referral services for employment, housing, and living arrangements. Health-related topics and protective and legal services are commonly furnished. Older adults gather in senior centers to receive information, meet and interact with friends, obtain services, and participate in planned and informal activities (Research reveals, 1992; Gillespie & Sloan, 1990).

In the early 1970s support for meal services was added to the Older Americans' Act. Since then, senior centers have become the usual location for delivery of nutritional services. These centers have expanded to include both congregate meals and home-delivered meals. Moreover, senior centers have evolved in focus and increasingly have assumed more responsibility for providing health-related services (Krout, 1989).

Psychosocial Support

The gerontological nurse strives to improve the quality of living for the older person. Support sessions may enable the nurse to help the older client achieve social and psychological growth. Groups are useful for encouraging interactions, nurturing friendships, offering support, and providing an accepting environment for expression of feelings. Many groups with older persons do not require an accomplished therapist; the registered nurse is well qualified to establish group sessions. Older people need encouragement from each other; they also need to offer encouragement.

Burnside (1984) describes four levels of group work that nurses have used successfully. In order of skills required, these are reality orientation, remotivation, reminiscing (including music, art, health teaching and many others), and group psychotherapy. A psychiatric nurse or other psychiatric health professional should do the group psychotherapy.

Reality orientation (RO) is a therapeutic modality used within a group setting or on a one-to-one basis. It uses repetitive activities to reinforce orientation to time, place, and person in moderately confused older people. To be most effective, RO techniques are used consistently throughout the day by everyone who comes in contact with the confused patient. This is called the 24-hour environment; conversation and activities reinforce reality and orientation to time, place, and person. Daily group sessions lasting about 30 minutes use simple educational materials including memory games and sensory training props. RO is helpful for some patients in encouraging independence and quality of life. A large body of literature describes and evaluates this psychosocial technique. Involvement of staff and family in providing caring human contact may partially explain positive results (Burnside, 1984; Scanland & Emershaw, 1993). The degree, type, and duration of confusion may all influence the effectiveness of an RO program. Its use can raise anxiety levels in severely cognitively- impaired persons, and therefore, is not appropriate.

Remotivation therapy is a highly structured type of therapy designed to encourage greater involvement between patients and staff. It stimulates and revitalizes uninvolved and confused persons and encourages communication skills. A specified number of sessions are scheduled over the course of several weeks. In half an hour to an hour the participants are encouraged to respond to the topic or prop of the meeting (e.g., animals or sports). The five basic steps for each meeting include introductions, reading to the group, discussion, the work world, and expressions of appreciation. The process can be shortened to eliminate reading and the work world. Studies show some successes (Burnside, 1984; Janssen & Giberson, 1988).

Many nurses are particularly skilled in leading health promotion groups. In addition to acquiring knowledge about specific health topics, the participants are encouraged to ask questions and contribute personal experiences that may be useful to others. These sessions provide a structure within which people can interact, socialize, and ask questions in a natural and nonthreatening atmosphere.

Music therapy provides a method of nonverbal communication for persons with all levels of function. It is particularly useful for persons who are unable to speak or interact meaningfully. Music is soothing and adds interest and pleasure to practically every situation. People can sing, listen, keep tempo, reminisce, and relax. Music often produces sensory and social stimulation (Bright, 1988).

Burnside (1988) distinguishes *reminiscence* from *life review* and cautions against using the terms interchangeably. Reminiscence is valuable in the psychosocial management of older persons. Although it often focuses on positive and happy events from the past, it can be painful. Free-flowing or structured, it focuses upon one or more recalled memories. Three suggested purposes of reminiscence include image enhancement, problem solving, and self-understanding. Participants in these groups may be alert or confused. Nurses, including neophytes and undergraduate nursing students, can encourage reminiscence by older persons in a one-to-one relationship or in a group setting. Reminiscence groups can be led by nonnursing caregivers. Other modalities such as music, pets, poetry, art, and movement are helpful when used concurrently with reminiscence. Pet therapy arouses many old memories. Older people often give these animals names of previous pets. Many share personal experiences with pets, often from childhood.

Conversely, life review brings to consciousness old unresolved conflicts. These are examined with the help of the psychiatric nurse or psychiatric therapist and then reintegrated. Successful accomplishment of life review gives a new meaning and significance to life. Through this psychoanalytically based modality the older person looks critically into the meaning of life, makes reassessments, and resolves and accepts the past. When problems are not resolved or accepted, regrets, depression, and suicide can result. Life review is done with one individual or in a group setting with cognitively intact clients (Burnside, 1988; Butler & Lewis, 1991).

Nurses in community and institutional settings have been successful in developing and providing *group psychotherapy* for older people. Within a group context, older persons learn to express and share feelings, gain new friendships, adapt to new lifestyles, experience a sense of belonging, receive social and sensory stimulation, and increase self-esteem. Researchers report increases in life satisfaction and an improvement in life quality (Abraham, Niles, Thiel, Siarkowski, & Cowling, 1991; Haight & Burnside, 1992; Moore, 1992).

The benefits of group therapy are often not objectively measured, although some researchers have documented significant results using validated instruments. Lack of sensitive instruments, inability to measure certain responses, difficulty in implementing control groups and random sampling, and problems with attrition are some problems with quantification and objective evaluation. Nevertheless, group leaders, involved staff, and participants are enthusiastic in their endorsements of support groups. Conducting a group session can be satisfying professionally and at the same time address a simple yet profound need of the older adult.

❖ *Summary*

Independence, decision making, positive self-esteem and activity involvement all contribute to positive mental health. According to the continuity theory of aging, life satisfaction is most likely to be achieved for the older person if the present remains consonant with the past. Successful progression through life's stages with satisfactory resolution of developmental tasks results in feelings of completeness and integration for the older adult. The nurse can initiate many interventions to counter the negative influence of societal ageism on the self-concept of the older person. Adequate finances, good health, and social relationships all contribute to life satisfaction in later life. Preretirement planning is believed to facilitate the financial, social, and emotional adjustments of retirement. Most people elect to retire, many before age 65. Part-time work can ease retirement trauma. Other options include educational activities, volunteerism, and creative pursuits.

Friendship and family relationships enhance life satisfactions by meeting social, psychological, and instrumental needs. Friendships are particularly important in the absence of family support. Women have more stable, intimate, and supportive friendships than men. Later life brings a higher degree of marital satisfaction. The three components of interpersonal relationships, belonging, interdependence, and intimacy, are major functions of a successful marriage. Confiding relationships, one form of intimacy, are associated with lower levels of loneliness and higher levels of self-esteem and mental and physical health. Most older people have one or more confidants. Sexual intimacy and loving are necessary and desirable at all ages. Many older persons are sexually active. Holding, touching, and closeness are means of sexual expression.

The spiritual aspects of care are sometimes ignored, yet research shows active religious involvement and commitment from many older persons. Companion animals raise the quality of life for many older people, particularly those who live alone. One's own home provides privacy and independence. Relocation adjustment occurs if the older person perceives the move as desirable, legitimate, voluntary, and reversible. A favorable environment enhances behavioral change and increases competence. The older person will be helped to maintain independence and autonomy through the use of environmental supports.

Chronic illnesses, common in old age, threaten independence and well-being. Quality of life diminishes when sensory deficits and physical problems deter participation in favorite activities. Although some decrements and physical problems cannot be prevented, the nurse can initiate measures to limit their negative impact and help the person adapt. Nurse-managed clinics and wellness programs involve older persons in positive health practices. These are often closely allied with multipurpose senior centers that offer social and nutritional services. Psychosocial support sessions grant older people an opportunity to share feelings, make new friends, and enhance feelings of self-esteem. Nurses are qualified to conduct these groups, and they report successful results.

❖ *References*

Abraham, I. L., Niles, S. A., Thiel, B. P., Siarkowski, K. I., & Cowling, W. R. (1991). Therapeutic group work with depressed elderly. *Nursing Clinics of North America, 26*(3), 635-650.

ACTION Annual Report. (1992). Washington: U.S. Government Printing Office.

Adams, R. G. (1989). Conceptual and methodological issues in studying friendships of older adults. In R. G. Adams and R. Bleiszner (Eds.), *Older adult friendship* (pp. 17-41). Newbury Park, CA: Sage.

Anderson, T. B., & McCulloch, B. J. (1993). Conjugal support: Factor structure for older husbands and wives. *Journal of Gerontology, 48*(3), S133-S142.

Atchley, R. C. (1994). *The social forces in later life* (7th ed.). Belmont, CA: Wadsworth.

Atchley, R. C. (1989). Continuity theory of normal aging. *The Gerontologist, 29*(2), 183-190.

Bensink, B. W., Godbey, K. L., Marshall, M. J., & Yarandi, H. N. (1992). Institutionalized elderly: Relaxation, locus of control, self-esteem. *Journal of Gerontological Nursing, 18*(4), 30-36.

Bengston, V., Rosenthal, C., & Burton, L. (1990). Families and aging: Diversity and heterogeneity. In R. H. Binstock & L. K. George (Eds.), *Handbook of aging and the social sciences* (3rd ed., pp. 263-287). New York: Academic Press, Inc.

Blazer, D. (1991). Spirituality and aging well. *Generations, 15*(1), 61-65.

Boldt, M. T., & Dellmann-Jenkins, M. (1992). The impact of companion animals in later life and considerations for practice. *Journal of Applied Gerontology, 11*(2), 228-239.

Bosse, R., Aldwin, C. M., Levenson, M. R., & Workman-Daniels, K. (1991). How stressful is retirement? Findings from the Normative Aging Study. *Journal of Gerontology, 46*(1), 9-14.

Bowers, I-C.H., & Bahr, S. J. (1989). Remarriage among the elderly. In S. J. Bahr & E. T. Peterson (Eds.), *Aging and the family* (pp. 83-95). Lexington, MA: Lexington Books.

Bright, R. (1988). *Music therapy and the dementias: Improving the quality of life.* St. Louis: MMB Music.

Brooke, V. (1989a). How elders adjust. *Geriatric Nursing, 10*(2), 66-68.

Brooke, V. (1989b). Your helping hand. *Geriatric Nursing, 10*(3), 126-129.

Brubaker, T. H. (Ed.). (1990). *Family relationships in later life* (2nd ed.). Beverly Hills: Sage.

Burnside, I. (1984). *Working with the elderly: Group process and techniques* (2nd ed.). Monterey, CA: Wadsworth Health Science.

Burnside, I. (1988). *Nursing and the aged: A self care approach* (3rd ed.). New York: McGraw-Hill.

Butler, R. N., Lewis, M. I. & Sunderland, T. (1991). *Aging and Mental Health* (4th ed.). New York: MacMillan.

Carter, J. S., Williams, H. G., & Macera, C. A. (1993). Relationships between physical activity habits and functional neuromuscular capacities in health older adults. *Journal of Applied Gerontology, 12*(2), 283-293.

Catlin, P. A., Milliorn, A. B., & Milliorn, M. R. (1992). Horticulture therapy promotes wellness, autonomy in residents. *Provider, 18*(7), 40.

Chin-Sang, V., & Allen, K. R. (1991). Leisure and the older black woman. *Journal of Gerontological Nursing, 17*(1), 30-34.

Coleman, P. B. (1992). Personal adjustment in late life: Successful aging. *Reviews in Clinical Gerontology, 2,* 67-78.

Comfort, A., & Dial, L. K. (1991). Sexuality and aging: An overview. *Clinics in Geriatric Medicine, 7*(1), 1-7.

Condie, S. J. (1989). Older married couples. In S. J. Bahr & E. T. Peterson (Eds.), *Aging and the family* (pp. 143-158). Lexington, MA: Lexington Books.

Connidis, I. A., & Davies, L. (1992). Confidants and companions: Choices in later life. *Journal of Gerontology, 47*(3), S115-122.

Cox, C. L., Kaeser, L., Montgomery, A. C., & Marion, L. H. (1991). Quality of life nursing care: An experimental trial in long-term care. *Journal of Gerontological Nursing, 17*(4), 6-11.

Cummings, E., & Henry, W. E. (1961). *Growing old: The process of disengagement.* New York: Basic Books.

Cusack, O. (1988). *Pets and mental health.* New York: Haworth Press.

Cutler, S. J., & Hendricks, J. (1990). Leisure and time use across the life course. In R. H. Binstock & L. K. George (Eds.), *Handbook of aging and the social sciences* (3rd ed., pp. 169-185). New York: Academic Press.

Daly, E. A., & Futrell, M. (1989). Retirement attitudes and health status. *Journal of Gerontological Nursing, 15*(1), 29-32.

Davidhizar, R., & Schearer, R. (1992). Humor: No geriatric nurse should be without it. *Geriatric Nursing, 13*(5), 276-278.

Elderhostel summer programs catalog (1993). Boston: Elderhostel.

Erikson, E. H. (1963). *Childhood and society* (2nd ed.). New York: Norton.

Erikson, E. H., Erikson, J. M., & Kivnick, H. Q. (1986). *Vital involvement in old age.* New York: Norton.

Exercise isn't just for fun. (1991). *Aging,* (362), 37-41.

Fagelson, P. S. (1990). Older Americans are becoming the newest students. *Aging Network News, 7*(12), 10.

Forbis, P. A. (1988). Meeting patients' spiritual needs. *Geriatric Nursing, 9*(3), 158-159.

Frey, D. E., Kelbley, M. A., Durham, L., & James, J. S. (1992). Enhancing the self-esteem of selected nursing home residents. *The Gerontologist, 32*(4), 552-557.

George, L. K. (1990). Social structure, social processes, and social-psychological states. In R. H. Binstock & L. K. George (Eds.), *Handbook of aging and the social sciences* (3rd ed., pp. 186-204). New York: Academic Press.

George, L. K., & Clipp, E. C. (1991). Subjective components of aging well. *Generations, 15*(1), 57-60.

Gillespie, A. E., & Sloan, K. S. (1990). *Housing options and services for older adults.* Santa Barbara, CA: ABC-CLIO.

Gillett, P., Johnson, M., Juretich, M., Richardson, N., Slagle, L., & Farikoff, K. (1993). The nurse as an exercise leader. *Geriatric Nursing, 14*(3), 133-137.

Goldmeier, J. (1986). Pets or people: Another research note. *The Gerontologist, 26,*(2), 203-206.

Gueldner, S. H., & Spradley, J. (1988). Outdoor walking lowers fatigue. *Journal of Gerontological Nursing, 14*(10), 6-12.

Haight, B. K., & Burnside, I. (1992). Reminiscence and life review: Conducting the processes. *Journal of Gerontological Nursing, 18*(2), 39-42.

Hamner, M. L. (1990). Spiritual needs: A forgotten dimension of care? [Editorial]. *Journal of Gerontological Nursing, 16*(12), 3-4.

Hamilton, G. P. (1992). Health care of the older adult. In S. C. Smeltzer & B. G. Bare (Eds.), *Brunner and Suddarth's Textbook of Medical-Surgical Nursing* (7th ed.). Philadelphia: Lippincott.

Hardy, C. C. (1989). *How to retire prosperously and gracefully.* New York: J. K. Lasser Institute.

Harris, M., & Gellin, M. (1990). Pet therapy for the homebound elderly. *Caring, 9*(9), 48-51.

Havighurst, R. J. (1968). Personality and patterns of aging. *The Gerontologist, 8*(3), 20-23.

Havighurst, R. J. (1972). *Developmental tasks and education* (3rd ed.). New York: McKay.

Healthy People 2000: National Health Promotion and Disease Prevention Objectives. (1991). (DHHS Publication No. PHS 91-50213.) Washington DC: U.S. Government Printing Office.

Hiatt, L. G. (1986). The future of aging and technology: Roles for gerontologists. *Generations, 11*(1), 4-9.

Hooker, K., & Ventis, D. G. (1984). Work ethic, daily activities, and retirement satisfaction. *Journal of Gerontology, 39*(4), 478-484.

Hubbard, P., Werner, P., Cohen-Mansfield, J. C., & Shusterman, R. (1992). Seniors for justice: A political and social action group for nursing home residents. *The Gerontologist, 32*(6), 856-858.

Huss, M. J., Buckwalter, K. C., & Stolley, J. (1988). Nursing's impact on life satisfaction. *Journal of Gerontological Nursing, 14*(5), 31-36.

Igou, J. F., Hawkins, J. W., Johnson, E. E., & Utley, Q. E. (1989). Nurse-managed approach to care. *Geriatric Nursing, 10*(1), 32-34.

Jameton, A. (1988). In the borderlands of autonomy: Responsibility in long term care facilities. *The Gerontologist, 28*(Suppl. June), 18-23.

Janssen, J. A., & Giberson, D. L. (1988). Remotivation therapy. *Journal of Gerontological Nursing, 14*(6), 31-34.

Jerome, D. (1991). Social bonds in later life. *Reviews in Clinical Gerontology, 1*(3), 297-306.

Kaakinen, J. R. (1992). Living with silence. *The Gerontologist, 32*(2), 258-264.

Kasper, J. D. (1988). *Aging alone: Profiles and projections.* New York: The Commonwealth Fund Commission on Elderly People Living Alone.

Kendig, H. L., Coles, R., Pittelkow, Y., & Wilson, S. (1988). Confidants and family structure in old age. *Journal of Gerontology, 43*(2), S31-S40.

Kerschner, H. K., & Butler, F. F. (1988). Productive aging and senior volunteerism: Is the U.S. experience relevant? *Ageing International, 15*(2), 15-19.

Kivnick, H. Q. (1993). Everyday mental health: A guide to assessing life strengths. *Generations, 17*(1), 13-20.

Koenig, H. G. (1993). Religion and aging. *Reviews in Clinical Gerontology, 3*(2), 195-203.

Koenig, H. G., George, L. K, & Siegler, I. C. (1988). The use of religion and other emotion-regulating coping strategies among older adults. *The Gerontologist, 28*(3), 303-310.

Koenig, H. G., Kvale, J. N., & Ferrel, C. (1988). Religion and well-being in later life. *The Gerontologist, 28*(1), 18-28.

Krout, J. A. (1989). *Senior centers in America.* New York: Greenwood Press.

Kunkel, S. (1989). An extra eight hours. *Generations, 13*(2), 57-60.

Larson, R., Zuzanek, J., & Mannell, R. (1985). Being alone versus being with people: Disengagement in the daily experience of older adults. *Journal of Gerontology, 40*(3), 375-381.

Lawton, M. P. (1986). *Environment and aging* (2nd ed.). Albany: Center for the Study of Aging.

Lee, G. R., & Sheehan, C. L. (1989). Retirement and marital satisfaction. *Journal of Gerontology, 44*(6), S226-S230.

Leitner, M. J., Leitner, S. F., & Associates. (1989). *Leisure Enhancement.* New York: Haworth Press.

Levin, W. C. (1988). Age stereotyping: College student evaluations. *Research on Aging,* *10*(3), 134-148.

Marriott Seniors Volunteerism Study. (1991). Commissioned by Marriot Senior Living Services and United States Administration on Aging. Washington, DC: Marriott Senior Living Services.

McCracken, A. L. (1988). Sexual practice by elders: The forgotten aspect of functional health. *Journal of Gerontological Nursing, 14*(10), 13-18.

Mikhail, M. L. (1992). Psychological responses to relocation to a nursing home. *Journal of Gerontological Nursing, 18*(3), 35-39.

Miller, M., & Lago, D. (1990). Observed pet owner in-home interactions: Species differences and association with the pet relationship scale. *Arthrozoos, 4*(1), 49-54.

Moore, B. G. (1992). Reminiscing therapy: A CNS intervention. *Clinical Nurse Specialist, 6*(3), 170-3.

Moore, S. R. (1989). Walking for health. *Journal of Gerontological Nursing, 15*(7), 26-28.

Mullins, L. C., & Mushel, M. (1992). The existence and emotional closeness of relationships with children, friends, and spouses. *Research on Aging, 14*(4), 448-470.

Nelson, P. B. (1990). Religious orientation of the elderly. *Journal of Gerontological Nursing,16*(2), 29-35.

Neugarten, B. L., Havighurst, R. J., & Tobin, S. S. (1968). Personality and patterns of aging. In B. Neugarten (Ed.), *Middle age and aging.* Chicago: University of Chicago Press.

Neuhs, H. P. (1991). Ready for retirement? *Geriatric Nursing, 12*(5), 240-241.

Noakes, E. H. (1988). Buildings that work for people, and not against them. *Perspective on Aging, 17*(5), 14-15.

Parnes, H. S. (1989). Postretirement employment. *Generations, 13*(2), 23-26.

Pelican, P., Barbieri, E., & Blair, S. (1990). Toe the line: A nurse-run well foot care clinic. *Journal of Gerontological Nursing, 16*(12), 6-10.

Penn, C. (1988). Promoting independence. *Journal of Gerontological Nursing, 14*(3), 14-19.

Pfister-Minogue, K. (1993). Enhancing patient compliance: A guide for nurses. *Geriatric Nursing, 14*(3), 124-132.

Preston, D. B., & Dellasega, E. (1990). Elderly women and stress: Does marriage make a difference? *Journal of Gerontological Nursing, 16*(4), 26-32.

Quinn, J. F., & Burkhauser, R. V. (1990). Work and retirement. In R. H. Binstock & L. K. George (Eds.), *Handbook of aging and the social sciences* (3rd ed., pp. 307-327). New York: Academic Press.

Reinardy, J. R. (1992). Decisional control in moving to a nursing home: Postadmission adjustment and well-being. *The Gerontologist, 32*(1), 96-103.

Reisman, J. M. (1988). An indirect measure of the value of friendship for aging men. *Journal of Gerontology, 43*(4), 109-110.

Research reveals tremendous growth in senior centers. (1992). *Aging Network News, 10*(7), 1, 6.

Roberts, S. L. (1980). Territoriality: Space and the aged patient in the critical care unit. In I. M. Burnside (Ed.), *Psychosocial nursing care of the aged* (pp. 195-210). New York: McGraw Hill.

Rosenkoetter, M. M., & Bowes, D. (1991). Brutus is making rounds. *Geriatric Nursing, 12*(6), 277-278.

Ruhm, C. J. (1989). Why older Americans stop working. *The Gerontologist, 29*(3), 294-300.

Ruxton, J. P. (1988). Humor intervention deserves our attention. *Holistic Nurse Practitioner, 2*(3), 54-62.

Scanland, S. G., & Emershaw, L. E. (1993). Reality orientation and validation therapy. *Journal of Gerontological Nursing, 19*(6), 7-11.

Schantz, P. M. (1990). Preventing potential health hazards incidental to the use of pets in therapy. *Anthrozoos, 4*(1), 14-23.

Schilke, J. M. (1991). Slowing the aging process with physical activity. *Journal of Gerontological Nursing, 17*(6), 4-8.

Schlenker, E. D. (1993). *Nutrition in aging* (2nd ed.). Philadelphia: Mosby.

Simon, J. M. (1988). The therapeutic value of humor in aging adults. *Journal of Gerontological Nursing, 14*(8), 8-13.

Sit, M. (1992). With elders in mind. *Generations, 16*(2), 73-74.

Steinbach, U. (1992). Social networks, institutionalization, and mortality among elderly people in the United States. *Journal of Gerontology, 47*(4), S183-S190.

Stevens, E. S. (1991). Toward satisfaction and retention of senior volunteers. *Journal of Gerontological Social Work, 16*(3/4), 33-41.

Sullivan, J. L., & Deane, D. M. (1988). Humor and health. *Journal of Gerontological Nursing, 14*(1), 20-24.

Thomas, A. M., & Morse, J. M. (1991). Managing urinary incontinence with self-care practices. *Journal of Gerontological Nursing, 17*(6), 9-14.

Thomas, B. L. (1988). Self-esteem and life satisfaction. *Journal of Gerontological Nursing, 14*(12), 25-30.

Thomasma, M. (1990). Moving day: Relocation and anxiety in institutionalized elderly. *Journal of Gerontological Nursing, 16*(7), 18-25.

Travis, S. S. (1987). Older adults' sexuality and remarriage. *Journal of Gerontological Nursing, 13*(6), 9-14.

U.S. Senate Special Committee on Aging. (1991). *Aging America: Trends and projections.* Washington, DC: Dept. of Health and Human Services.

Utley, Q. E., Hawkins, J. W., Igou, J. F., & Johnson, E. E. (1988). Giving and getting support at the wellness center. *Journal of Gerontological Nursing, 14*(6), 23-27.

Verschueren, J. (1993). When older learners take charge. *Aging Network News, 10*(10), 1, 6.

Vinick, B. H., & Ekerdt, D. J. (1989). Retirement and the family. *Generations, 13*(2), 53-56.

Weinrich, S. P., & Boyd, M. (1992). Education in the elderly: Adapting and evaluating teaching tools. *Journal of Gerontological Nursing, 18*(1), 15-20.

Weinrich, S. P., Boyd, M., & Nussbaum, J. (1989). Continuing education: Adapting strategies to teach the elderly. *Journal of Gerontological Nursing, 15*(11), 17-21.

Weisberg, J., & Haberman, M. R. (1992). Drama, humor, and music to reduce family anxiety in a nursing home. *Geriatric Nursing, 13*(1), 22-24.

Weisberg, J., & Pack, M. (1991). Hannah Katz: Resident tabby. *Geriatric Nursing, 12*(3), 117-118.

Willits, F. K., & Crider, D. M. (1988). Health rating and life satisfaction in the later middle years. *Journal of Gerontology, 43*(5), S172-176.

Wilson, R. W., Patterson, M. A., & Alford, D. M. (1989). Services for maintaining independence. *Journal of Gerontological Nursing, 15*(6), 31-37.

Chapter *3*

❖ *Resources*

Mildred O. Hogstel
M. Kathryn Nichols

There will be an increasing emphasis on additional resources for the mental health care of older adults in the future as older people and their families need and seek more mental health care. Resources include governmental resources, both federal and state, in the form of legislation and finances, special physical facilities, and personnel prepared in the areas of gerontology and mental health.

Governmental funding for mental health care of older adults has been very limited, but some small improvements are being made in this area. Nursing homes and adult day care centers, especially those that have special units for patients with Alzheimer's disease, have started to revise their physical structure and design to meet the special needs of these types of clients.

One of the major problems in mental health care of older adults is the fact that there are very few nurses or other health care personnel with adequate preparation in geriatric psychiatry. This is particularly true in nursing homes, where a large percentage of the residents have some type of mental, emotional, or behavioral problem, and where most of the direct nursing care is given by nurse assistants who have minimal educational preparation in the psychosocial and emotional aspects of nursing care (see Chapter 11). Professional nurses face a major challenge in improving their own knowledge and skills in geropsychiatric nursing as well as teaching and supervising others in the care of mentally ill older adults.

❖ *Governmental Resources*

Protection and Advocacy

Mentally ill older adults are particularly vulnerable to abuse and neglect in institutional settings. The Protection and Advocacy for Mentally Ill Individuals Act was passed in 1986 as a result of reports of abuse and neglect of patients in state mental hospitals. This law allows each state advocacy agency to:

Investigate incidents of abuse and neglect of people with mental illnesses and pursue administrative, legal and other appropriate remedies to protect individuals who are in hospitals, nursing homes, group homes, board and care homes, half-way houses and similar facilities, or jails" (The 100th Congress and Mental Health, 1988, p. 8).

This amendment also defines neglect as "the failure to provide a safe environment or the failure to maintain adequate numbers of appropriately trained staff" (pp. 8-9). Additional funds have become available "for advocacy services to protect existing state, federal and constitutional rights" (p. 8).

Older Americans Act

The Older Americans Act, originally enacted in 1965, was reauthorized for a 4-year extension in 1992. New provisions of the law include "non-medical services for frail elderly individuals, including victims of Alzheimer's disease, and clarifies that mental health services should be among those health services authorized under the Act" (The 100th Congress and Mental Health, 1988, p. 18). These provisions also include coordinating ombudsman services for older people with the Protection and Advocacy agencies (p. 18), encouraging the provision of mental health services to older people, authorization of funds for training, research and other projects, and requiring local area agencies on aging to coordinate mental health services they provide with community mental health services (p. 19).

Legislation Affecting Nursing Homes

Several changes in the Nursing Home Reform Amendments of the Omnibus Budget Reconciliation Act (OBRA) of 1987 affect nursing homes. Although OBRA is comprehensive, its primary purpose was to improve the lives and care of nursing home residents. Some of the specific guidelines relate to mental health. Individuals whose primary or secondary diagnosis is mental illness or mental retardation cannot be admitted to nursing homes because the state is responsible for the care of those persons, and Medicaid, which pays for most nursing home care, is partially federally funded. However, many older persons with mental illness or mental retardation also have one or more physical problems and therefore qualify for nursing home care. This guideline, therefore, requires a preadmission and annual mental health screening of all nursing home residents. Few individuals are denied admission based on these criteria except for those with major psychoses. Because states differ considerably in their resources and philosophy about the care of the mentally ill, the future possibilities for overall treatment and care of chronically mentally ill older adults remain bleak.

Other guidelines of OBRA are that residents should be involved in their care planning and treatment options and that the use of physical and chemical restraints should be reduced. For example, restraints cannot be used simply to prevent wandering, and psychotropic medications can be used only for a specific condition and in a reduced dose (usually one third to one half the standard adult dose). See Chapter 11 for more details of OBRA on nursing home care.

❖ *Financial Resources*

Insurance Coverage

Insurance coverage for mental health services has always been less than for other health problems. The patient often has to pay 50% of the costs instead of the 20% to 30% for physical illnesses, especially for outpatient care. Some of the reasons are "rising health care costs, the absence of consumer demand for mental health coverage, and insurers' continuing fear of the potential cost of this coverage" (Sharfstein and Koran, 1990, p. 227). Other reasons for this lack of coverage include several myths related to psychiatric care, such as that (1) cost of treatment is unpredictable and uncontrollable, (2) coverage encourages excessive use, (3) mental health care is not cost effective, and (4) treatment is not accountable to the insurance companies (pp. 227-228).

Custodial care for persons with chronic long-term illnesses such as Alzheimer's disease and other dementias "is not covered by Medicare, Medicaid, or private insurers" (Svetlik, 1991, p. 225), which places a heavy burden on families to seek assistance of various kinds in the community (see Chapter 13). Because of the increasingly high costs of health care, older people are more likely to spend their health care dollars on what they consider to be essential care and medications. Many older people perceive mental health care as unnecessary and sometimes unwanted.

Medicare

Medicare Part A (hospital insurance) will pay for up to 190 days of inpatient treatment in a participating psychiatric hospital over a lifetime. If the patient is treated for a psychiatric condition in a certified general hospital, the benefits are the same as for any other kind of medical care. Thus some older people who need periodic psychiatric care over several years are treated in general hospitals.

Medicare payment for outpatient treatment of mental illness is limited. According to *The Medicare 1994 Handbook* (1994, p. 28),

When furnished on an outpatient basis, mental health treatment services are subject to a payment limitation that is called the "outpatient mental health limitation." In effect, once the annual deductible is met, Medicare Part B pays only 50 percent (not 80 percent) of the approved amount for these services. On assigned claims, beneficiaries are responsible for paying the remaining 50 percent. For unassigned claims, beneficiaries may have to pay more.

Outpatient treatment may be in a physician's office or a psychiatric hospital in a partial hospitalization (day treatment) program, a trend that reduces costs and may be satisfying to older patients, although transportation to these services may be a problem.

Medicaid

Medicaid is a combined federal and state welfare program that provides health care to the indigent of all ages. It is even more limited than Medicare in paying for mental health care. Each state differs in the amount of care it provides because of state administration of the budget and the need to match federal funds. Traditionally, state mental hospitals have provided mental health care for the indigent of all ages. Even that care today is limited because most patients are only given 30 days of inpatient care per calendar year. Many patients are discharged into the community, where there are limited resources for treatment and support. This practice increases the number of homeless mentally ill.

Medicaid is becoming more and more restrictive because of the decreasing availability of federal and state funds. The criteria are more intense for admission to a psychiatric facility (for example, present danger to self or others) and the number of days are being decreased. Inpatient care is often restricted to stabilization with a maximum five-day stay. In an effort to hold down costs, some states have initiated a Medicaid waiver that will allow these funds to be used for specified home-based care (private home or adult foster home) for clients who qualify. This type of care would be appropriate, for example, for clients diagnosed with Alzheimer's disease. Medicaid does help pay for much of the custodial care of residents with Alzheimer's disease in long-term care facilities *if* they qualify and also have the need for skilled 24-hour nursing care. There is much controversy about the extent to which mental health care will be included in any future health care reform proposals.

Private for-profit psychiatric hospitals can be paid for the care of clients on Medicaid, but most do not choose to participate because of the low reimbursement. Medicaid pays a limited amount for outpatient psychiatric care and none for partial hospitalization. Most outpatient care will be given in a public hospital or clinic.

❖ Physical Facilities

Psychiatric Hospitals

Private for-profit psychiatric hospitals, like many other types of hospitals, expanded in number and size during the 1980s. Insurance coverage for psychiatric care was expanding, and psychiatric hospitals were not subject to the prospective payment system (PPS) legislation that was passed in 1983 in an attempt to decrease health care costs (Kovner, 1990), especially for patients on Medicare. However, in the early 1990s abuses began to surface as the hospitals, which were overbuilt, attempted to keep their occupancy rates high. In one state "at a series of public hearings concerning several hospital chains, former patients gave sometimes shocking testimony about being kept in hospitals against their will, receiving treatment for ailments that had not be [sic] diagnosed and being hospitalized until their insurance had expired" (Madigan, 1993, p. 22). Various marketing strategies such as kickbacks to school counselors and physicians for referring patients to the hospital were considered unethical by many. In one instance a lonesome 83-year-old woman who had called a local telephone number advertising counseling found herself admitted to a psychiatric hospital for clinical depression for three weeks at a cost of $20,235.75 (Price, 1991).

Most of these problems have been resolved through the legal system, but many psychiatric hospitals have been closed for lack of patients, and the public has become more wary of psychiatric care. This is especially true for many older persons, who have a negative view of psychiatric care anyway, probably because of the old concept of state "insane asylums."

This reform movement has reinforced the need for more outpatient psychiatric care, hospital day treatment programs (see Chapter 13) and geropsychiatric units in general hospitals (see Chapter 10) where older patients can receive medical as well as psychiatric care.

Geropsychiatric Units in Psychiatric Hospitals

The number of geropsychiatric units in psychiatric hospitals increased in the early 1990s as the number of geriatric psychiatrists increased and the need for special psychiatric care for older clients became recognized. However, because of decreasing Medicare and private insurance payments to all hospitals, including psychiatric hospitals, some for-profit psychiatric hospitals are not expanding their geropsychiatric programs. In some states Medicaid does not pay for treatment in for-profit psychiatric hospitals, which limits their services to patients who are private payers or those who have Medicare and private insurance.

Although specialty hospitals such as psychiatric hospitals are exempt from the Prospective Payment System under Medicare (Knickman and Thorpe, 1990), there is a tendency for Medicare to limit payment for hospital stays for psychiatric care. However, the hospital and/or family can ask for a review through the official state peer review organization if they believe that further hospitalization is essential.

Geropsychiatric patients usually do not fit into existing therapeutic programs such as group therapy because of differences in age, discussion topics, and problems of communication (for example, vision and hearing deficits). One older man who had participated in a group therapy session refused to continue because the primary topics of discussion were divorce, drugs, and sex, which were not problems for him. There were not enough older patients to have separate group sessions for them. Also, many older people do not feel comfortable talking about their problems and feelings in a group setting. However, older adults are being admitted more frequently to psychiatric hospitals and administrations are working to improve their services for this age group.

A geropsychiatric unit in a psychiatric hospital must be designed for a specific clientele. For example, most psychiatric units are designed for ambulatory patients who usually have no major medical problems and who can meet most of their daily physical needs (e.g., eating and toileting) with minimal assistance. However, many geropsychiatric patients have one or more chronic health problems that require specific physical arrangements.

Structure and Design

The physical structure and design of geropsychiatric units should address the special sensory, mobility, and safety needs of older patients. Suggestions to consider in the design of such units are listed below.

- Handrails should be firmly attached to the walls of halls and bathrooms.
- Handrails should be attached to both sides of the commode.
- Side rails should be on each bed.
- Wheels on beds and wheelchairs should lock securely.
- "Chairs should be padded, firm, with nonskid legs, arms to grip while rising, and a fairly high seat" (Keen-Payne, 1994.)
- All letters and numbers on direction signs, rooms, dietary cards, and printed instructions should be in large type or print.
- The colors red, yellow, and orange should be used instead of blue, pink, purple, or brown.
- "Clear demarcations should be visible between wall and floor, linens and bed, and buttons, knobs, and handles. This color scheme assists the older person with diminished sight to note differences in contours and levels in the room" (Keen-Payne, 1994).
- Wall and floor coverings should have a plain solid design instead of figures or prints.
- The use of white on walls and floors should be limited (especially bright glaring white).
- Room televisions should be on shelves at eye level instead of attached to the ceiling.
- Bathrooms and lavatories should accommodate wheelchairs.
- Room telephones should have large numbers.
- Cords to signal lights should be able to be attached to the patients' clothing so that if a confused patient tries to get out of bed, the light for that room will come on at the nurses' station immediately. (White women of small stature in their 80s are at extremely high risk for a hip and/or wrist fracture if they should fall.)
- The rooms of patients who are at high risk for crawling over side rails or falling should be labeled in a specific manner on the doors of the rooms and on the signal light system at the nurses' station.
- Two or more rooms should have a closed monitor TV with a screen at the nurses' station for severely confused or disoriented older patients.
- Colorful vest restraints should be available but used *only* if absolutely necessary.
- Air, water, gel, or other special types of mattresses should be available for all mobility-impaired patients.
- A large clear calendar and clock with large Arabic numbers should be in each patient's room.
- A reality orientation board should be kept up-to-date in the hall.

Geropsychiatric Units in General Hospitals

Some general hospitals have special units for the care of older patients who have both mental and physical health problems. These units are ideally suited for the total interdisciplinary assessment and care of older persons (see Chapter 10).

Emergency Care Facilities

Mentally ill persons can be difficult to care for when they enter an emergency department in a general hospital because of severe disruptive and possibly combative behavior that the family, friends, or neighbors cannot manage. Emergency department personnel often do not consider a psychiatric problem a high priority because they are used to caring for patients with major physical trauma such as hemorrhage. Also, the emergency department staff are not prepared to assess and treat these patients, so the patients often have to wait for hours before being seen. Older persons often leave and wander out on the street if no one is with them. Therefore, a psychiatrist should be available 24 hours a day for immediate assessment and treatment for these patients. Otherwise, harm could come to the patient, the staff, and others in the department.

Alzheimer's Disease Facilities

Nursing Homes

"Long-term care facilities have been the major resource for care of persons with [Alzheimer's disease], but it is recognized that their design and approaches to care may not be the best for persons with dementia" (Sand, Yeaworth, & McCabe, 1992, p. 28). Some nursing homes have units for residents with Alzheimer's disease and related disorders. Sometimes these units are simply one locked wing that is designated for all residents with Alzheimer's disease. There may be no special activities or programs for these residents, and staff are not trained to meet their needs. Also, they usually cost more than a regular unit and may not have any better outcomes because there are no specific standards for such units (Sand et al., 1992).

Other facilities have excellent units where activities such as exercise and programs such as music are designed to meet the special needs of those with Alzheimer's disease. Also, the staff are especially selected and trained to communicate with and care for residents in various stages of Alzheimer's disease.

In a descriptive study comparing the care of residents with Alzheimer's disease in nursing homes with and without special units, Sand et al. (1992) noted some interesting results. The homes with special units for Alzheimer's residents had more staff than the facilities without special units and found daytime wandering less of a problem. Most of the homes with special care units had specific admission criteria, had made physical environmental changes, provided special activities that included families, and used distraction, redirection, and reminiscing more than reality orientation. Staff did not use restraints for daytime wandering, as did staff of the homes without special units. Overall, the special Alzheimer's disease units "used fewer chemical and physical restraints, reported a decrease in the number of problem behaviors, and indicated that environmental changes provided a personal sense of freedom and dignity" (Sand et al., 1992, p. 34).

These units should have all of the safety and orientation factors just listed. In addition, a protected patio is very helpful to allow patients to walk outside when weather permits. Planned and guided walks should also be implemented. Walking helps to prevent wandering, increase the appetite, aid sleep, maintain mobility, and prevent premature physical problems. The environment, services, schedules, and personnel in these units should be as consistent as possible from day to day. See Chapter 7 and Appendix D for other suggestions regarding the environment for patients with Alzheimer's disease.

Special Care Centers

A \$9.3 million special care center in Fort Worth, Texas, is exclusively for the care of persons with Alzheimer's disease and related disorders. The funding was provided by a charitable trust from a local businessman who died of Alzheimer's disease. This facility provides inpatient care, adult day care, and all of the personnel and ancillary services needed to provide the best care and support possible for persons with Alzheimer's disease and their families. For more information on adult day care centers see Chapter 13.

❖ *Human Resources*

An increasing number of health care providers are combining their educational preparation, knowledge, and skills in caring for older adults with mental, emotional, and behavioral problems. These types of personnel include geropsychiatric nurses, geriatric psychiatrists, geriatric social workers, and other categories of mental health workers with a background in gerontology.

Geropsychiatric Nurses

According to Fox (1987, p. 6), "There are slightly more than 50,000 professional psychiatric nurses in the United States at this time. Unfortunately, a very small number of these nurses specialize in geropsychiatric nursing." In 1993, there were 23,537 nurses certified by the American Nurses' Association in psychiatric and mental health nursing and 11,626 nurses certified in gerontological nursing (American Nurses' Association, 1994). Nurses provide most of the daily care for older adults in general hospitals, nursing homes, and day care centers and are the largest group of professionals in the field of mental health care. Yet few of them have special preparation in geropsychiatric nursing.

Geropsychiatric nurses are unique because they need special preparation and expertise in several areas of nursing: gerontological nursing, psychiatric and mental health nursing, medical and surgical nursing, and community health nursing. General knowledge and skills in all of these areas are important in assessing the problems and meeting the needs of geropsychiatric clients. A basic understanding of gerontological nursing is necessary to recognize patient behaviors that do not fit the growth and development norms for a specific age group. The geropsychiatric nurse should be able to diagnose and meet the physical and psychosocial needs of older adults. The geropsychiatric nurse also should be familiar with the psychiatric diagnoses most common in older adults, as well as the treatment, including medications and nursing care for patients with these diagnoses. Because almost all clients 65 years of age and older have one or more chronic medical problems (e.g., arthritis, hypertension, diabetes, cataracts, glaucoma), the nurse caring for gero-psychiatric patients should be comfortable providing nursing care based on the patient's physical needs. Since most older clients live in the community and return to the community after treatment and care, the nurse also needs to know the community resources available to help maintain the older client at home (see Chapter 13).

Geropsychiatric nurses should be able to operate a glucometer and administer insulin accordingly, immediately recognize the symptoms of an impending myocardial infarction or cardiovascular accident, and use nursing skills to care for or supervise the care of an immobile patient (e.g., how to prevent pneumonia and contractures and how to implement bowel and bladder training). There will be patients who use walkers and who are in wheelchairs on geropsychiatric units. Safety factors are essential. A 95-year-old patient with mental problems who is in a wheelchair will have much different needs from those of a 35-year-old ambulatory patient. All these situations can occur on a geropsychiatric unit. There may be as much need for physical care as for mental and emotional care and support. A holistic approach to nursing care is essential when caring for geropsychiatric patients.

Geriatric Psychiatrists

When older people have a mental or emotional health problem, they usually visit their primary care physician instead of a psychiatrist, psychologist, or other mental health care provider, because they seek help for a physical problem even though a mental health problem is present.

However, an increasing number of geriatric psychiatrists are beginning to focus on the mental health needs of older adults. Two of the pioneers in geriatric medicine are Robert N. Butler (1975), first director of the National Institute on Aging of the National Institutes of Health, and Carl Eisdorfer, who has held workshops throughout the country and written many articles in the medical and gerontological literature related to geropsychiatry. Some medical schools have fellowship programs in geriatric psychiatry. Physicians may become nationally certified in general psychiatry and, with added qualifications, become certified with a sub-specialty in geriatric psychiatry (American Medical Association, 1994). Also, the American Association for Geriatric Psychiatry is a professional organization of psychiatrists who have a special interest in the mental health care of older people. They have more than 1300 members (American Association for Geriatric Psychiatry, June 4, 1993).

Geriatric Social Workers

Most social workers working in geriatric psychiatry have taken one or more courses in gerontology in their social work programs but no special preparation in courses specifically related to geriatric psychiatry. Social workers in the field of geriatric psychiatry suggest that programs interested in preparing social workers for this area include more courses or course content in gerontology, psychotropic drugs, and family support and therapy.

Other Mental Health Care Providers

Other health care providers who work with mentally ill older adults and their families in hospitals and the community are psychologists with masters and doctoral degrees who have had special education and experience in gerontology, abnormal and clinical psychology, and individual, family, and group therapy. Mental health workers who work with patients in individual and group therapy may be sociologists, occupational therapists, and recreational therapists.

An Interdisciplinary Approach

Geropsychiatry is unique because it requires an interdisciplinary approach, perhaps more than any other area of health care. Older people who have mental problems often also have chronic medical problems because of their age. Children and grandchildren or sisters and brothers are often involved in identifying and reporting mental problems of an older family member and in providing care and support during the period of treatment and rehabilitation. The following family situation describes the use of an interdisciplinary approach with a family that had many problems related to the mental health problems of an older family member.

Case Study **Sandwich Generation Family**

Mrs. Barton, who was 49 years old, sought help for her mother, Mrs. Callan, who was 69 years old and very depressed. Mrs. Callan had been caring for *her* mother, Mrs. Henry, aged 89, for several years. Mrs. Barton had six children, three teenagers who lived at home, and three grandchildren whom she cared for occasionally. She also was employed full-time. She was in the middle of a five-generation family, called the *sandwich generation*. She was under heavy stress trying to manage her numerous responsibilities. Her husband was withdrawing from family relationships, and the teenagers' lives were being disrupted by their severely depressed grandmother. Mrs. Barton finally sought professional help. She explained her problem to a geriatric social worker in a psychiatric hospital whom she had learned about from the local mental health association. A gerontological mental health nurse visited

Continued.

Case Study **Sandwich Generation Family—cont'd**

---

the home to assess Mrs. Callan. Because Mrs. Callan had periods of severe depression, staying in bed for days at a time and eating very little, she was referred to a geriatric psychiatrist, who admitted her to a local psychiatric hospital. Mrs. Barton had previously found it necessary to place Mrs. Henry in a nursing home when Mrs. Callan was no longer able to care for her. Then Mrs. Barton, her husband, and their teenage children had several counseling sessions with a clinical gerontological psychologist to help them explore their feelings and return to a more normal lifestyle. After several weeks of treatment and care in the hospital, Mrs. Callan improved greatly, and the geriatric social worker helped her to choose and move to a retirement center. Therefore a very difficult and potentially explosive family situation was helped by a team of health providers working in geropsychiatry, both in the hospital and in the community.

❖ Education

Baccalaureate Degree Programs

The integration of gerontological nursing into baccalaureate degree nursing programs has been slow, with more emphasis being placed on specific medical diagnoses common in older adults and clinical practicum assignments in nursing homes and community settings (Hogstel, 1988).

Specific content and clinical experiences in geropsychiatric nursing are considered important and are being implemented in some baccalaureate degree nursing programs. In one program a 2-hour lecture by a geriatric psychiatrist and planned clinical assignments with older adults in several community settings have been initiated. Students also are being assigned more often to older patients in psychiatric hospitals where they have their major clinical practicum. Students should be able to use facts and theories learned about geriatric psychiatry in their clinical practicums in medical-surgical and community health nursing, which have large numbers of older clients, as well as in psychiatric nursing.

Master's Degree Programs

In 1993, Hoeffer conducted a survey of National League for Nursing accredited master's programs with a major in psychiatric/mental health nursing and/or gerontological nursing. She found that "Geropsychiatric nursing is offered by the psychiatric/mental health nursing specialty, most often in a graduate nursing program with both psychiatric/mental health nursing course work and gerontologic nursing specialties" (Hoeffer, 1994, p. 37). Also, she noted that psychiatric/mental health programs "with a geropsychiatric nursing focus offered preparation for advanced practice as a clinical nurse specialist" (p. 37).

❖ *Professional Journals*

At present no journal is dedicated exclusively to geropsychiatric nursing, although the *Journal of Gerontological Nursing, Geriatric Nursing,* and the *Journal of Psychosocial Nursing* all contain articles on geropsychiatric nursing from time to time, as does the *American Journal of Nursing* (see Appendix H for addresses). The *American Journal of Geropsychiatry,* the official publication of the American Association for Geriatric Psychiatry, began a quarterly publication in 1992. The *Journal of the American Geriatrics Society* contains many articles on geropsychiatric issues in addition to those about geriatrics in general. Its publisher, the American Geriatrics Society, admits nurses as members.

❖ *National Certification*

Professional certification of nurses in specific functional or clinical areas of nursing was initiated by the American Nurses' Association in 1973. This national voluntary certification program recognizes individual nurses who meet certain criteria. This type of national "certification is reserved for those nurses who have met requirements for clinical or functional practice in a specialized field, pursued education beyond basic nursing preparation, and received the endorsement of their peers" (American Nurses Association, 1994, p. 3).

Criteria differ according to the type of certification that is sought. Nurses in geropsychiatric nursing might have the option of receiving certification in one or more of the following areas:

- ◆ Gerontological Nurse (generalist)*
- ◆ Psychiatric and Mental Health Nurse (generalist)*
- ◆ Clinical Specialist in Gerontological Nursing (requires a master's or higher degree)
- ◆ Clinical Specialist in Adult Psychiatric and Mental Health Nursing (requires a master's or higher degree)[†]

❖ *Standards of Practice*

Nurses who care for geropsychiatric clients should apply the standards of nursing practice for both gerontological nursing (see Box 3-1) and psychiatric and mental health nursing (see Box 3-2). These standards, prepared and published by the American Nurses' Association, serve as guidelines for quality nursing care for individual nurses. They should be used as a basis for the nursing process in assessing, diagnosing, planning, implementing, and evaluating nursing care. They can also be used for peer review and performance evaluation. These standards have evolved over a period of years and will undoubtedly be revised as nursing changes in the future.

---

* Beginning with the 1998 test administration, all generalized certifications will require a baccalaureate or higher degree in nursing.

[†]Interested nurses should call 1-800-284-CERT or write the American Nurses' Credentialing Center, 600 Maryland Avenue, S.W., Washington, DC 20024-2571, for a detailed catalog with application forms, testing dates, and locations.

Box 3-1 **Standards and Scope of Gerontological Nursing Practice***

Standard I. *Organization of Gerontological Nursing Services*
All gerontological nursing services are planned, organized, and directed by a nurse executive. The nurse executive has baccalaureate or master's preparation and has experience in gerontological nursing and administration of long-term care services or acute care services for older clients.

Standard II. *Theory*
The nurse participates in the generation and testing of theory as a basis for clinical decisions. The nurse uses theoretical concepts to guide the effective practice of gerontological nursing.

Standard III. *Data Collection*
The health status of the older person is regularly assessed in a comprehensive, accurate, and systematic manner. The information obtained during the health assessment is accessible to and shared with appropriate members of the interdisciplinary health care team, including the older person and the family.

Standard IV. *Nursing Diagnosis*
The nurse uses health assessment data to determine nursing diagnoses.

Standard V. *Planning and Continuity of Care*
The nurse develops the plan of care in conjunction with the older person and appropriate others. Mutual goals, priorities, nursing approaches, and measures in the care plan address the therapeutic, preventive, restorative, and rehabilitative needs of the older person. The care plan helps the older person attain and maintain the highest level of health, well-being, and quality of life achievable, as well as a peaceful death. The plan of care facilitates continuity of care over time as the client moves to various care settings, and is revised as necessary.

Standard VI. *Intervention*
The nurse, guided by the plan of care, intervenes to provide care to restore the older person's functional capabilities and to prevent complications and excess disability. Nursing interventions are derived from nursing diagnoses and are based on gerontological nursing theory.

Standard VII. *Evaluation*
The nurse continually evaluates the client's and family's responses to interventions in order to determine progress toward goal attainment and to revise the data base, nursing diagnoses, and plan of care.

* American Nurses' Association (1987). *Standards and scope of gerontological nursing practice.* Washington, DC: Author; with permission.

Continued.

Box 3-1 **Standards and Scope of Gerontological Nursing Practice—cont'd**

Standard VIII. *Interdisciplinary Collaboration*
The nurse collaborates with other members of the health care team in the various settings in which care is given to the older person. The team meets regularly to evaluate the effectiveness of the care plan for the client and family and to adjust the plan of care to accommodate changing needs.

Standard IX. *Research*
The nurse participates in research designed to generate an organized body of gerontological nursing knowledge, disseminates research findings, and uses them in practice.

Standard X. *Ethics*
The nurse uses the code for nurses established by the American Nurses' Association as a guide for ethical decision making and practice.

Standard XI. *Professional Development*
The nurse assumes responsibility for professional development and contributes to the professional growth of interdisciplinary team members. The nurse participates in peer review and other means of evaluation to assure the quality of nursing practice.

❖ *Summary*

To meet the special mental health needs of an increasing older population, more resources will be needed in the future. These resources include federal and state programs and funding, specially designed physical facilities, and a variety of personnel who are prepared and interested in the field of geropsychiatry. Government standards and funding for mental health programs for older adults are beginning to improve. Psychiatric hospitals are evaluating their geropsychiatric units. Adult day care centers are providing special facilities for older patients with Alzheimer's disease.

Geropsychiatric nurses are unique because they must possess general knowledge and skill in four areas of nursing: gerontological nursing, psychiatric and mental health nursing, medical and surgical nursing, and community health nursing. Specific educational programs to prepare geropsychiatric nurses are limited. Four types of national certification are available in gerontological and psychiatric and mental health nursing. Perhaps some day there will be American Nurses' Association certification for the specialty of geropsychiatric nursing. Nurses working with geropsychiatric patients should apply both the American Nurses' Association Standards of Gerontological Nursing Practice and the Standards of Psychiatric and Mental Health Nursing Practice in their care of older patients with mental health problems.

Box 3-2 **Standards of Psychiatric and Mental Health Nursing Practice: Standards of Care***

Standard I. *Assessment*
The psychiatric-mental health nurse collects client health data.

Standard II. *Diagnosis*
The psychiatric-mental health nurse analyzes the assessment data in determining diagnosis.

Standard III. *Outcome Identification*
The psychiatric-mental health nurse identifies expected outcomes individualized to the client.

Standard IV. *Planning*
The psychiatric-mental health nurse develops a plan of care that prescribes interventions to attain expected outcomes.

Standard V. *Implementation*
The psychiatric-mental health nurse implements the interventions identified in the plan of care.

Standard V-A. *Counseling*
The psychiatric-mental health nurse uses counseling interventions to assist clients in improving or regaining their previous coping abilities, fostering mental health, and preventing mental illness and disability.

Standard V-B. *Milieu Therapy*
The psychiatric-mental health nurse provides, structures, and maintains a therapeutic environment in collaboration with the client and other health-care providers.

Standard V-C. *Self-Care Activities*
The psychiatric-mental health nurse structures interventions around the client's activities of daily living to foster self-care and mental and physical well-being.

Standard V-D. *Psychobiological Interventions*
The psychiatric-mental health nurse uses knowledge of psychobiological interventions and applies clinical skills to restore the client's health and prevent further disability.

* Reprinted with permission from *A Statement on Psychiatric-Mental Health Clinical Nursing Practice and Standards of Psychiatric-Mental Health Clinical Nursing Practice,* © 1994, American Nurses Association, Washington, DC.

Continued.

Box 3-2 **Standards of Psychiatric and Mental Health Nursing Practice: Standards of Care—cont'd**

Standard V-E. *Health Teaching*
The psychiatric-mental health nurse, through health teaching, assists clients in achieving satisfying, productive, and healthy patterns of living.

Standard V-F. *Case Management*
The psychiatric-mental health nurse provides case management to coordinate comprehensive health services and ensure continuity of care.

Standard V-G. *Health Promotion and Health Maintenance*
The psychiatric-mental health nurse employs strategies and interventions to promote and maintain mental health and prevent mental illness.

Standard V-H. *Psychotherapy*
The certified specialist in psychiatric-mental health nursing uses individual, group, and family psychotherapy, child psychotherapy, and other therapeutic treatments to assist clients in fostering mental health, preventing mental illness and disability, and improving or regaining previous health status and functional abilities.

Standard V-I. *Prescription of Pharmacological Agents*
The certified specialist uses prescription of pharmacological agents in accordance with the state nursing practice act to treat symptoms of psychiatric illness and improve functional health status.

Standard V-J. *Consultation*
The certified specialist provides consultation to health-care providers and others to influence the plans of care for clients and to enhance the abilities of others to provide psychiatric and mental health care and effect change in systems.

Standard VI. *Evaluation*
The psychiatric-mental health nurse evaluates the client's progress in attaining expected outcomes.

❖ *References*

American Association for Geriatric Psychiatry. (1993). Personal communication, June 4.

American Medical Association. (1994). Personal communication, August 17.

American Nurses' Association. (1987). *Standards and scope of gerontological nursing practice.* Washington, DC: Author.

American Nurses' Association. (1994). *A statement on psychiatric-mental health clinical nursing practice and standards of psychiatric-mental health clinical nursing practice.* Washington, DC: Author.

American Nurses' Association. (1994). *American nurses credentialing center certification catalog.* Washington, DC: American Nurses' Credentialing Center.

Butler, R. N. (1975). *Why survive? Being old in America.* New York: Harper & Row.

Fox, J. C. (1987). Mental health manpower in aging. *Aging Network News, 3*(12), 6-7.

Hoeffer, B. (1994). Essential curriculum content. *Journal of Psychosocial Nursing, 32*(4), 33-38.

Hogstel, M. O. (1988). Gerontological nursing in the baccalaureate curriculum. *Nurse Educator, 13*(3), 14-18.

Keen-Payne, R. (1994). Hospitalized older adults. In M. Hogstel (Ed.). *Nursing care of the older adult* (3rd ed.). New York: Delmar.

Knickman, J. R., & Thorpe, K. E. (1990). Financing for health care. In A. R. Kovner (Ed.), *Health care delivery in the United States* (4th ed.). New York: Springer.

Kovner, A. R. (Ed.) (1990). *Health care delivery in the United States* (4th ed.). New York: Springer.

Madigan, T. (1993, January 1). Hospitals, state reach agreement. *Fort Worth Star Telegram,* pp. 21A, 22.

Price, D. M. (1991, November 24). $20,000 treatment can't cure loneliness. *Fort Worth Star Telegram*, Section A, p. 35.

The Medicare 1994 Handbook. (1994). U.S. Department of Health and Human Services Pub. No. HCFA 10050. Baltimore, MD: U.S. Government Printing Office.

The 100th Congress and Mental Health. (1988). Alexandria, VA: National Mental Health Association.

Sand, B. J., Yeaworth, R. C., & McCabe, B. W. (1992). Alzheimer's disease special care units in long-term care facilities. *Journal of Gerontological Nursing, 18*(3), 28-34.

Sharfstein, S. S., & Koran, L. M. (1990). Mental health services. In A. R. Kovner (Ed.). *Health care delivery in the United States* (4th ed.). New York: Springer.

Svetlik, D. (1991). Mobilizing community resources. In M. F. Weiner (Ed.). *The dementias: Diagnosis and management.* Washington, DC: American Psychiatric Press.

Chapter 4

❖ *Assessment*

Janis M. Campbell

Assessment of older adults is more complex than evaluating younger persons because of the many physical, psychological, social, and spiritual changes related to aging. The increasing number of adults aged 65 and older means greater use of health care facilities and interactions with health care providers. Fundamental changes in all areas reshape older adults' perceptions of life and affect their mental health. Physical stamina and capabilities tremendously influence an individual's outlook. Therefore, assessment as an individual ages is an ongoing process. Meeting the health care challenges of more than 32 million older Americans requires well-informed health care providers.

Mental health and mental illness in older adults is a broad area to assess. A geropsychiatric nursing approach assesses clients in all areas of functioning to determine their level of cognitive functioning. Mental health problems of older adults are affected by the complex interrelationship of psychological, biological, sociological, and spiritual factors. Individual assessment includes all aspects of a person's life.

Only 5% of the older population are institutionalized; the majority of older adults are in some kind of independent living arrangement. Persons in independent living manage their own health with some assistance from health care providers. These older persons provide their health history and are the main source of a complete and accurate database.

Older adults are the main consumers of health care and have more interaction with health care providers than any other age group. Any change in their health status could affect their lifestyles, living arrangements, or ability to carry out activities of daily living. Advancing years bring physical, psychological, and social change. A major consideration of older adults is the maintenance of independence through good health as changes occur.

Older people usually do not dwell on their health while they are mobile. It has been found that they are happy and consider themselves well as long as they can carry out activities of daily living, even when they have multiple chronic health problems.

Restricted mobility affects all aspects of a client's life and leads to rapid deterioration of physical and mental health.

❖ *General Assessment Considerations*

Assessment of older adults requires a thorough and complete collection of information on all aspects of an individual's life. The assessment process is an integration of data on a person's biological, psychological, and social functioning and their interrelated aspects. Any change in one aspect of an individual's life affects the entire well-being of an individual.

Older adults are a diverse group. A systematic mental health assessment includes emotional and cognitive functioning and age-related physical changes. This assessment must also include socioeconomic, cultural, and gender-related beliefs, values, attitudes, customs, and health care practices. Any dominant culture contains subculture groups. Members of subcultures share characteristics that may be distinguished by age, gender, ethnicity, religion, and health practices. Cultural factors may influence health beliefs, communication patterns, living styles, and values. Individual differences related to subcultures may affect communication patterns that include verbal and nonverbal communication.

Gender roles affect individual perceptions of developmental milestones. Gender socialization diversity contributes to emotional and psychological reactions to life events. A mental health assessment should include opportunities to discuss gender and emotional needs. An important consideration is the coping patterns used by individuals during transitions from one developmental phase to another.

Assessment is divided into logically sequenced segments. Each segment includes any life-threatening problems, client concerns, and the health care provider's objective examination. Although assessment is logical and systematic, some assessments can be combined to reduce repetition and fatigue to the client. To collect data simultaneously, the health care provider will have to be natural, listen carefully, and be observant. When clients are filling in portions of a questionnaire, the interviewer can observe such things as eyesight, coordination, fine muscle movement, and comprehension.

The Aging Process

Assessing older individuals requires skill, patience, and a thorough knowledge of the aging process. Nurses cannot confine assessment to one aspect of an individual's life or limit assessment to physical and mental functioning. An older adult's social relationships, the amount and quality of contact with support persons, the number of social roles compared with previous roles at a younger age, economic resources to meet changing needs, and capability to perform activities of daily living are all important considerations in the overall assessment of current and potential future functioning.

Assessing an older population requires a knowledge of the universality of aging, its progression, and the irreversibility of its effects. Although there is a commonality among all older adults, each person uniquely ages according to genetics, culture, nutrition, and factors still being researched. A thorough and *total* individualized assessment is required to determine adequate nursing intervention strategies. Care in a home setting will include assessing mobility and safety, counseling, teaching, home health maintenance, review of medications, individualized care, and coordination of community services.

Older adults exhibit symptoms of aging at differing rates that affect all aspects of their lives. The assessment process provides the database necessary for making accurate nursing diagnoses. Nursing intervention strategies must include a multidisciplinary approach to the many challenges presented in assessing an older population.

Health problems in the aged are complex, characterized by multiple and overlapping chronic illnesses. It is difficult to differentiate the normal aging process from pathology. In addition, multiple presenting symptoms are often confusing and mask many underlying health problems. Assessment should include the client's adaptive style regarding health problems and functional capacity, support systems, living situation, economic situation, recent life events, and disease versus illness.

Respect for Older Adults

Often clients feel as though their lifestyles and health habits are being negatively evaluated and will make excuses for their way of life or illnesses. An older person may feel intimidated by a younger, educated person asking personal and invasive questions. Older adults may feel that sharing health concerns will cause the interviewer to view them negatively or to be judgmental about their past lifestyles and health habits. Clients will observe the interviewer carefully for any signs of negative response or concerns and will often ask the interviewer whether their responses were all right. Older individuals may become concerned that the interviewer has additional information about their health problems that is not being shared. It is important to make the client feel at ease and have a nonjudgmental attitude. Keeping clients informed about their responses reduces their anxiety and increases willingness to participate in the total assessment process.

Clients will respond more readily and openly to an interviewer whom they perceive to be interested and concerned and not rushed. The interviewer must listen carefully to clues clients give relative to the extent of their health problems and the effects such problems have on their lifestyle.

Self-reporting by an older adult may not be accurate and may require exploration and clarification on the part of the interviewer. It is important to allow time for remembering details and rephrasing questions that are not answered adequately. Sometimes a person does not understand the extent of information needed or does not understand the relevance of the questions. It may be helpful to read the questions with the client to make sure the terminology is clear and that the information requested is understood.

Response to verbal requests may take time because one of the normal aging symptoms is the slowing of response time. This slowing is related to how impulses are sent to the brain and responses transmitted. Allowing sufficient time for response will elicit the information needed. By not allowing time for this normal process to occur, the interviewer conveys to the client a lack of understanding of aging. Slowed responses may also be related to confusing, unclear, or unfamiliar language or terminology (especially medical terminology) used by the interviewer.

Most older persons do not like being called condescending or familiar names such as "honey," "dearie," "grandma," or "grandpa." They may resent the assumption that they are grandparents, or the terms may make them feel old. Older adults may resent the assumption of familiarity. The clients should be spoken to on an adult level and in a nonthreatening manner.

Interviewers should carefully assess the person's need for touch. Some older adults enjoy being touched because it conveys warmth; however, some do not like being touched because such contact implies familiarity that they are not experiencing. As an individual ages, there is a decline in the ability to feel light touch, especially on the extremities.

Most older persons are acutely aware of their physical and psychological changes and try to hide the signs of this decline from others. They develop compensatory social mechanisms for any physical or mental deficiencies to protect their egos and prevent detection. Initial assessment should include assessment of vision, hearing, and mental status in order to determine needed changes or alterations in the assessment of or approach to clients.

Awareness of cultural, ethnic, gender, and socioeconomic differences among different groups of people prevents misinterpretation of assessment findings. Also, a thorough knowledge of differences prevents judging older adults' health perceptions, mental health, and health management on stereotypical perceptions. Specific differences related to age, gender, and ethnic group are normal, but assumptions that members of groups practice specific beliefs may be erroneous. Culture and ethnicity may influence appearance, behavior, and attitudes toward ways health and illness are experienced. During an assessment, objectivity avoids imposing personal values on another individual.

Reminiscence

Since most of an older person's opportunities for life's work have been attempted or accomplished, an important task is to conduct a life appraisal through reminiscing (Smith, Buckwalter, & Albanese, 1990). *Reminiscence* is common and gives the interviewer insight into lifestyles and health histories. Encouraging reminiscence demonstrates interest in the person and provides valuable information. Data gleaned from past and present concerns serve as background for the diagnosis of health problems. As a person discusses his or her life and reminisces about the past, the interviewer gathers data about memory, decision making, preferences, patterns of living, reactions to life situations, and developmental stage accommodation. Efforts have to be made to balance an older person's need to engage in reminiscence and an interviewer's need to collect data.

Focusing the conversation on the task at hand will keep the client on the topic. The vast experience of older adults leads many times to long explanations of the events leading to a situation. The very nature of the chronicity of health conditions requires a long time for explanation of the development of the condition, course of the problems, and the treatment regimen.

Family Support Systems

Family or significant other support systems have been shown to be a factor in the mental health of the aged. A family history revealing relatives or significant others who are still living will give clues to the client's mental health status by providing information about the client's coping mechanisms, life events, and available support systems.

Support systems are critical to the health of older adults, affecting them physically and emotionally. Persons who are institutionalized and have interested persons visiting them, spending time with them, and offering support have been found to have a better psychological outlook. Research has not identified the exact reason support systems have such a positive effect on life; but it has been found that they are a buffer against life's stressful events (Stillman, 1986).

Understanding family functioning sheds a great deal of light on a client's life views. An assessment of social functioning includes interviewing family or significant others. The Family APGAR test was developed to measure adaptation, partnership, growth, affection, and resolve (Smilkstein, 1978). The author of this instrument selected these factors based on common themes found in social science literature. Each of the five areas in the acronym APGAR contains questions relative to that area. A closed-ended questionnaire gives an overview of family function. Clients check one of three choices, which allows the interviewer to make a qualitative measurement of family satisfaction. Smilkstein suggested that this instrument should be used when families are involved in client care, clients are new to a system, or information is needed to manage a family in a dysfunctional state.

Understanding family functioning may assist in understanding and resolving the client's health problems. Evidence of dysfunction alerts health care providers to areas of conflict and possible health-related problems.

❖ Health History

All good assessments begin with an interview and health history. There are also many standardized tools available to obtain data about the client, several of which will be discussed where appropriate in this chapter. (Appendix A contains a sample health history.)

The health history provides information about clients' perceptions of their life stressors and the ways they coped with stressors, changes in lifestyle, and ability to adapt to change. Changes brought about by normal aging require alterations in an individual's approach to life. Adaptation, compensation, and continued changes become a norm. A health history provides insight into ways clients have dealt with life events, feelings about these events, and preparation for the inevitable changes. As an interviewer takes a nursing history, clients may reveal feelings about the aging process and adjustments to activities of daily living.

Assessment should include determining an individual's assets as well as areas in which the person would benefit from assistance, referral, or institutionalization. Assessment provides a systematic and complete method for collecting information needed to develop a nursing diagnosis. Good assessment techniques include subjective and objective data collection methods. The measurement instruments should be used to collect data, document areas of strengths and concerns, and provide direction so that nurses can focus on problems amenable to intervention strategies.

Clients who are unable to communicate or who have limited communication capabilities should have a significant other with them during health assessment. Additional sources of data may be other health care personnel who have provided the client with health care. Information useful for a holistic assessment must be gathered from family members or support persons. Clients should always be present during questioning of significant others or caregivers so that the interviewer may observe their reactions to the responses.

Health care providers should share information to prevent repetition of data collection and as a way to be cost-effective. The data collection can be beneficial in identifying nursing needs in the community or institutional setting.

Nursing interaction with this age group can occur in a variety of settings including nursing homes, extended care facilities, independent living apartments for older persons, and health care agencies the client enters from private living arrangements. Regardless of the type of living arrangement, clients should always be treated respectfully and with dignity. Major considerations in assessing an older adult population are level of mobility and living arrangements. Both of these factors have a profound effect on the cognitive and emotional functioning of older clients and influence their physical and mental health. Older adults seek medical consultation to maintain an independent lifestyle; many have a repugnance for institutional living. They make every effort to maintain an independent living arrangement.

Time for Assessment

The accuracy of the interview and health history will depend to a great extent on health providers' willingness to be patient with clients' needs to expound on their life events. Interviews and life histories take time. Approximately 30 minutes should be allocated for the initial gathering of data. Older clients tire easily, and the accuracy of their responses may be questionable when a complete history is taken all at one time.

Some older adults may be able to tolerate only relatively short periods of the time needed for a full assessment, and the entire process may have to be spread over several assessment periods. Allowing time for rest and relaxation will promote a more accurate picture of the total functioning capability of an individual. Fatigue reduces older individuals' ability to function at their best. The best time for an interview and history is during the morning hours. Cognitive functioning tends to decrease in the late afternoon and evening (Carnevali, 1992). The majority of older persons are happy to comply with the assessment process and are willing and able to participate as long as certain adaptations are made.

Every effort should be made to make the client comfortable and at ease with the interviewer. It is worth the effort to devote an initial time period to develop rapport and allow the client to become comfortable with the interviewer. Clients will be less reticent to discuss personal matters with someone who is willing to share time developing a relationship.

The client and interviewer should be physically comfortable, and enough time should be set aside for establishing rapport through casual conversation. After the initial introduction the interviewer should state the purpose of the appointment, time allocated, and disposition of data gathered. This method of assessment is time consuming, but the accuracy of the information obtained will outweigh any loss of time.

Initial Database

An initial total assessment provides a database for comparing later assessments and suspected changes in the holistic functioning of an older client. A normal aging progression can be documented and then compared with baseline data when the information is clear and concise. Individuals within this age group face a variety of developmental tasks, including the following (Farrell, 1990):

- Changes in physical strength and health
- New family roles
- Participation in age-related activities
- Retirement and income adjustments
- Useful activities to enhance self-worth
- Evaluation of living arrangements
- Loss of spouse, family members, and friends
- Life review
- Facing mortality

During the assessment the nurse should focus on the client's self-care and any concerns. Many times direct questions will elicit answers that do not disclose the client's complete history. Asking clients to discuss a typical day, from awakening through bedtime and overnight, will elicit details about their lifestyle and habits. Exploring additional details with the client will provide the interviewer with an enormous amount of information. Typical questions should include the following:

- What is your typical day like from the time you get up until you go to bed, and what is your night like from the time you go to bed until you get up the next morning?
- What do you eat in a 24-hour period and how many times a day do you eat?
- Where do you live and what are your living arrangements?
- What changes have you noticed in your life?
- What type and how much exercise do you get?
- How do you describe your beliefs about the meaning or purpose of life?
- Is religion or a belief in a higher being important to you?
- What changes have you noticed in your health patterns?
- Have you noted changes in your response time? In your ability to react? In your coordination?
- How do you feel about yourself sexually?
- Have you experienced any problems with urination or changes in your bowel movements?
- How do you use your leisure and recreation time?
- What changes have you noticed in your body?

Additional data from persons in a hospital or nursing home facility can be obtained with questions such as the following:

- Have there been behavioral changes in the client?
- Are there changes in his or her appearance and hygiene habits?
- Has the client developed annoying behaviors?
- Have sudden or gradual changes occurred in physical, cognitive, or mental functioning?
- Has the client been unable to make sound decisions or care for himself or herself?

Initial assessment may be in a hospital setting, community agency, or the client's home. Contrary to popular myths, older adults can respond to and participate in a health history at a high level provided certain considerations are kept in mind. People in this age group respond best when one stimulus is presented at a time and when sufficient time for response to stimuli or questions is given. An individual's coping mechanisms influence the history he or she gives, as well as the way questionnaires are answered. Anxiety reduces performance and contributes to lower scores on memory tests (Deptula, Singh, & Pomara, 1993). A combination of anxiety and depression further contribute to poor memory performance. Therefore, anxiety reduction techniques by an interviewer promote recall performance.

A thorough assessment enables nurses to plan health care with clients and their significant others by determining priorities of need. Family or support persons may be able to provide background information about the client's daily activities, interaction with support persons, changes in health and coping ability, decision-making capabilities, and response to emotionally laden situations. They may also provide insight into the level of independence the client enjoys.

In addition, family members or support persons can provide information about the client's satisfaction with life. Nurses should be alert to any signs of physical and/or psychological abuse of the older person. Careful observation of the client's interaction with family members or support persons can help determine whether abuse is occurring. Older individuals may be very reluctant to share information about abuse for fear of losing their homes, affection, or support from their families. The possibility of abusive behavior must always be thoroughly investigated before any action is taken or accusations are made.

❖ General Health Screening Tools

Instruments designed to screen multiple dimensions of a client's life reveal areas of strength or of concern. The accuracy of data collection can assist in identifying health care services needed and areas where the quality and quantity of care should be improved. Instruments should not only be accurate but sensitive enough to reveal hidden problem areas.

There are many assessment tools available to collect data from the client. Kane and Kane (1981) have developed a comprehensive review of assessment tools appropriate for older clients. Instruments that have been developed and standardized in research settings provide accurate and easily accessible methods for garnering information from clients that will lead to planned intervention. Tools should be selected carefully based on their various strengths and weaknesses. Examples of several tools for screening are found in Table 4-1 on p. 88.

The Psychogeriatric Nursing Assessment Protocol (PNAP) developed by Abraham, Smullen, & Thompson-Heisterman (1992) guides health care providers in assessing patients and their support systems in a comprehensive and accepted method through a multidimensional approach. The PNAP is a framework that enables the user to assess patients and their family in detail. To use the PNAP to the fullest extent, the practitioner must understand geropsychiatric concepts, aging, and biopsychosocial interactions as well as possess good interviewing skills. The major areas covered by the PNAP are the reasons for the visit to a health care facility: functional assessment, mental assessment, geriatric behavioral assessment, caregiver assessment, family functioning assessment, social functioning assessment, previous nursing care received, and a supplemental environment assessment (Abraham et al., 1992).

Data collection is focused on the patient but may include family or caregivers. Clinical strategies are geared to the needs of an older adult. The PNAP is a valuable assessment tool that can be used for collaboration with other disciplines in planning health-promoting interventions.

Some assessment tools have been developed for specific types of facilities. Long-term care tools provide guides for determining appropriate levels of care for clients in long-term care facilities. The Long-Term Care Information System (LTCIS) has been used to determine level of care in many institutions and classifies clients according to the assessment information collected (Falcone, 1981). This instrument focuses the data collection on the assessment phase to plan quality health care services. The client data provide direction for placement and program planning to meet individual health care needs. The institutional assessment assists in the identification of areas in which the quality and efficiency of services to clients needs improvement.

❖ *Difficulty in Making Diagnoses*

Diagnosing an older person's health problems presents a challenge to health care providers. Recognizing the degree of overlap in psychological and physiological problems is an important initial step for arriving at accurate diagnoses and nursing interventions. Determining the exact problems an older person has is often confounded by the very changes that accompany aging. The aging process has an impact on the manifestation of diseases. For example, an older person with a hyperthyroid condition can present with confusion similar to that in dementia but not demonstrate any of the symptoms of hyperthyroidism found in a younger person. Symptoms of hypothyroidism may be similar to those of depression.

Biological and psychological changes do occur as an individual ages. However, extensive deterioration of cognitive functioning does not normally occur with aging. Physiological and sociological factors may mediate the changes experienced by older adults and affect the interviewer's observations. Such factors as nutrition, health, emotions, environment, educational level, and culture play a role in cognitive functioning. Actual behavior should be described objectively instead of being labeled.

Many chronic and metabolic conditions cause changes in behavior and are manifested by disturbances in behavior and cognitive functioning. Misdiagnosis of physical problems or mental changes can create an enormous problem for clients and caregivers. The intricate interrelationship of physical and psychological behavior makes identification of health problems difficult.

Normal effects of aging on the central nervous system result in changes in intellectual and nervous system functioning. As the brain and central nervous system age, anatomical and biochemical changes occur that retard the transmission of impulses and delay reaction and thinking time. Aging affects the nervous system at various levels. A decrease in dopamine levels in the corpus striatum may cause loss of dopaminergic neurons. The decrease in dopamine may explain tremors of the extremities seen in older adults. Changes at the neurotransmitter synapses lead to decreased efficiency of turnover, release, and binding with neuromodulator substances. Coupled with biochemical changes, neurotransmitter imbalances, membrane alterations, and metabolic disturbances are intracellular and intercellular imbalances. These changes have regional selectivity that partially explains the differences in the aging process on individuals, but they do occur throughout the lifespan (Davis-Sharts, 1989).

A frame of reference is needed for accurate identification of differences in psychological and physiological changes. Baseline data or data obtained from a reliable source provide pertinent information. Baseline data should include an older person's functionings; methods of communication; thoughts and feelings; adaptation and adjustments to aging; relationships with others, especially significant others; use of time; cultural and ethnic patterns, beliefs, and attitudes; health beliefs and habits, and general life orientation. Certain considerations must be kept clearly in mind when attempting to distinguish between psychological and physiological problems:

1. There is a well-documented linear decline in the function of various tissue and organ systems associated with aging.
2. Symptoms of depression are of epidemic proportion in the older population and have a deleterious impact on physiological functioning.
3. Pathophysiological changes are potential causative factors in decreasing cognitive functioning, so that psychological changes accompany pathophysiology (Foreman & Gradowski, 1992).

Older persons may have multiple health problems. Additionally, many of the older person's physical and psychological adaptive systems are already operating on reserve capacities. Any additional burdens placed on them will result in symptoms that are not always distinguishable from each other or able to be easily diagnosed.

Sudden changes in behavior can denote physical illness, medication reactions, or a combination of physical problems and mental or emotional problems. Behavioral and cognitive dysfunction usually have long-standing developmental patterns; but sudden behavioral change can signal a life-threatening problem. Everyone experiences periods of hostility, aggression, forgetfulness, and confusion at times. It is the sudden change without provocation that concerns health care providers. Such behavioral changes can result from dehydration, electrolyte imbalance, drug interactions, malnutrition, infectious conditions, other pathologies, or a combination of or interaction of any of these conditions. Pathological symptoms in older adults are too often attributed to aging. A combination of aging, body responses, and pathology presents a confusing picture. Exploring all possible causes for a behavioral change can save the person and significant others enormous problems and embarrassment.

Multiple health problems usually require medications to control. Medications can alter an individual's physical and cognitive functioning and responses to an interviewer. A complete history is needed of all prescribed medications, over-the-counter medications, and home remedies. The interviewer should determine medication names, dosage, time and method of administration, and possible side effects. Older persons often have different physicians for different health problems and may be taking medications that counteract, interact with, or inhibit each other's effect.

Accurate data are crucial in determining the nature of a sudden behavioral change. Family and significant others are invaluable in providing information about history and manifestations of such a sudden change. Interviewing will take on the focus of detective work as the nurse leads the family through the client's lifestyle and life events.

❖ *Physical Assessment*

Knowledge about basic physical assessment and the changes occurring during normal aging are important. Physical assessments are best done on a yearly basis, because changes can occur rapidly. Changes in physiological functioning occur more rapidly in older adults than in younger age groups and have long-term effects. Age-related changes in sensory perception can affect mental status. Older people react to disease processes with a slower healing time than in younger age groups.

Because an older person fatigues and chills quickly, physical examination should be in a warm, well-lighted, comfortable room and conducted expeditiously. Time should be allowed for slower movements and reaction time. The physical should be completed as quickly as possible, taking into consideration the older adult's decreasing strength and energy, though not at the expense of collecting accurate data.

Physical examination techniques for older adults differ from approaches used with younger adults; however, inspection, palpation, percussion, and auscultation are still essential. The most noteworthy differences are related to structural integrity and changes resulting from aging. Physical losses are evident in the older person's reliance on supportive devices such as eyeglasses, hearing aids, and walking devices. A systematic physical assessment should be congruent with a health history and reflect the statements made by the client.

Physical examination begins with an assessment of general appearance, behavior, motor activity, and body language. The client's appearance gives clues to his or her success at adapting to and coping with physical problems. Physical aspects of activities of daily living, such as respiratory functioning, circulation, nutrition, elimination, mobility, and sleep patterns, can be evaluated easily.

The physical examination includes determining the client's present health concerns, especially problems that have had an impact on his or her lifestyle. An examination can reveal potential problem areas as each organ system is evaluated. Study of the family history and the client's medical history leads to identification of areas at high risk for potential problems.

As sensory organ functions diminish, older adults demonstrate slower response time and decreased sensitivity that may inappropriately be labeled as a decrease in intellectual functioning (Jarvis, 1992). The decline in sensory organ functions is embarrassing to older adults, and they tend to try to mask a hearing or eyesight deficit until the physical examination reveals deficiencies. The majority of people over age 40 require glasses to read at close range. Presbyopia, or loss of the ability of the eyes to accommodate to near vision, is one of the most common changes in aging eyes.

Cataracts or glaucoma are commonly found in older eyes, and the ability of the eye to adapt to dim light and darkness is decreased as the size of the pupil decreases to let in less light (Ebersole & Hess, 1994). Therefore, examination rooms should be well lighted so that clients can read any questionnaires or forms easily. Any printed material should have large print so that it can be read easily. The best interview format is verbal interaction between client and interviewer rather than a questionnaire the client must fill out in writing.

Neurosensory hearing loss gradually occurs in older adults, making high-frequency sounds difficult to hear. Ability to hear higher vocal pitches decreases with age. Neurosensory hearing loss is the most common cause of conductive hearing problems. Keeping the voice at a lower pitch is helpful for comfortable communication. The interviewer should face the client and speak clearly and slowly in a slightly louder tone of voice. It is not necessary to shout at the client with a hearing loss because this will intensify his or her anxiety and discomfort. Shouting does not help the situation and tends to embarrass the client. Difficulty hearing causes frustration, suspicion, and social isolation, as well as making the person look confused.

All such sensory problems may be accentuated during a time of stress such as an interview; therefore, the interviewer should find a quiet, private, and comfortable room with few distractions. This will minimize the client's fears about discussing physical problems and enhance his or her self-esteem by not exposing any masked health problems to persons other than the interviewer. Clients should be encouraged to wear any sensory augmentation devices they have in order to enhance the quality of the interaction.

Skin changes occurring as a result of sun exposure over many years include wrinkling and loss of turgor. Older persons are also subject to changes in muscular density, distribution of fatty tissue, and neuromuscular sensation. These changes require alteration in the examination technique. Most older clients have loose abdominal skin, which needs to be assessed for dehydration, a common problem with this age group. Palpation must be deep to elicit any pain a client may be experiencing. Reaction time is decreased in abdominal muscles when the client relaxes.

Percussion changes will be noted in the quality of the tone. The liver span may change from 5 to 7 centimeters in the young adult to 6 to 12 centimeters in the older adult. The upper liver border is located at the fifth to seventh intercostal space.

Auscultation of the lungs will elicit a softer vesicular sound. Atrophy of muscle tissue and a common change in structure to a thin and emaciated chest wall will intensify sounds. With aging, abdominal sounds change to more prominent bowel sounds, and there are more gurgling sounds.

❖ *Functional Assessment*

Functional assessment is a systematic and objective process aimed at determining a client's level of performance. The information gained from functional assessment gives needed data about an individual's daily adaptation.

Pfeiffer (1974) developed a functional care assessment called Older Americans

Research and Service Center Instrument (OARS). This tool allows collection of data on mental, physical, social, and economic aspects of daily living from a multidisciplinary approach. Pender (1987) developed an assessment tool called Lifestyle and Health Habits that individualizes assessment techniques. This tool was developed to focus on clients' personal lifestyles and their impact on health. The focus is on self-care, nutrition, physical and recreational activity, sleep patterns, stress management, self-actualization, goal setting, relationships, environment, and health care systems (Miller, 1990).

Because mobility has a profound effect on an individual's perception of well-being, a careful assessment of activities of daily living (ADL) must be made. Clients often consider themselves well as long as they do not require personal care. Evaluating ADL can be done with the use of specially designed instruments. These assessment tools are valuable regardless of the setting in which the nurse is seeing the client. The tools measure ADL indirectly by evaluating the clients' perceptions of their capabilities instead of by behavioral observation. Often clients will intentionally skew answers to questions about their ADL out of a fear of being placed in a nursing home. Asking them to perform simple tasks will assist in more accurately evaluating their ability to perform ADL tasks. Verbal or written reports require validation. Some older persons are frightened of making mistakes and will respond in ways they think will please the interviewer. Alleviating the client's anxiety will help him or her to relax. This may be accomplished with a short conversation.

Instrumental activities of daily living (IADL) assess task performance at a higher level. These tasks are more complex than ADL and focus on clients' abilities to interact with their environment. The tasks include (1) shopping, (2) cooking, (3) housekeeping, (4) doing laundry, (5) using transportation, (6) managing money, (7) managing medications, (8) using the telephone, (9) reading, (10) maintaining a home, (11) communicating, and (12) using time (Kane & Kane, 1981). Because many of these tasks are usually performed by women, some men may be at a disadvantage. This instrument is useful for individuals living in an independent arrangement and assists health care providers to identify services that may prolong independent living arrangements.

❖ *Mental Status Assessment*

Mental health in older adults encompasses a multitude of considerations and requires a comprehensive assessment. Serious mental disturbances may be prevented or their effects reduced if diagnosed and treated early. The aging process does not affect mental health and leaves the parameters of mental status mostly intact. Problems with chronic illness coupled with changes in mental capabilities and losses during aging all add to the stress on the older population.

Testing for memory is an important function of health care providers. A person's basic intellectual level affects the quality of information recalled. The health care provider tests for immediate, recent, and remote memory. Immediate memory can easily be tested by digit recall. Problems in this area are indicators of early cognitive loss. Recent memory can be tested by asking what foods the patient had for breakfast because this meal was found to be easily remembered, since it is a lifelong practice. Tests of remote memory focus on past events that should be familiar, such as date of marriage or who was president 40 years ago.

Physical changes manifested in appearance are more apparent than mental status changes. Whether an older adult resides in the community or a long-term care facility, planned mental status evaluation should be included in routine examinations. Assessment of mental status changes must be viewed in the context of the entire clinical picture.

Approximately 80% of nursing home residents suffer from mental illness or cognitive disorders. Unaffected residents have a significant risk of developing mental health or behavioral problems because of physical comorbidity and the environment in long-term care facilities (Smith, Buckwalter, & Albanese, 1990). Therefore, regular mental status assessment is essential to identify mental health problems early. A mental status assessment should be completed on admission to any inpatient facility and continued throughout the individual's stay within the institution (Hogstel, 1991). Since mental status changes can be subtle, assessments should be done weekly or monthly in long-term care facilities.

Cognitive impairment in older adults may be the result of depression, organic brain disorders such as delirium causing sudden onset of impaired cognition, or dementia that develops as a slow degeneration in cognitive functioning, or any combination of the three. Each condition has a different onset, course, progression, and clinical features (Foreman & Gradowski, 1992). The primary clinical features of cognitive impairment differentiating the three conditions are the chronicity and increasing difficulty with abstract thought processes found in dementia. Since each condition has an identifiable clinical feature, health care providers' prompt identification may improve the client's condition or significantly slow the progress of the problem, resulting in less negative consequences to the older adult.

A number of the cognitive tests listed in Table 4-1 can be used to assess the cognitive ability of patients. Pfeiffer's (1975) Short Portable Mental Status Questionnaire (SPMSQ) is the easiest to administer to individuals with short attention spans. This instrument is brief and can easily be used with acutely ill older adults who tire easily, contributing to errors in evaluation (Foreman, 1990). The SPMSQ, which contains only 10 questions, tests remote memory, knowledge of current events, and mathematical ability. It is scored on the number of errors an individual makes and measures levels of mental impairment. This test can be administered in conjunction with the Older Americans Research and Service Center Instrument (OARS) test or as a separate test. Scores run from 1 to 10, with 10 indicating severe intellectual impairment. Scores are adjusted to clients' educational levels. The SPMSQ and its scoring method may be found in Appendix B.

Mental status tests evaluate neuropsychiatric problems with sensory acuity, short-term and long-term memory, judgment, and problem-solving ability. The results of mental status tests are often confused with information gained from intelligence tests that are administered to evaluate an individual's ability to perceive

Table 4-1   Sample Assessment Tools

Name	Author	Category
Older Americans Research and Service Center Instrument (OARS)	Pfeiffer (1974)	Functional
Health Assessment Guide for an Elderly Person	Yurick et al. (1984)	Functional
Program for an Integrated System of Community Elderly Services (PISCES)	Robinson et al. (1984)	Functional
Long-Term Care Information System (LTCIS)	Falcone (1981)	Long-term
Beck Depression Inventory	Beck (1972)	Depression
Self-Rating Depression Scale (SDS)	Zung (1965)	Depression
Lifestyle and Health Habits	Pender (1987)	Lifestyle
Family APGAR	Smilkstein (1978)	Family
Instrumental Activities of Daily Living (IADL)	Lawton (1971)	IADL
Index of Activities of Daily Living (ADL)	Katz et al. (1963)	ADL
Short Portable Mental Status Questionnaire	Pfeiffer (1975)	Memory
Mini-Mental Status Exam	Folstein et al. (1975)	Cognitive
Functional, Reasoning, Orientation, Memory, Arithmetic, Judgment, and Emotion (FROMAJE)	Libow (1981)	Mental
Psychogeriatric Nursing Assessment Protocol (PNAP)	Abraham et al. (1992)	Mixed

relationships, recognize relationships, and develop logical plans. The use of mental status tests in geropsychiatry assists the health care provider to determine present levels of functioning. Intelligence tests allow the health care provider to determine ability to use perceived information to manipulate the environment.

Many of the sophisticated intelligence tests must be administered and evaluated by someone familiar with the testing who is able to interpret the results. To administer and evaluate an intelligence test without the necessary credentials to evaluate the results accurately would be a disservice to the client.

Assessing intelligence in an older adult can be done accurately and may provide valuable information when the assessment is conducted by a qualified health care professional. The most important aspect of assessment is allowing an individual time to complete required tasks. Intelligence seems to be affected only when physiological limitations become excessive or extreme changes in social roles occur.

Many intelligence tests do not consider the vast differences in socioeconomic conditions and cultural development among older adults. The effects of educational background and life experiences affect the test outcome. Intelligence tests are not free of cultural influences. Physiological, genetic, and environmental influences vary in individuals. For example, a lifetime rich in experiences such as education, occupation, travel, and mental stimulation affects an individual's verbal skills and abilities.

There is a clear relationship between poor health, intelligence test scores, and cognitive functioning (Brown, 1988). Individuals with chronic illness tire easily and do not concentrate well on tasks. Psychological distress may be manifested in altered mood states, changes in self-perception, or decreased motivation to perform. Physiological and psychological factors are interactive and negatively affect psychological functioning. Cardiovascular and central nervous system functioning play a major role in problems related to psychological decline.

The interaction between emotional and cognitive functioning and physiological decline are an important consideration in the assessment of older adults. A cerebrovascular accident has catastrophic effects on cognitive functioning.

Institutionalized clients should be evaluated for level of consciousness, alertness, and awareness of internal and external stimuli. An individual's level of attention can be assessed by noting the ability to maintain concentration on an assigned task. The arousal center in the brain stem interacts with higher cortical functioning affecting consciousness (Eisdorfer & Cohen, 1982). There are no impairments to these centers during the normal aging process.

❖ Psychological and Emotional Assessment

Screening of cognitive functioning is a valuable tool for assessing deficits and determining the need for further evaluation of mental status and capabilities. The screening tools used by the nurse are not intended to be diagnostic but to determine progression of changes in the mental status of an individual. Additional testing by other health care professionals provides more detailed and in-depth information. Such data provide a continuity for nursing diagnosis and assist the client by identifying changes in cognitive functioning. Assessment of cognitive functioning is concerned with evaluation of conscious processes, present thoughts, memory, judgment, comprehension, reasoning, and problem-solving strategies used in daily living.

Approximately "2%-4% of the population over age 65 have Dementia of the Alzheimer's Type" (American Psychiatric Association, 1994, p. 137). Dementia is the term used for a host of conditions that includes, for example, dementia of the Alzheimer's type, dementia due to Parkinson's disease, dementia due to Huntington's disease, and dementia due to other general medical conditions (APA, 1994). These types of conditions are characterized by impaired memory and judgment, problems with intellectual functioning, and accompanying behavioral disturbances. The incidence of dementia increases dramatically with increasing age; 20% for those age 85 and older (APA, 1994). Researchers have found that individuals who are highly educated and those who keep themselves intellectually stimulated have a lower incidence of dementia (Bender, 1992). The difference between reversible and irreversible dementia lies in the cause of the problems.

Cognitive Assessment

Cognitive changes occur most rapidly in the very old age group. It has been suggested that intelligence and cognitive functioning steadily decline about 5 years before the client's death (Riegel & Riegel, 1972). This decline may be related to the numerous problems associated with chronic illnesses as daily life becomes a preoccupation with the pursuit of physical comfort. Therefore, mental and psychological evaluation should be done more frequently as a person ages and should become an integral part of the yearly physical examination.

Cognitive deficits have been found to be positively related to the amount of brain damage. Older persons have greater brain impairment than those in younger age groups. Neuropathology extensively affects cognitive functioning. The clock test was developed to screen cognitively impaired older adults and individuals suffering specifically with Alzheimer's disease. The clock test consists of drawing, setting, and reading a clock. These three components of the clock test require abstract conceptualization that remains intact with normal aging (Tuokko, Hadjistavropoulos, Miller, & Beattie, 1992). This test reflects generalized disturbances in conceptualization of time and is particularly useful as a screening and research tool. An individual who develops adaptive abilities earlier in life performs better during old age than an individual with a premorbid personality who does not develop adaptive or coping skills. There is evidence that cognitive functioning is intertwined with emotions and motivation. Activities conducted throughout life that enhance self-worth and feelings of usefulness are valuable assets for older adults. Most intellectual and learning studies on older adults have failed to take into account the individual's educational level, occupation, or lifelong learning habits.

The cognitive functions of learning and memory decline with age, resulting in decrements in performance of many learning tasks (Kermis, 1986). This decrease in cognitive functioning is related to an increase in anxiety and in performing tasks that are not part of an individual's usual way of functioning. Increased stress and anxiety lead to decreased performance.

Deptula et al. (1993) suggest that many older adults do not perform well on learning and memory tests because the testing situation is stressful and anxiety producing. Older adults do well on learning and memory tests when stress is reduced and enough time is allowed for mental processing of information. Older adults have a slowed reaction time related to the physiological effects of aging. In addition, they may have decreased ability for complex decision making and decreased speed of performance, but there is no decrease in general knowledge (Baily, 1992). Allowing more time for mental processing decreases autonomic arousal, which enhances test performance abilities. Reduction in the number of stimuli and increased requests for familiar retrieval information reduce stress and lead to normal reaction time.

Aging modulates the relationship between emotional states and memory functions in older adults. Negative emotional states adversely affect older adults' performance. Anxiety and worry reduce memory performance in older adults. Deptula et al. (1993) suggest that learning behavioral relaxation techniques improves memory in older adults with high anxiety. Careful assessment of physiological functioning has to be made before a clear assessment can be made of the cognitive performance of an individual. There is a linear decline in the physiological functioning during the aging process. The constant and consistent nature of the loss of physiological functioning affects cognitive functioning. The brain tissue and nervous system decay is paralleled by decline in all the organs. Cognitive functioning is affected by decline in both the nervous system and other organs.

Impact of Physiological Problems

The impact of pathophysiological changes causes a decrement in cognitive functioning. Major physiological problems affecting an older adult's cognitive functioning are cardiovascular problems, metabolic disorders, hematological disorders, neurological disorders and deficits, and iatrogenic disorders.

Cardiovascular changes lead to problems with cognitive functioning. A reduction in cardiac stroke volume leads to a decrease in cardiac output of 30% to 40% from ages 25 to 65. Blood volume perfusion to the central nervous system decreases by 0.35% per year in older adults. Myocardial infarctions and congestive heart failure reduce cardiac perfusion and lead to cognitive impairment.

Metabolic dysfunctions are associated with mental aberrations. A confusional state results from chemical imbalances. Hematological disorders cause problems because of reduced blood flow to the brain.

Iatrogenic disorders are caused by a combination of drugs given for treatment of multiple illnesses reaching toxic levels. Drugs given for physiological and psychological problems often exceed the tolerance limits of an individual and interact to cause a confused state. Medications can cause an imbalance in normal body functions, reduce blood flow, alter impulse transmission, and interfere with chemical balances, all of which lead to confusion.

Sleep disturbances or excessive sleeping should be investigated because sleep problems can be medically or psychologically important to the client and significant others. Sleep pattern alterations in older adults arise from a 40% decrease in the number of catecholaminergic neurons in the locus coeruleus. Age-related changes contribute to sleep pattern alterations. Older adults spend less time in delta sleep, the stage leading to feelings of restfulness. The complaints of not feeling rested, not sleeping well, and daytime sleepiness can be attributed to a decrease in delta sleep and an increase in the number of awakenings during a sleep period (Davis-Sharts, 1989). Older persons need the same amount of sleep as younger persons; however, they have a diminished ability to achieve stages 3 and 4, or deep sleep, and are unable to maintain a deep level of sleep. Consequently, they awake feeling tired and as though they had not slept. Disturbance in sleep patterns may be age related and may occur in combination with physiological problems, psychological problems, neurological changes, or drug-induced changes in sleep patterns. Additionally, breathing disorders, poor sleep habits, or changes in sleep patterns such as sleeping more during the daytime hours can cause sleeplessness at night. The environment may not be conducive to sleeping if it is too noisy, too light, uncomfortable, or anxiety producing. Information about the patient's lifestyle and sleep patterns is important regardless of the living arrangement in assessing whether the changes are related to aging or disease, or are drug induced.

A subjective sleep history should also be accompanied by a sleep-wake log, record of sleep behaviors, and a thorough physical and psychological history. Disturbances in sleep-wake patterns can lead to severe depression in older people.

Psychological Performance

Controversial studies have suggested that intelligence may remain stable over a lifetime and that any psychological changes may be related to life events or physical deterioration. An outcome of the studies has been a recognition of the considerable variation and differences that exist in the ways aging affects various abilities. Individuals age at differing rates. Many research investigations have failed to consider the differing levels of education, occupation, recreation, and activity (Kermis, 1986).

Research study findings indicate that older adults do not do well on intelligence tests, primarily because they are not interested in the content areas and the subject matter does not pertain to their life situation (Burnside, 1988). An older adult functions well on psychological tests when given the time and appropriate information for the task.

Structural, physiological, and electrophysiological changes in later life are well documented, leaving little doubt about the changes that occur in an individual's ability to function. Research is still needed on the rate and pattern of changes and the irreversibility of any psychological changes.

A widespread problem with older adults is depression caused by psychological or physical problems, or both. Depression may be a manifestation of physical illness, losses experienced, or organic changes in the brain (Dellasega & Shellenberger, 1992). A vicious cycle is set in motion when the individual becomes acutely aware of physical decline, causing depression to set in. Depression has a deleterious effect on physiological functions, and the cycle begins.

Many instruments are available to evaluate the depression experienced by an older adult. A widely used instrument developed by Beck and Beck (1972) has been used to detect and measure depression. Their instrument, The Beck Depression Inventory, is a 13-item questionnaire that examines aspects of mood, self-image, and somatic complaints commonly experienced by depressed persons. Scores may range from 0 to 16. A score of 16 indicates a severe depression (Beck and Beck, 1972). This self-administered instrument has been tested for reliability and validity worldwide.

Another well-known instrument that measures depression in an older population was developed by Zung. The Zung Self-Rating Depression Scale (SDS) was developed specifically to measure depression in older adults (Zung, 1965). This instrument contains 20 items that evaluate the areas of mood, well-being, optimism, and somatic problems. It is scored on a four-point scale, and scores are summed and divided by 20 to arrive at a percentage. This widely used test has proved reliable and valid worldwide.

❖ Summary

All forms of information obtained through subjective and objective means have to be analyzed in a systematic, logical manner. Ordering data in a logical sequence simplifies this work. At times, intervention strategies must be initiated before the total assessment has been completed. Action must be taken when a life-threatening problem has been identified.

Data summarization should include information about a client's assets and deficits. Information should be collated to reflect the interrelationship of physical, psychological, cognitive, and social aspects of an individual's life. An important part of the data is a record of the client's reactions to and perceptions of assets and losses and his or her available adaptation and coping mechanisms. Since each person's life is unique, coping and adaptation mechanisms reflect life experiences and patterns. Any area impacts and affects all other systems.

Sorting data into meaningful and individualized information culminates in nursing diagnoses. Nursing diagnoses reflect the accuracy, completeness, and thoroughness of the total assessment. Nursing intervention strategies can be individualized and priority given to the most life-threatening concerns as well as the client's immediate concerns. A comprehensive plan can then be developed.

Most mental health problems in older adults are treatable. A careful and accurate assessment of mental illness can lead to successful intervention strategies. Growing old requires a great deal of adjustment as an individual faces the challenges of a new and different stage of life.

❖ References

Abraham, I. L., Smullen, D. E., & Thompson-Heisterman, A. A. (1992). Geriatric mental health: Assessing geropsychiatric patients. *Journal of Psychosocial Nursing, 30*(9), 13-19.

American Psychiatric Association. (1994). *Diagnostic and statistical manual of mental disorders* (4th ed.) Washington, DC: Author.

Baily, J. (1992). To find a soul. *Nursing 92, 22*(7), 63-64.

Beck, A. T., & Beck, R. W. (1972). Screening depressed patients in family practice: A rapid technique. *Postgraduate Medicine, 52*(6), 81-85.

Bender, P. (1992). Deceptive distress in the elderly. *American Journal of Nursing, 92*(10), 29-33.

Brown, M. D. (1988). Functional assessment of the elderly. *Journal of Gerontological Nursing, 14*(5), 13-17.

Burnside, I. (1988). *Nursing and the aged.* New York: McGraw-Hill.

Carnevali, D. (1992). *Nursing management for the elderly* (3rd ed.). Philadelphia: Lippincott.

Davis-Sharts, J. (1989). The elder and critical care: Sleep and mobility issues. *Nursing Clinics of North America, 24*(3), 755-767.

Dellasega, C., & Shellenberger, T. (1992). Discharge planning for cognitively impaired elder adults. *Nursing and Health Care, 13,* 526-531.

Deptula, D., Singh, R., & Pomara, N. (1993). Aging, emotional states, and memory. *American Journal Psychiatry. 150*(3), 429-434.

Ebersole, P., & Hess, P. (1994). *Toward healthy aging* (4th ed.). St. Louis: Mosby.

Eisdorfer, C. & Cohen, D. (1982). *Geriatrics for the primary care physician.* Menlo Park, CA: Addison-Wesley.

Falcone, A. R. (1981). *Synopsis of long-term care information system programs.* New York: Assessment Training Center, Cornell University Medical Center, Department of Public Health.

Farrell, J. (1990). *Nursing care of the older person.* Philadelphia: Lippincott.

Folstein, M. E., Folstein, S. E., & McHugh, P. R. (1975). Mini-mental state: A practical method for grading the cognitive state of patients for the clinician. *Journal of Psychiatric Research 12,* 189-198.

Foreman, M. D. (1990). Complexities of acute confusion. *Geriatric Nursing, 11*(3), 136-139.

Foreman, M. D., & Gradowski, R. (1992). Diagnostic dilemma: Cognitive impairment in the elderly. *Journal of Gerontological Nursing, 18*(9), 5-12.

Hogstel, M. O. (1991). Assessing mental status. *Journal of Gerontological Nursing, 17*(5), 42-43.

Jarvis, C. (1992). *Physical Examination and Health Assessment.* Philadelphia: Saunders.

Kane, R. A., & Kane, R. L. (1981). *Assessing the elderly.* Lexington, MA: Lexington Books.

Katz, S., Ford, A. S., Moskowitz, R. S., Jackson, B. A., & Jaffe, M. W. (1963). Studies of illness in the aged. The Index of ADL: A standardized measure of biological and psychosocial function. *Journal of the American Medical Association, 185,* 94-98.

Kermis, M. D. (1986). *Mental health in late life.* Boston: Jones & Bartlett.

Lawton, M. P. 1971). The functional assessment of elderly people. *Journal of the American Geriatrics Society, 19*(6), 465-481.

Libow, L. A. (1981). A rapidly administered, easily remembered mental status evaluation: FROMAJE. In L. S. Libow & F. T. Sherman (Eds.). *The core of geriatric medicine.* St. Louis: Mosby.

Miller, C. A. (1990). *Nursing care of older adults: Theory and practice.* Philadelphia: Lippincott.

Pender, N. (1987). *Health promotion in nursing practice.* Norwalk, CT: Appleton-Century-Crofts.

Pfeiffer, E. A. (Ed.) (1974). *Multidimensional functional assessment: The OARS methodology.* Durham, NC: Duke University Center for the Study of Aging and Human Development.

Pfeiffer, E. A. (1975). A short portable mental status questionnaire for assessment of organic brain deficit in elderly patients. *Journal of the American Geriatrics Society, 23*(10), 433-441.

Riegel, K. F. & Riegel, R. M. (1972). Development, drop, and death. *Developmental Psychology, 6*(2), 306-319.

Robinson, C., Combs, D., Pierson, S., Roberts, J., Hagesfeld-Bohinc, J., & Venesy, B. (1984). *The PISCES assessment process and manual.* Akron, OH: Infoline/PISCES Project.

Smilkstein, G. (1978). The family APGAR: A proposal for a family function test and its use by physicians. *The Journal of Family Practice, 6*(6), 1231-1238.

Smith, M., Buckwalter, K. C., & Albanese, M. (1990). Gerophychiatric education program: Providing skills and understanding. *Journal of Psychosocial Nursing, 28*(12), 9-12.

Stillman, R. A. (1986). Social stress and social support. *Generations, 10*(3), 18-20.

Tuokko, H., Hadjistavropoulos, T., Miller, J. A., & Beattie, B. L. (1992). The clock test: A sensitive measure to differentiate normal elderly from those with Alzheimer disease. *Journal of the American Geriatrics Society, 40*(6), 579-584.

Yurick, A. G., Spier, B. E., Robb, S. S. & Ebert, N. J. (1984). *The aged person and the nursing process.* Norwalk, CT: Appleton-Century-Crofts.

Zung, W. K. (1965). A self-rating depression scale. *Archives of General Psychiatry, 12*(1), 63-70.

Chapter 5

❖ *Psychotropic Drugs*

Edward A. Luke, Jr.

Americans age 65 and older constitute approximately 12.7% of the population (American Association of Retired Persons, 1993). This group receives approximately 25% of all prescription drugs (O'Brien & Kursch, 1987; Baum, Kennedy, Knapp, Faich, & Ariello, 1987; Sloan, 1981). Clients over 65 average 13 prescriptions per year (Lamy, 1980). Of the ambulatory patients over 65, as many as 80% may receive some type of medication (LaVange and Silverman, 1987). Older adults age 60 and over "make up one-sixth of the population, they use almost 40% of the prescription drugs, an average of 15.4 prescriptions filled a year" (Wolfe & Hope, 1993, Overview p. 2). Although cardiovascular drugs, analgesics, sedatives, and hypnotic drugs are the most common medications taken by older patients, psychotropic medications make up a significant portion of prescriptions used by this group (Lamy, 1980).

❖ *Clinical Implications*

In prescribing medications for the older client, it is important to remember that altered psychodynamics and psychokinetics will play an important role in how these drugs affect the client and interact with other medications (Box 5-1). Absorption, distribution, protein binding, hepatic metabolism, and renal excretion all affect drug metabolism. Central nervous system neurotransmitter and drug receptor site changes that occur with aging are being reported. These alterations may not only affect medication doses but also may require some changes in specific medications indicated or contraindicated in older adults. Since most drugs are administered orally, alterations in the gastrointestinal tract in older people can have numerous and far-reaching consequences. A decrease in the amount of stomach acids may alter the bioavailability of drugs at the site of absorption in the intestine. Changes in blood

---

Box 5–1 **Factors Affecting Medications in the Older Patient**
Gastrointestinal absorption alterations

> Increase in body fat
> Decrease in muscle mass
> Decrease in total body water
> Decrease in plasma albumin
> Changes in neurotransmitters and receptor sites
> Decrease in hepatic metabolism
> Decrease in hepatic blood flow

---

flow to the gastrointestinal tract may decrease the rate of absorption. Changes in motility may actually increase the amount of some drugs that is absorbed. Peak time of absorption and rate of absorption may alter the amount of drug available and blunt the blood level that is reached by some medications (Calkins, Davis, & Ford, 1986).

The volume of distribution of drugs is altered in older adults. As the normal body ages, there tends to be an increase in total body fat, whereas the amount of muscle mass and total body water present decreases (Swift, 1988). This translates into clinical implications for elimination half-life. If the medication is more easily absorbed into body fat, more will be distributed through the body and will take longer to be eliminated, as in diazepam (Valium). The elimination half-life can be well over 100 to 150 hours. Because of a decrease in total body water, more of a highly water-soluble medication will be absorbed into a smaller amount of water and will be eliminated more quickly, thus decreasing the time it takes to eliminate that drug from the body. Most psychotropic medications, with the exception of lithium, tend to be more soluble in fatty tissues.

Plasma albumin levels tend to decrease with age. Because most drugs are protein bound, they tend to adhere to the albumin in the plasma. Only the amount of free drug, that is, the amount of drug not bound to protein, will produce the clinical effect. If the amount of albumin decreases, then less of the drug will be able to be bound to the decreased amount of protein, allowing an increase in free drug amounts. As the amount of free drug increases, so will the therapeutic and the toxic effects. Therefore, an older patient receiving the same level of drug as a younger patient will have a greater risk of toxic effects because of the increased amount of free drug in the plasma.

Many of the psychotropic medications are metabolized by the liver. When a medication is taken orally and absorbed through the intestinal tract, the initial blood flow is through the liver before entering the systemic circulation. In the first pass 40% to 80% of the drug may be eliminated before reaching the systemic circulation. Liver impairment brings about an increase in drug blood levels.

The elimination half-life of the drug also increases. The half-life of a drug is the time required for half of the drug to be eliminated from the body. As the time for elimination of the drug lengthens, the elimination half-life will increase. It normally takes four to five half-lives to eliminate 90% of a drug. In older adults, this can be increased to days and even weeks and thus may have far-reaching consequences for the clinical effects of medication as well as its elimination once it has been discontinued. In taking a drug history, the interviewer should not only ask about current medications, but also any medications that have been taken and discontinued within the past month or two.

With normal aging in healthy individuals, renal filtration may drop about 30% (Everitt & Avorn, 1986). The clinical effect of this change is an increase in the time needed to eliminate drugs that are filtered out and eliminated through the kidneys and thus an increase in the elimination half-time for such drugs. Elimination half-time, of course, will be further lengthened in patients with renal impairment caused by trauma or disease. It becomes highly critical to monitor blood levels of medication in renally impaired patients as well as many older patients receiving drugs such as lithium. Therapeutic blood levels may be reached with smaller doses of medications, and doses may be reduced to every other day and achieve the same therapeutic effect.

Medication dosages in older adults should be critically evaluated. Many times dosages that are appropriate in younger patients will cause toxic effects in older people because of the changes in the pharmacokinetics of the drug in the body. This may mean that lower doses of medication will be sufficient to achieve the same blood level and therefore therapeutic effect in older patients. It also may mean that the elimination half-life of a drug is greatly increased and reducing the dosage frequence, such as to every other day, may achieve the same therapeutic effect as daily doses in a younger client. Checking blood levels of medications in older clients may become more important and necessary in monitoring clinical effects.

❖ *Common Clinical Concerns*

Interactions

Drug-Drug Interactions

Half of all nonprescription drugs bought over the counter are purchased by people over 65 years of age. Of these purchases, 21% are taken regularly for at least 6 months (David, 1981). Surveys of drug usage in older adults indicate that cardiovascular drugs are the most frequently prescribed medications for older patients, followed by psychotropic drugs and gastrointestinal agents. Nolan and O'Malley (1988) found that between 3% and 10% of hospital admissions of older patients were for adverse drug reactions. Twelve percent of all patients admitted had some kind of adverse drug reaction. It has been shown that with an increase in the number of prescriptions per person, there is a concomitant increase in the frequency of adverse drug reactions. These begin with 4% in 1 to 5 prescriptions and increase to 54% with 16 to 20 prescriptions (May, Stewart, & Cluff, 1977; Pucinof et al., 1985).

Drug-Food Interactions

The effects on medications of nutrients in specific foods often go unrecognized. Previously, it was thought that taking medications on an empty stomach was the most appropriate schedule for administration. It has since been reported that a number of drugs, such as antimicrobials, bronchodilators, diuretics, and vasodilators are best taken on an empty stomach but that the bioavailability of certain drugs is enhanced when they are taken with foods. Also, some medications should or should not be taken with specific kinds of food (Osis, 1986). Lamy (1982) described the effects of drugs on the gastrointestinal system; for example, malabsorption problems can deplete the bioavailability of certain medications.

Noncompliance

Noncompliance with medical regimens is certainly well documented as a problem in all age groups. This is especially true in the older population. Parkin, Henney, Quirks, and Crooks (1976) found that in a study of clients with a mean age of 66.2 years, only 49.2% were taking their drugs correctly, 34.4% did not understand the drug regimen and therefore made errors, and 23.4% were noncompliant, even though they understood the drug regimens. One of the most frustrating experiences for health care providers is listening to an older patient talk about taking the "little yellow pill" or using similar descriptions. Labeling each prescription with its use can help patients understand their drug regimen. Asking the druggist to put nonchildproof caps on prescription containers can add to the ease of taking the medications. Clients have often complained of not taking the medication because they could not open the bottle. The financial status of the patient should also be a consideration. Clients who have a pharmacy bill of several hundred dollars a month and are on a limited income may pick and choose which prescriptions they will fill. Trading medications and using old, outdated, and unused prescriptions are common practices that can create problems for older people. Failing to coordinate medications with other physicians or failing to ask patients what other medications have been prescribed for them by other physicians can cause compliance problems that may only be detected through lack of therapeutic effect or untoward side effects. The client who is paranoid may have to have medication administration witnessed by family members to ensure compliance. Doing the brown bag biopsy, that is, having the family bring in all of the patient's medications, may be the only sure way of determining the exact medications the patient is taking or has in his possession. The family of one client brought in 75 different medications prescribed by 6 different doctors and filled by 9 different pharmacies.

Nursing Implications

The nurse should do a careful drug history as part of the total assessment in every clinical setting. Many older people do not consider over-the-counter (OTC) products as drugs, so the nurse should specifically ask about them and include them in the history. In an out-patient, home, or other community setting, the nurse should ask about availability of prescribed drugs. The cost of drugs is one of the major complaints of older persons, and some of them have to choose between purchasing drugs and food.

Teaching is another important nursing intervention. Clients should be taught the essential information about the drugs they are taking, such as the name, purpose, dose, time, method of taking, and possible side effects. A clearly prepared list of all this information in large bold print should be given to the client to take home, with a phone number to call the physician or nurse if questions or problems arise. Side effects of some psychotropic drugs can be particularly distressing (i.e., tardive dyskinesia), and clients should be warned about this possibility at the beginning of treatment. Mental changes such as confusion may also occur, and older clients need to know that these changes may be due to the drugs and not their condition.

In acute care and long-term care settings such as nursing homes, all oral drugs should be scheduled at appropriate intervals (not all given at one time), with adequate fluids (at least 6 to 8 ounces), and the clients observed carefully for swallowing difficulties. If clients have problems swallowing capsules or tablets, the nurse should request that the physician order the drug in a liquid form if available or choose another drug. If neither is an option, some drugs must be crushed completely and mixed with a substance that can easily be swallowed. It is best not to use foods that the client frequently eats and enjoys because it may cause the client to develop a dislike for the food. Applesauce, although frequently used, is not a good choice because particles of the applesauce can be easily aspirated. Smooth junior level baby fruits, such as plums or prunes, are possible alternatives. Some drugs, such as spansules and enteric coated tablets should never be crushed. Some oral drugs dissolve completely in water for nasal gastric or gastrostomy tube administration, but others will never dissolve even though crushed well and can easily obstruct the tube and require a replacement. Again, the nurse should request a different order from the physician.

❖ *Major Drug Categories*

Antidepressants

Antidepressants are a major class of neuroleptic medications. This class includes heterocyclics, monoamine oxidase inhibitors (MAOI), and psychostimulants. Antidepressants first came into use in the 1950s. They represented a major breakthrough in the treatment of major depressive disorders, both unipolar and bipolar, including delusional depression, depression secondary to other causes such as alcohol abuse and prescribed medications, panic disorder, obsessive-compulsive disorder, bulimia, attention deficit disorder, posttraumatic stress disorder, and chronic pain syndromes. The mechanism of action of these medications is still in question, although there is pharmacological evidence that they affect monoamine neurotransmitter systems in the brain. The tricyclic antidepressants block the reuptake of norepinephrine and/or serotonin, while the MAOIs are thought to potentiate the action of monoamines by inhibiting their breakdown and metabolism.

Tricyclic and Heterocyclic Antidepressants

CLINICAL USE.   The efficacy or clinical effect of these medications is all equal. There is not one best drug to use. The choice of medication is based on the following:

- Thorough diagnostic evaluation leading to appropriate patient selection
- Selection of drug through side effect profiles that are appropriate for each patient
- Adequate dosage for appropriate trial of medication for at least 3 to 4 weeks
- Assured patient compliance

Thorough patient evaluation for appropriate diagnostic considerations should be given to any patient selected to receive any medication. The selection of patients meeting the appropriate criteria will help ensure better patient response. Indiscriminate use of antidepressants for patients who may be suffering from a reactive depression to a specific emotional trauma unnecessarily exposes these patients to toxicity and clinical side effects of these medications.

An adequate and appropriate dose of these medications is necessary to ensure a good response. Most of the tricyclic antidepressants, as listed in Table 5-1, require a dose of 150 mg. Trazodone (Desyrel), one of the heterocyclic medications, has an adequate dose of 250 mg, whereas protriptyline (Vivactil) and nortriptyline (Pamelor) require a lesser dose. The adequate trial of fluoxetine (Prozac) requires a dosage of 20 mg per day. These are doses for young and middle-aged adult patients, not geriatric patients. A geriatric client will require a dose that is approximately half the dose for a normal younger adult. Starting most of these medications at 50 mg per day and increasing the dosage over a 5- to 10-day period to the normal maintenance dose would be an appropriate clinical plan. Fluoxetine may be started at 10 mg per day or 20 mg every other day and continued at this dose for a trial of 3 to 4 weeks.

The initial response to these medications will typically not be seen for 7 to 10 days. The initial adequate response may take another 10 to 14 days to evaluate. These medications typically give an up-and-down course of one good day following a bad day, with the patient experiencing more good days as the treatment progresses. Approximately 6 to 8 weeks will be needed to have a full adequate response for most clients (Fig. 5-1). It may be necessary to test blood levels to judge the adequacy of compliance in some patients.

SIDE EFFECTS.   Typical side effects of antidepressants include anticholinergic effects, sedative side effects, cardiovascular effects, and orthostatic hypotension. The anticholinergic effects include tachycardia, dilated and sluggish pupils, blurred vision, dry mouth, warm dry skin, constipation, and urinary retention. Central anticholinergic effects may be manifested by confusion, delirium, possible hallucinations, and seizures. Sedation is a major side effect of most antidepressants. Patients with more agitation in their depression may be given one of the more sedative

Table 5-1 Antidepressants

Cyclic agents	Geriatric dose/day (mg)	Sedation	Anticholinergic	Cardiac toxicity	Hypotension
Amitriptyline (Amitril, Endep, Elavil)	10-75	High	Very High	High	Medium
Imipramine (SK-Pramine, Tofranil)	10-75	Medium	Medium-high	Medium	Medium
Doxepin (Adapin, Sinequan)	10-75	High	Medium	Medium	Medium
Desipramine (Norpramin, Pertofrane)	10-75	Low	Low	Low	Low
Nortriptyline (Aventyl, Pamelor)	10-50	Low	Medium	Low	Low
Trimipramine (Surmontil)	10-75	High	Medium-high	High	Medium
Protriptyline (Vivactil)	5-20	Low	High	Medium	Medium
Maprotiline (Ludiomil)	10-75	Medium	Low-medium	Low	Medium
Amoxapine (Asendin)	10-100	Medium	Low	Medium	Medium
Fluoxetine (Prozac)	10-20 daily/or every other day	Unusual	None	None	None
Sertraline (Zoloft)	25-50	Unusual	None	None	None
Paroxetine (Paxil)	10-20	Unusual	None	None	None
Atypical Agents					
Trazodone (Desyrel)	75-150	High	None	Low	Medium
MAOIs:					
Phenelzine (Nardil)	15-45	Medium	Low	None	Medium-high
Tranylcypromine (Parnate)	10-40	Medium	Low	None	Medium-high
Isocarboxazid (Marplan)	10-40	Medium	Low	None	Medium-high

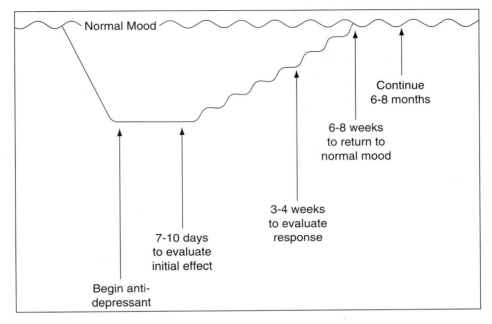

Figure 5-1 Timeline for treatment with an antidepressant.

antidepressants, whereas a more retarded, sluggishly depressed patient may be given one of the less sedating medications. Cardiovascular effects may be due to blocking of the Purkinje fibers in the heart; they may be manifested by tachyventricular and supraventricular arrhythmias. For a patient with preexisting cardiac arrhythmias or recent myocardial infarction, tricyclic antidepressants are typically contraindicated. Orthostatic hypotension is a potentially dangerous side effect, especially in older adults. Prescribing medications that have milder orthostatic side effects may lead to better compliance and safety.

Monoamine Oxidase Inhibitors (MAOIs)
Monoamine oxidase inhibitors work through the prevention of breakdown of the monoamines. Tyramine is a substance in many foods that is not broken down when the MAOIs are present. Tyramine may produce a profound α-adrenergic activation that may lead to a hypertensive crisis with systolic blood pressure rising to well over 200. This has been called a cheese reaction, since tyramine is present in relatively high concentrations in aged cheese. Tyramine is found in many other foods. Therefore, patients receiving MAOIs must be placed on a special low-tyramine diet. This diet should be explained to the client before initiation of treatment. A substantial number of medications also may lead to hypertensive reactions in clients taking MAOIs. Clients should be warned of this and should be told to inform their physicians and pharmacists any time a drug is prescribed or an over-the-counter medication is

considered for purchase. This interaction should not deter clinicians from prescribing MAOIs, since they have no cardiovascular side effects. MAOIs are often the drug of choice, especially in older patients who have preexisting cardiac arrhythmias. Older adults who are following a fresh meat, potato, and vegetable diet can safely use MAOIs; however, MAOIs are still a second-line drug for most clients unless one of the other medications is contraindicated.

Serotonin Selective Reuptake Inhibitors

Fluoxetine (Prozac), sertraline (Zoloft), and paroxetine (Paxil) are new types of antidepressants known as serotonin selective reuptake inhibitors (SSRIs). They are pure serotonergic agents, which typically have few side effects. They usually are not sedative, and fluoxetine may cause insomnia, which necessitates administering it in the morning rather than at night. The most common side effects are usually gastrointestinal distress such as nausea, vomiting, and diarrhea. They also may cause anxiety or headaches. They carry a low risk of death and overdose. Because of the low side effect profile for this class of medication, these antidepressants are replacing the tricyclic antidepressants as first-line medications in the treatment of major depression. Because of the serotonergic mechanism, they may also be useful in the treatment of obsessive-compulsive disorder, although they are not as yet approved for this usage.

Psychostimulants

Methylphenidate (Ritalin), dextroamphetamine (Dexedrine), and pemoline (Cylert) are psychostimulants that may be used in physically ill clients to help initiate antidepressant response when one of the other antidepressants is contraindicated. Starting these medications at low doses such as 5 mg of methylphenidate twice a day may be helpful. Because these medications may cause insomnia, schedules for administration should be twice a day with an early morning and a noon or afternoon dose. Doses should rarely be given after 6 PM. These medications may cause tachycardia, and proper cardiac evaluation of these clients should be included in the treatment plan.

Termination of Treatment

Once the depression lifts, indicating an adequate response, these antidepressants should be continued for 6 to 8 months. Stopping medications before this may put the client at a high risk for relapse. When the client and the physician have concurred that treatment should be terminated, tapering these medications off over a period of 2 to 4 weeks may be initiated. If the symptoms of depression recur, reinstating medications at the former maintenance level is indicated. A client who has a recurrent unipolar depression may be treated for an indefinite period to help prevent relapse.

Electroconvulsive Therapy

For treatment-resistant depression, when a client has had previous adequate response, or in life-threatening depressive situations such as acute suicidal reaction or profound melancholia with dehydration, electroconvulsive therapy (ECT) may be the treatment of choice. Although ECT has a significant social stigma, it has proved at least as or more efficacious than the antidepressant medications and should be included in a treatment plan for depression, acute schizophrenia, or resistant mania. Today ECT is given only with an adequate anesthetic and a muscle relaxant to prevent broken bones, compression fractures, and chipped teeth, which were common in the past. Client response to 10 to 14 ECT treatments given every other day is typically much quicker than the 6- to 8-week response for antidepressants. ECT should be undertaken only by trained clinicians in an appropriate setting, and only if the patient's needs coincide with well-recognized indications.

Antimanic Medications

Bipolar affective disorder, or manic-depressive disorder as it is sometimes called, plagues clients with unstable moods. Moods will range from severely depressed to hypomanic and full mania. In manic episodes, patients will demonstrate grandiosity, increased psychomotor activity, decreased judgment, easy distractibility, irritability, decreased need for sleep (the person may not sleep for several days in a row), elevated moods, pressured speech, and racing, intrusive thoughts. This disorder was difficult to treat until John Cade, an Australian physician, discovered the calming effects of lithium in 1949 (McEnany, 1992). Lithium treatment for bipolar affective disorder has become the mainstay of treatment.

Lithium

Lithium was first used as a salt substitute, and its toxic effects were often fatal. Because of this, its acceptance in the medical field was delayed for a long time. It was not until the 1960s and early 1970s that lithium carbonate was fully accepted in the United States for treatment of bipolar disorder.

Lithium has proved to be an effective drug of choice for both treating and preventing manic and depressive episodes in bipolar illness. However, for rapidly cycling clients (those cycling more than three times per year), lithium may not prove effective. Other medications such as anticonvulsants, calcium channel blockers, alpha-adrenergic agonists, and beta-blockers have been tried with varying success. All of these drugs have problematic side effects and require close supervision and management by a physician trained in their use. The precise mechanism of action of these medications in the treatment of bipolar disorder remains unknown. It is hypothesized that the regulation of calcium through the normal membrane may be a critical element. Their possible effect on various neurotransmitters has also been hypothesized.

CLINICAL USE.   Before treatment with any of these medications is begun, a thorough medical evaluation should be performed, including an electrocardiogram and evaluation of complete blood count, renal function, thyroid function, and liver function. Lithium is typically begun in older clients in lower doses. The starting dose should be 300 mg per day. Evaluation of blood levels should be done every 3 or 4 days. Blood levels should be drawn 12 hours after the last lithium dose. This should be done twice weekly until an appropriate blood level is reached. Lithium may be increased every 3 or 4 days by 150 to 300 mg per day. Because the half-life of lithium is approximately 24 hours, once-a-day dosing may be used. Divided doses may be used initially until the blood level is reached and to help minimize toxic effects in some clients. Blood levels between 0.4 and 1.5 mEq/L are the parameters for therapeutic plasma levels. Clients should be treated with the lowest possible effective dose of lithium, although clinical effects may be reached outside these general parameters. A client's blood level should be monitored every month during the first 6 months. Once the therapeutic level has been achieved, blood levels should be checked every 2 to 3 months for as long as the client is taking lithium.

SIDE EFFECTS.   Lithium is known to be toxic to both the thyroid and the kidneys. Evaluation of both renal function and thyroid function every 6 months is indicated while the client is receiving lithium. If a hypothyroid state develops, a thyroid supplement may be prescribed. If diabetes insipidus develops with concomitant polydipsia and polyurea, discontinuation of lithium must be considered.

Clients taking lithium may also experience fine hand tremors and gastrointestinal disturbances such as diarrhea, nausea, and vomiting. Neurological difficulties such as ataxia may also develop at higher blood levels. Weight gain is a frequent side effect of lithium, and some clients may develop dermatological reactions, including acneiform and follicular eruptions or psoriasis. Lithium can cause benign flattening or inversion of T waves but may also cause sinoatrial blocks. Cardiac status should be evaluated before initiating lithium; in older clients with preexisting arrhythmias, lithium may be contraindicated. In clients who have preexisting renal dysfunction, lithium should be begun only after evaluation of the clinical risk to the client. Alternate drug treatment should be considered.

Lithium toxicity is typically seen with blood levels over 1.5 mEq/L. Moderate to severe toxicity is seen in blood levels over 2.0 mEq/L, and convulsions and death can occur with blood levels greater than 2.5 mEq/L.

Lithium may interact with many other drugs, which can raise or lower lithium levels. Nonsteroidal antiinflammatory drugs may increase lithium levels, and theophylline may decrease lithium levels.

Alternate Antimanic Medications

In clients who are unable to tolerate lithium or for whom it has either been contraindicated or proved ineffective, a number of medications can be used in the treatment and prevention of bipolar mood swings. Carbamazepine (Tegretol), clonazepam (Clonopin), and valproic acid (Depakene) are anticonvulsant medications that have been shown to have some efficacy in the treatment of bipolar disorder. Verapamil (Isoptin, Calan), a calcium channel blocker, has also been used. Clonidine (Catapres), an alpha-adrenergic agonist, and propranolol (Inderal), a beta-adrenergic receptor blocker, have been prescribed in difficult-to-manage patients. Carbamazepine has been known to cause aplastic anemia, which can be fatal, and persistent leukopenia as well as thrombocytopenia in some patients. Verapamil, clonidine and propranolol may cause hypotension, so these medications should be initiated slowly and blood pressure monitored as therapeutic efficacy is evaluated.

When these medications are given to older adults, lower blood levels and doses may prove effective. Bipolar affective disorder typically begins at a younger age and persists throughout life. A patient who has been adequately maintained at a higher blood level may develop toxic symptoms; therefore, lowering the medication dosage should be considered. Occasionally individuals develop a bipolar disorder in later years; therefore the possibility of this disease should be considered in clients who meet diagnostic criteria even if they have no history of bipolar disorder.

Antipsychotics

Medications for the treatment of acute psychosis, chronic schizophrenia, and agitation in demented clients have been termed antipsychotics, neuroleptics, and major tranquilizers. Chlorpromazine (Thorazine) was introduced in 1950. Since that time there has been clear and dramatic improvement in clients who have been treated with all three types of medications. The term *major tranquilizer* has probably been the major misnomer given these medications, because their principal use has been in the treatment of psychotic thinking. Antipsychotics should typically be avoided in the treatment of clients with severe anxiety disorder. The benzodiazepines or other antianxiety medications termed *minor tranquilizers* are certainly the drugs of choice for these disorders. The antipsychotic medications may be categorized as phenothiazines, thioxanthenes, butyrophenones, dibenzoxazepines, and indole derivatives. The prevailing theory regarding the mechanism of action of these medications is that they are dopamine blocking agents. They are thought to block the postsynaptic dopamine receptors in the brain. Antipsychotics have far-reaching effects on other neurotransmitters; as we learn more about their actions, we may find that their antipsychotic potential is due to the regulation of other neurotransmitter systems.

CLINICAL USE.   The antipsychotic medications (Table 5-2) have been the mainstay of treatment for clients with chronic schizophrenia. They may also be used for clients with acute psychosis and delirium (nighttime confusion, intensive care unit psychosis, postoperative psychosis, and medication toxicity). In clients with dementia, antipsychotic medications have proved useful in the management of agitation and aggressive behavior. In older adults, antipsychotic medications should be started at lower doses. The management of the medications is based on the side effects paired with the clinical presentation of the patient. In the older client, high-potency medications such as haloperidol (Haldol), thiothixene (Navane), and trifluoperazine (Stelazine) have proved very useful because of their lower incidence of side effects, including sedation, anticholinergic effects, and cardiovascular effects. These medications do tend to have a higher rate of extrapyramidal effects, but at the lower doses at which these drugs are initiated, such extrapyramidal problems may be seen at a

Table 5-2 Antipsychotic Agents

Phenothiazines	Dose equivalent (mg)	Sedation	Hypotension	Anticholinergic	Extrapyramidal problems
Chlorpromazine (Thorazine)	100	High	High	Medium	Low
Mesoridazine (Serentil)	50	Medium	Medium	Medium	Medium
Thioridazine (Mellaril)	95	High	High	High	Low
Acetophenazine (Tindal)	15	Low	Low	Low	Medium
Fluphenazine (Prolixin)	2	Medium	Low	Low	High
Perphenazine (Trilafon)	8	Low	Low	Low	High
Trifluoperazine (Stelazine)	5	Medium	Low	Low	High
Thioxanthenes					
Chlorprothixene (Taractan)	75	High	High	High	Low
Thiothixene (Navane)	5	Low	Low	Low	High
Dibenzoxazepine					
Loxapine (Loxitane)	10	Medium	Medium	Medium	High
Butyrophenones					
Haloperidol (Haldol)	2	Low	Low	Low	High
Indolone					
Molindone (Moban)	10	Medium	Low	Medium	High

much lower rate than in younger clients. Dosage in the range of 0.5 to 1 mg 2 to 3 times a day may be effective in the management of agitation in older clients. Higher doses may be necessary, and these medications should be titrated for clinical effect. Typically, in geriatric clients doses that are approximately half of what is required in younger clients may prove efficacious. The lower-potency medications such as chlorpromazine and thioridazine (Mellaril) may be highly sedating, and the client may become oversedated at doses that are subtherapeutic. These medications are also highly anticholinergic and may cause significant problems. The lower-potency medication should be considered; again, their usage should be based on their side effects and the clinical presentation of the client. The lowest possible dose necessary to control the illness should be used.

Long-acting forms of both haloperidol and fluphenazine hydrochloride (Prolixin) are available. These are deconoate forms and typically may be given once a month to once a week, depending on the needs of the client. In an older client, they should be used only in case of lack of compliance. Most older clients who need such medications are in settings where their medications are supervised, and the use of these medications should be a last resort. Once these medications are injected, their half-lives can be 1 to 4 weeks or longer, and their side effects can be difficult to manage. The use of these medications simply for the convenience of the staff should be avoided.

Side effects. The antipsychotic medications may produce serious side effects because of their effect on the postsynaptic dopamine receptors. These effects may include extrapyramidal symptoms (EPS) such as acute dystonic reactions, pseudoparkinsonian syndrome, akathisia, akinesia, and rabbit syndrome. Tardive oral dyskinesia may also be a permanent neurological side effect. The neuroleptic malignancy syndrome is a rare and serious side effect that may lead to death.

EPS may include acute dystonic reaction such as an oculogyric crisis, in which the eyes become deviated and fixed. An acute dystonic reaction in which there is rigidity of the muscles may also be seen. This can be evaluated with the development of cogwheel rigidity. The patient with akathisia may complain of a feeling of "drivenness" and inability to sit still. Pseudoparkinsonism will manifest itself as a Parkinson-like tremor of the extremities. Akinesia is a decrease in psychomotor movements (often termed the *Thorazine shuffle*). Rabbit syndrome consists of fine rapid movements of the lips that mimic the chewing movements of a rabbit. These side effects are often treated with anticholinergic drugs such as benztropine (Cogentin), biperiden (Akineton), diphenhydramine (Benadryl), or trihexyphenidyl (Artane). Dopamine agonists such as amantadine (Symmetrel) may also be used. The anticholinergic drugs may exacerbate anticholinergic side effects such as dry mouth, blurred vision, constipation, urinary retention, anticholinergic delirium. Amantadine may be a better choice for older adults because of their higher sensitivity to anticholinergic side effects.

Tardive dyskinesia (TD) is a serious neurological side effect of the antipsychotic medications. It may become permanent; therefore clients for whom these medications are prescribed should always be warned about the possible development of these side effects, and this warning should be documented in the client's chart. TD is characterized by involuntary movements of the face, trunk, or extremities. These may express themselves as only minor fasciculations of the tongue but can develop into extremely bothersome choreoathetoid movements of the extremities. Clients taking neuroleptic medications should be evaluated at each appointment for the development of TD. If TD develops in a patient, discontinuation of the medication has to be considered. If there is a substantial risk of redevelopment of psychotic symptoms, the patient and/or the family should be included in a discussion of the clinical risk to benefit ratio of continuing the medication. There is at the present time no reliable treatment of TD other than discontinuation of the antipsychotic medication because there is an increased risk with long-term use of these drugs. The client should be maintained on the lowest possible antipsychotic dose while the necessity of continuing these medications is evaluated.

Neuroleptic malignant syndrome (NMS) is a rare side effect that may be life threatening. This syndrome is seen more frequently with the use of high-potency antipsychotic medications. Typical initial symptoms are hypothermia, severe extrapyramidal effects, autonomic dysfunction, delirium, mutism, stupor, and coma. Discontinuation of the antipsychotic medication should be followed by the use of dantrolene sodium or bromocriptine, which appear to be the most successful agents in the treatment of NMS. These medications should be continued until all symptoms resolve. Dantrolene has a significant potential for liver toxicity and should not be administered to clients with hepatic dysfunction.

Clozapine

Clozapine (Clozaril) is a breakthrough drug in the class atypical antipsychotic agents. It first became available in the United States in 1990. This medication is a highly effective treatment for schizophrenia. It has an extremely low incidence of acute EPS and TD. This medication has shown itself to be very effective with patients in whom other antipsychotic medications have had limited benefit. The most dangerous side effect is agranulocytosis, which can be fatal (1% to 2%). Clozapine should be used only with carefully selected patients whose blood counts can be carefully monitored weekly. The experience with clozapine on older patients is very limited. It is not a first-line drug, and the option of using it should be weighed carefully for patients in whom severe EPS or TD has been demonstrated with the use of other antipsychotic medications.

Antianxiety Agents

Anxiety disorders are some of the most frequently diagnosed mental illnesses. Examples of the DSM-IV subtypes are panic disorder with and without agoraphobia, social phobia, agoraphobia, specific phobia, obsessive-compulsive disorder, post-traumatic stress disorder, generalized anxiety disorder, and anxiety disorder due to a general medical condition (American Psychiatric Association, 1994). Barbiturates were the mainstay of treatment before 1950. Later the benzodiazapines, because of their increased safety, replaced the barbiturates. Other classes of drugs have been developed that may be effective in the treatment of anxiety disorders. One consequence of the long-term use of these drugs is dependency, and certain types may be problematic when used in geriatric clients.

Benzodiazepines

Benzodiazepines as a class represent a much safer anxiolytic medication with a high therapeutic index. The danger of respiratory suppression is increased when these medications are taken with other sedative drugs, especially alcohol.

These medications affect the gamma-aminobutyric acid (GABA) system, the major inhibitory neurotransmitter in the brain. They can be divided into long-acting and short-acting medications because of their metabolic pathways. Long-acting benzodiazepines have active metabolites. Diazepam (Valium) is metabolized into desmethyldiazepam, the half-life of which may range from 50 to 200 hours. The long-acting benzodiazepines have a propensity for buildup in the bloodstream, which may lead to sedation and depression, especially in older adults.

The short-acting benzodiazepines are preferred for use in older patients. Because of their shorter half-life, accumulation is avoided with multiple daily doses. The long-acting benzodiazepines include chlordiazepoxide (Librium), chlorazepate (Tranxene), clonazepam (Klonopin), diazepam (Valium), halazepam (Paxipam), and prazepam (Centrax). The short-acting benzodiazepines include lorazepam (Ativan), oxazepam (Serax), and alprazolam (Xanax) (Table 5-3).

CLINICAL USE.   Benzodiazepines are very effective for treating anxiety disorders. They should be used at the lowest possible dose and titrated for clinical effect. Short-term use is preferred as an adjunct to therapy, which may include psychotherapy, behavior modification, and biofeedback.

Alprazolam (Xanax) has been shown to be efficacious in the treatment of panic disorder. Its long-term use may be indicated for the treatment of this crippling disorder.

Table 5-3   Benzodiazepines for the Geriatric Patient

Agent	Half-life (hours)	Daily dose (mg)
Alprazolam (Xanax)	6-15	0.125-0.5
Lorazepam (Ativan)	10-20	0.25-1.5
Oxazepam (Serax)	5-15	5-30
Chlordiazepoxide (Librium)	36-200*	2.5-25
Clonazepam (Klonopin)	36-200*	0.25-2
Diazepam (Valium)	36-200*	1-10
Prazepam (Centrax)	36-200*	2.5-10

*Not recommended for older adults because of the extremely long half-life.

Long-term use of benzodiazepines for the treatment of anxiety disorders other than panic disorder should be avoided; short-term use (approximately 4 to 8 weeks) should be the typical prescribing time. Remember, anxiety symptoms in older adults may be precipitated by a number of physical illnesses and by medications used to treat these disorders.

WITHDRAWAL OF BENZODIAZEPINES. Discontinuation of the benzodiazepines after 30 to 60 days may lead to withdrawal syndrome. The most dangerous consequence may be seizures. Benzodiazepines should be decreased slowly at approximately 10% per week, especially in clients who have been treated for more than 3 months.

Buspirone (BuSpar) is one of the newer anxiolytic medications. Its mechanism of action has been theorized to be its effect on serotonin and dopamine receptor systems. Buspirone is important because it does not lead to dependency and does not cross-react with benzodiazepines and alcohol. Its efficacy has not been statistically different from that of the benzodiazepines, but its onset of action is much slower, taking up to 2 weeks to demonstrate clinical response.

The effective dose range for buspirone is 15 to 60 mg daily. The typical effective daily dose is 5 to 10 mg tid. Initial dosage should be 5 mg tid, increased by 5 mg every 2 or 3 days until an optimal clinical response is observed. Because of its lack of cross-reactivity, it is not a useful medication in the treatment of alcohol withdrawal syndrome.

Other Anxiolytic Agents

For clients who meet the criteria for major depression, that is, in whom an anxious depressive response is noted, antidepressants are the drugs of choice. They should be initiated in low doses and titrated to the typical antidepressant dose. Subtherapeutic dosing may expose the client to the side effects of the drug without producing any therapeutic response.

Beta-adrenergic blocking agents such as propranolol (Inderal) have been effective in treating the peripheral manifestations of anxiety such as tachycardia, sweating, and palpitations. Use of less lipophilic beta-blockers may be helpful and cause fewer depressive side effects.

❖ *Medications for Memory Problems*

Severe cognitive impairment is one of the most troublesome disorders in older adults, affecting 5% of the population over 65 years of age. The cost is over $5 billion per year. Over half of all dementia is caused by Alzheimer's disease (AD), for which there is no cure yet. A number of classes of medications have been explored. Compounds affecting the neurotransmitter acetylcholine have been tried; tetrahydro-5-aminoacridine (THA) is one of the latest (Summers, Majovski, Marsh, Tachiki, & Kling, 1986). THA (Tacrine, tacrine cognex), along with physostigmine, bethanechol, and lecithin, have all had mixed results. Other drugs affecting other neurotransmitters, such as serotonin, GABA, and dopamine, do not appear to be promising medications. Altering neuropeptides, adrenocorticotrophic hormone, thyrotropin-releasing hormone, and vasopressin such as synthetic ACTH 4-9, Organon 2766, and TRH analogues have had negative results reported. The opiate receptor antagonist naloxone failed to support improvement in controlled trials. Nootropics, compounds to increase metabolism in the brain, such as piracetam, have demonstrated equivocal or negative results. New strategies that affect calcium channels, the angiotensin-renin system, "neurotrophic factors," glucocorticoids, and sex hormones are being researched.

❖ *Obsessive-Compulsive Disorder*

Obsessive-compulsive disorder is particularly difficult to treat. Fluoxetine in high doses has helped some patients. Clomipramine (Anafranil) has been shown to be helpful and is marketed for this disorder in the United States. Its side effects are typical of the tricyclic antidepressants such as imipramine (Tofranil)—cardiac toxicity, sedation, anticholinergic effects, and hypertension. The typical daily dose is 25 to 150 mg.

❖ *Sleep Disorders*

Sleep apnea and periodic leg movements in sleep (PLMS), or nocturnal myoclonus, are frequently seen at sleep disorder centers. Sleep apnea is the periodic cessation of breathing during sleep. Sleep apnea may be exacerbated by the benzodiazepines. They should be avoided in clients who have symptoms such as snoring or in whom sleep apnea is suspected or has been diagnosed. PLMS may be exacerbated by the use of tricyclic antidepressants used for sleep. Clients with PLMS often give histories of kicking their covers off the bed or have partners who complain of thrashing or kicking during the night. Sedative medications may not be indicated, especially in older adults. Careful diagnosis and evaluation of agents should be carried out rather than cavalier use of sedative hypnotics in the geriatric client.

Sedative-Hypnotics

Sleep disturbances in geriatric clients are common. Normal age-related changes include a decrease in quality sleep time, increase in sleep latency, decrease in REM sleep, and increased nighttime awakenings. Simple client education about the usual changes in normal sleep patterns that occur with aging may help reduce inappropriate use of sedative agents in the older population. Sedative-hypnotics should be used when the client's daytime functioning is impaired but not when the client's only complaint is "not sleeping well." Differentiation of initial insomnia from middle or terminal insomnia is also important. Initial insomnia may be more indicative of anxiety or difficulty initiating sleep because of simple arthritis or other underlying physical causes, whereas middle or terminal insomnia is often more indicative of an underlying depressive disorder for which an antidepressant may be needed. Long-term use of sedative-hypnotics will further disrupt sleep-wakefulness cycles and cause dependency on sleeping agents, resulting in less restful sleep. Once the normal age-related changes in sleep are explained to clients, many older adults report actually enjoying the need for less sleep and having more wakeful hours for activities.

Clients who are having difficulty sleeping and for whom a physical cause or underlying mental illness has been ruled out should first be given simple education to improve their sleep hygiene. Suggestions for improving sleep hygiene include not lying in bed attempting to sleep. The bed should be used only for sleep, not for other activities. If a client has difficulty initiating sleep, reading a boring novel may be helpful. Light exercise such as walking around the block may help, as well as taking a warm bath before bedtime. Eating a light snack before bedtime may also be suggested. Decreasing daytime napping and waking up at the same time each day may help regulate day-night wakefulness periods. If these suggestions fail to help, a short trial of a sedative hypnotic for 2 to 4 weeks may be indicated to help regulate the sleeping cycle. Withdrawing clients from long-term use of sedative agents may disrupt the sleep cycle for 2 to 8 weeks. These clients should be warned that a disruptive period may follow before the sleeping medication is withdrawn.

CLINICAL USE.   A variety of medications may aid sedation (Tables 5-4 and 5-5). In a client for whom arthritic pain is a problem, a simple aspirin at bedtime may alleviate the pain enough that normal sleep will ensue without the aid of a sedative agent. In clients for whom a sedative hypnotic is indicated, simple use of L-tryptophan, an amino acid that is the precursor of serotonin, may be helpful. Serotonin is theorized

Table 5-4   Sedative-Hypnotic Agents

Benzodiazepines	Half-life (hours)	Daily dose (mg)
Estrazolam (Pro-som)	10-20	0.5-2
Triazolam (Halcion)	1.6-5.4	0.125-0.25
Temazepam (Restoril)	10-20	15-30
Quazepam (Doral)	20-150*	7.5-15
Flurazepam (Dalmane)	40-150*	15-30

*Not recommended for older adults because of the extremely long half-life.

Table 5-5   Other Sedative Medications

Agent	Daily dose
L-Tryptophan	500 mg-2g
Chloral hydrate	500 mg-2g
Diphenhydramine (Benadryl)	25 mg-50 mg
Amobarbital sodium (Sodium Amytal)	50 mg-300 mg

to increase in sleep, and use of a precursor may be efficacious. Doses of 500 to 3000 mg of tryptophan may be useful in helping clients achieve a normal sleep pattern without the use of addictive agents such as benzodiazepines.

The benzodiazepines are currently the most commonly used sedative hypnotics. Three medications are presently approved for use: triazolam (Halcion), temazepam (Restoril), and flurazepam (Dalmane). Triazolam has the shortest half-life and a rapid onset. The half-life of this agent is approximately 6 hours. For those clients who have initial insomnia, triazolam may be an effective agent. Rebound insomnia has been observed in clients using this medication. Temazepam has an intermediate half-life of approximately 12 hours. This agent has a slower onset time, so that the medication should be taken 30 minutes to an hour before bedtime. Because of its longer half-life, it may also be useful in clients with middle or terminal insomnia and can be used concomitantly with an antidepressant when middle or terminal insomnia is a symptom of major depression. Flurazepam has the longest half-life, which may extend up to 200 hours in older adults. Clients who take flurazepam may experience daytime drowsiness. Since this can be a problem for clients, this drug cannot be recommended for use in older adults.

Antihistamines such as diphenhydramine (Benadryl) may be very useful in older clients. A dose of 25 to 50 mg at bedtime is recommended. Antihistamines may have untoward side effects and may be of limited benefit with specific clients.

Chloral hydrate is an old-line sedative hypnotic. The dose should be 500 to 1000 mg at bedtime. Chloral hydrate has some properties that may create irritability of the cardiac muscle. Its use may not be indicated in clients with preexisting cardiac arrhythmias.

Intermediate-acting barbiturates such as amobarbital sodium (Amytal sodium) may be useful for the client whose sleep cycles have been seriously disrupted. For clients with Alzheimer's disease who are awake for days at a time, amobarbital in doses of 50 to 300 mg may provide sedation, thus allowing the caregiver to sleep also. Higher doses may be required in demented clients with severe agitation. This drug should be carefully monitored and used only after other sleeping agents have been given an adequate trial.

❖ *Summary*

Older adults receive 25% of all prescription drugs. They are prone to multiple side effects because of possible drug-drug and food-drug interactions and altered psychodynamics and psychokinetics. Medications should be carefully prescribed and dosages carefully monitored for the older population. Noncompliance is also a major problem when older clients do not fully understand complicated drug regimens.

The most common psychotropic drugs prescribed for older adults are antidepressants, antimanic medications, antipsychotics, antianxiety agents, and sedative hypnotics. Several new drugs are being researched for use with older clients who have memory problems, particularly those associated with Alzheimer's disease. Some of these drugs have shown modest results, but much more research is needed in this area.

❖ *References*

American Association of Retired Persons and Administration on Aging. (1993). *A profile of older Americans.* Washington DC: US Department of Health and Human Services.

Baum, C., Kennedy, D. C., Knapp, D. E., Faich, G. A., & Ariello, C. (1987). Drug utilizations in the U. S. (1986). Springfield, VA: Office of Epidemiology and Biostatistics, Center for Drug Evaluations and Research, National Technical Information Service.

American Psychiatric Association. (1994). *Diagnostic and statistical manual of mental disorders.* (4th ed.) Washington, DC: American Psychiatric Association.

Calkins, E., Davis, P. J., & Ford, A. B. (Eds.). (1986). *The practice of geriatrics.* Philadelphia: Saunders.

David, J. (1981). Do it yourself medicine:3. *Nursing Times, 77*(9), 371-372.

Everitt, D. E., & Avorn, J. (1986). Drug prescribing for the elderly. *Arch Intern Med, 146*(12), 2392-2396.

Lamy, P. P. (1980). *Prescribing for the elderly.* Littleton, MA: PSG Publishing.

Lamy, P. P. (1982). Effects of diet and nutrition on drug therapy. *Journal of the American Geriatrics Society, 30,*(11s), s99-s112.

LaVange, L., Silverman, H. (1987). Outpatient prescription drug utilization and expenditure patterns of non-instituted aged Medicaid beneficiaries. *National Medical Care Utilization and Expenditures Survey, Series B.* Report II, DHHS Publication No. 86-20212. Health Care Financing and Administration. Washington, DC: U.S. Government Printing Office.

May, F. E., Stewart, R. B., & Cluff, L. E. (1977). Drug interactions in multiple drug administration. *Clinical Pharmacology Therapeutics, 22,* 322.

McEnany, G. (1992). Biologic therapies. In H. S. Wilson & C. R. Kneisl (Eds.). *Psychiatric Nursing* (4th ed.). Menlo Park, CA: Addison-Wesley.

Nolan, L., & O'Malley, K. (1988). Prescribing for the elderly: 2. Prescribing patterns: Differences due to age. *Journal of the American Geriatrics Society, 36*(3), 245-254.

O'Brien, J. C., & Kursch, J. E. (1987). Healthy prescribing for the elderly. *Postgraduate Med, 82*(6), 147-57.

Osis, M. (1986). Scheduling drug administration: Drug and food interactions. *Gerontion, 1,* 8-10.

Parkin, D. M., Henney, C. R., Quirks, J., & Crooks, J. (1976). Deviation from prescribed drug treatment after discharge from hospital. *British Medical Journal, 2,* 686-688.

Pucinof, F., Beck, C. L., Seifert, R. L., Gordon, L. S., Sheldon, P. A., & Silbergleit, I. L. (1985). Pharmacogeriatrics. *Pharmacotherapy, 5,*(6), 314.

Sloan, R. W. (1981). Geriatric drug therapy. *Family Practice, 13,* 599.

Summers, W. K., Majovski, L. V., Marsh, G. M., Tachiki, K., & Kling, A. (1986). Oral tetrahydroaminoacridine in long-term treatment of senile dementia, Alzheimer's type. *New England Journal of Medicine, 315*(20), 1241-45.

Swift, C. G. (1988). Prescribing in old age. *British Medical Journal, 296,* 913-15.

Wolfe, S. M., & Hope, R. E. (1993). *Worst pills best pills II.* Washington, DC: Public Citizen Health Research Group.

Chapter 6

❖ *Depression, Suicide, and Bereavement*

Marta Askew Browning

❖ Depression

Depression is a pervasive disorder that extinguishes the spark of life. It is often unrecognized in the older adult and has the potential to destroy the quality of life, if not life itself. Depression eliminates joy, laughter, empathy, happiness, and love. Finally, it slams the gates to the outside world, leaving its victim alone and isolated.

Significance of the Problem

Depression in older adults appears to be less frequent than in younger adults. The National Institute of Health Epidemiology Catchment area study reports a 6-month prevalence of depression in 2% of older adults who were surveyed. This contrasts with a rate four times as high for those aged 25 to 44 years (Meyers & Alexopoulas, 1988). This is encouraging because it indicates that most older adults remain free of crippling depressive symptoms.

However, depression is the most common functional psychiatric disorder among older adults (Meyers & Alexopoulas, 1988; Mignogna, 1986). Estimates of depressed older adult populations in combined community and institutional settings range from 5% to 65% (St. Pierre, Craven, & Bruno, 1986). A longitudinal study of normal older volunteers resulted in identification of 30% of the sample as suffering from mild depressive symptoms (Meyers & Alexopoulas, 1988). Blazer (1986) reported that approximately 15% of older adults mentioned significant depressive symptoms. Of that 15%, 7% to 8% suffered from bereavement or adjustment disorder; 3% to 4% suffered from atypical depression; 2% to 3% suffered from dysthymic disorder, and 1% to 2% suffered from major depression.

Depression in the general population is estimated to be twice as common in women as in men (American Psychiatric Association, 1994). Older women are likewise disproportionately represented among depressive diagnoses. However, this may partially be a function of survivability and the higher female to male ratios that exist in advanced age. Krause's (1986) study of older adults in Galveston, Texas, indicated that older women report more symptoms associated with depressed affect, such as somatic complaints and retarded activities, than men do. Women in his sample were identified as having greater vulnerability to depression, which he attributed to chronic financial strain. Economic status was linked to depression by other researchers. In a study (Goldsmith et al., 1986) of 3332 noninstitutionalized older adults in the city of Baltimore, it was found that older adults residing in low-status residential areas were three times as likely to have had recent depressive symptoms as older adults living in a middle-status area.

Rates of depression are higher in the recently bereaved, those with poor physical health, and in family members caring for frail, demented older persons (Thompson & Gallagher, 1986). Poor health is identified by older adults as the problem that most concerns them (Burnside, 1988), and poor health is clearly linked to depression. Some 40% to 50% of physically ill older adults and those in nursing homes are clinically depressed (Mignogna, 1986). Decline in functional independence and ability to perform activities of daily living (ADL) are closely associated with the emergence and/or exacerbation of depression in older adults (Parmelee, Katz, & Lawton, 1992; Kennedy, Kelman, & Thomas, 1990).

The study by Parmelee et al. (1992) of depression in long-term care settings found that a significant number of older adults with major depression showed no categorical improvement in their level of depression over time. They further found that almost one in five older adults who suffered from minor depression progressed to an episode of major depression. Thus, minor depression is a risk factor for the development for major depressive episodes. These researchers identified a subset of individuals in long-term care settings who have persistent depressive episodes. The recidivism of depression among these persons may be the result of incomplete compliance with medical regimens or, more alarmingly, the manifestation of an intractable tendency for depression to recur once short-term therapy is concluded.

Causes of Depression in Older Adults

Other Mental Illnesses
Depression may be associated with or secondary to other psychiatric disorders such as schizophrenia (catatonic), schizophreniform disorder, and dementia.

Loss
The older adult may experience multiple losses with insufficient time between losses to grieve. Each loss triggers a grief reaction, and each period of bereavement brings

about change. These changes may cause confusion, disorientation, and subsequent withdrawal (Garrett, 1987). Each loss may increase the individual's vulnerability to the next loss or precipitate a new loss. The impact of this accumulation of losses may be greater in the older adult because, unlike the young, older adults do not often have losses offset by gains or opportunities such as new jobs and creation of new families (Matteson & McConnell, 1988). Losses that commonly occur in the life of older adults include the following:

- ◆ Loss of job at retirement
- ◆ Loss or change in social role (for example, worker to retiree, wife to widow)
- ◆ Loss of significant others (for example, spouse, siblings, friends, adult children, pets)
- ◆ Loss of strength and agility
- ◆ Loss of sexual prowess
- ◆ Loss of health
- ◆ Loss or decline in economic stability
- ◆ Loss of or relocation from home
- ◆ Loss of personal freedom (particularly a problem for family caregivers of the physically ill)
- ◆ Loss of mental ability
- ◆ Loss of dreams
- ◆ Alterations in self-image
- ◆ Decrease in acuteness of senses

Physical Illness

Physical illnesses may precipitate depressive symptoms as biological and physiological outgrowths of these disorders, or depression may be a response to living with chronic disability or facing terminal illness. Table 6-1 lists physical disorders associated with depression in older adults. It is important for the clinician to rule out physical conditions before diagnosing depression as a psychiatric disorder. The underlying physical disorder must be treated first to reduce the depressive symptoms. For example, estimates of depression in patients with chronic obstructive pulmonary disease (COPD) approach 42% of the affected population (Gift & McCrone, 1993). Depression in these clients may be associated with chronic hypoxemia, stress precipitated by dyspnea, role losses, sexual impairment, and erosion of functional ability and independence. In some cases, mental health interventions will still be required or may be used concurrently with medical therapies.

Medication, Drugs, and Substance Abuse

Many older people have one or more chronic diseases. They generally take several prescription medications to treat these conditions, thus increasing the risk of drug interactions. In addition to prescription medications, the older adult may take a number of nonprescription medications for minor ailments (headaches, constipation, indigestion) or practice folk remedies such as purging once a week. Because

Table 6-1 Physical Disorders Associated with Depressive Symptomatology in Older Adults

Body system affected	Disorder
Cardiovascular	Congestive heart failure Myocardial infarction
Endocrine	Diabetes mellitus Hyperadrenalism (Cushing's disease) Hyperinsulinism Hyperparathyroidism and hypoparathyroidism Hypoadrenalism (Addison's disease) Hypoglycemia Hypopituitarism Menopause
Hematological	Infectious mononucleosis
Hepatic and pancreatic	Amyloidosis Cirrhosis Hepatitis Pancreatitis Wilson's disease
Immunological	Acquired immunodeficiency syndrome Giant cell arteritis Gout Rheumatoid arthritis Systemic lupus erythematosus
Integumentary	Psoriasis
Gastrointestinal	Inflammatory bowel disease
Metabolic	Hyperkalemia or hypokalemia Hypocalcemia Hyponatremia Hypomagnesemia Increased or decreased bicarbonate levels Uremia
Miscellaneous infections	Brucellosis Malaria Viral infections
Neoplastic	Lymphoma Oat cell carcinoma Pancreatic carcinoma Lung cancer Breast cancer Temporal lobe tumor

Table 6-1   Physical Disorders Associated with Depressive Symptomatology in Older Adults—cont'd

Body system affected	Disorder
Neurological	Chronic subdural hematoma
	Encephalitis and postencephalitic states
	Head injury
	Huntington's disease
	Multiinfarct dementia
	Multiple sclerosis
	Alzheimer's disease
	Parkinson's disease
	Seizure disorder
	Stroke
	Tertiary syphilis
Nutritional	Avitaminosis
	Decreased levels of ascorbic acid, folate, iron, niacin, pyridoxine, thiamine, or zinc
	Dehydration
	Pernicious anemia
	Protein deficiency
Renal	End-stage renal disease
Respiratory	Chronic obstructive pulmonary disease
	Influenza
	Pneumonia
	Sarcoidosis
	Sleep apnea
	Tuberculosis

Based on data from the following:

Black, J., and Matassarin-Jacobs E. (1993). *Luckman and Sorenson's medical-surgical nursing: A psychophysiologic approach* (4th ed). Philadelphia: Saunders.

Field, W. E. (1985). Physical causes of depression. *Journal of the American Geriatrics Society, 33*(6), 446-448.

Goff, D. C., & Jenike, M. A. (1986). Treatment-resistant depression in the elderly. *Journal of the American Geriatrics Society, 34*(1), 63-70.

Mignogna, M. (1986). Integrity vs. despair: The treatment of depression in the elderly. *Clinical Therapeutics, 8*(3), 248-259.

health care is often fragmented, older adults may see several physicians who are all prescribing medications. Each physician may be unaware of the drugs that have been prescribed by the others, with the result that the medications may have fatal interactions. Finally, physiological changes in absorption, metabolism, and excretion of medications caused by aging may potentiate the effects of medications and cause toxic side effects.

Careful medication histories should be obtained from older adults. The nurse who has access to the client's home environment should ask to see all medications, both prescription and nonprescription. Table 6-2 identifies some drugs commonly associated with depression in the older adult. In addition, alcohol and substance abuse pose particular danger to older adults and are often used as a method of blunting or blocking feelings associated with depressed mood. Therefore the nurse should be alert for the presence of these disorders.

Drugs that cause depressive symptoms should be discontinued unless their medical benefit outweighs the mental health risk. Physicians are often unaware of the

Table 6-2   Drugs and Medications Associated with Depressive Symptoms

Drug class	*Examples*
Amebicides and trichomonacides	Metronidazole
Antianxiety agents	Benzodiazepines, meprobamate
Antiasthmatics	Theophylline derivatives
Antibiotics	Sulfonamides, chloramphenicol
Antiemetics	Trimethobenzamide hydrochloride
Antineoplastic agents	Mercaptopurine, methotrexate, asparaginase, vincristine
Anorexiants/amphetamines	Caffeine, amphetamine sulfate, dextroamphetamine sulfate
Antiinfectives	Ethionamide
Antimalarials	4-Aminoquinolines
Antiparkinson agents	Levodopa, bromocriptine, amantadine hydrochloride
Antipsychotic	Phenothiazines, molindone
Barbiturates	Phenobarbital
Cardiovascular	Digitalis, clonidine, guanethidine, hydralazine, methyldopa, propranolol, reserpine
Hormones	Estrogen, progesterone, cortisone, prednisone
Narcotics/analgesics	Meperidine
Recreational drugs	Alcohol, LSD (lysergic acid diethylamide), cocaine, heroin
Urinary germicides	Acetohydroxamic acid

Based on data from the following:

Dreyfus, J. K. (1987). The prevalence of depression in women in an ambulatory setting. *Nurse Practitioner, 12*(4), 34-50.

Field, W. E. (1985). Physical causes of depression. *Journal of the American Geriatrics Society, 33*(6), 446-448.

Goff, D. C., & Jenike, M. A. (1986). Treatment-resistant depression in the elderly. *Journal of the American Geriatrics Society, 34*(1), 63-70.

Loebl, S., & Spratto, G. R. (1986). *The nurses drug handbook.* New York: Wiley.

Mignogna, M. (1986). Integrity vs. despair: The treatment of depression in the elderly. *Clinical Therapeutics, 8*(3), 248-259.

complex decisions to be made when prescribing for older adults. A study of Pennsylvania physicians (Ferry, Lamy, & Becker, 1985) revealed that fewer than 30% of the participating physicians indicated adequate knowledge of prescribing for older adults. The study indicated that older physicians scored lower on knowledge of geriatric pharmacology and should be encouraged to update skills. The nurse cannot assume that the physician understands the problem caused by polypharmacy and may have to become an active advocate for the patient to obtain a change in medication orders.

Failure to Thrive

Failure to thrive in older adults has been defined as a condition of frailty marked by progressive decline preceding cachexia. Verdery (Osato, Stone, Phillips, & Winne, 1993, p. 29) distinguishes between failure to thrive due to organic causes (e.g., malignancy, heart failure, uremia) and failure to thrive with an inorganic basis (e.g., neglect, abuse, immobility, depression). Confusion and depression may manifest themselves as loss of appetite (Groom, 1993). Thus, these disorders may be identified as an interactional syndrome involving diagnostic states of malnutrition, depression, and dementia.

Loneliness and Isolation

Loneliness occurs when the client experiences feelings of separation from another, perceives or actually has a disruption of social relationships, and experiences a discrepancy between relationships desired and those actually experienced with others (Copel, 1988). Loneliness affects 12% to 40% of the population aged 65 and above. It is identified as the fourth major concern of the older adult, outranked only by poor health, financial difficulties, and crime (Burnside, 1988). Loneliness is not a desirable state. It is nonproductive because the individual must expend energy to protect himself or herself from the dreaded feeling of being isolated (de la Cruz, 1986). Social isolation is seen by the victim as an external threat (de la Cruz, 1986). Loneliness occurs when needs for intimacy with others are not met. It renders its victims emotionally paralyzed and helpless (Copel, 1988). In older adults, forced separation from others has been identified as the major reason for loneliness; the loneliest older adults are those who have lost a spouse within the previous 5 years. Lack of contact with children and old friends and isolation imposed by lack of transportation, phone calls, and accessible social activities can also precipitate loneliness (Ryan & Patterson, 1987). Depression caused by underlying loneliness can often be relieved by involving older adults in social activities or support groups without the necessity of progressing to medications or other somatic treatments.

Caregiving Roles

Individuals who serve as caregivers for physically or cognitively impaired family members often feel anger, anxiety, and depression as a part of what has been termed *caregiver burden*. Clinical depression has been found to be more common in family caregivers than in the general population; therefore, performance of the caregiver role must be considered a risk factor for depression (Gallagher, Rose, Rivera, Lovett, & Thompson, 1989).

Missed Diagnosis

Diagnosis of depression in the older adult is difficult because of atypical symptom expression, which occurs in masked depression, in the presence of physical illness with associated depressive symptoms, and in drug- or medication-induced depression. In addition to these difficulties experienced by the diagnostician, several others warrant discussion. Normal changes in aging such as decreased appetite, alterations in sleep patterns (specifically, the increase in the number of nightly awakenings and decreases in stage 4 sleep), declining activity levels, and perceptual motor changes are confusing to clinicians (St. Pierre et al., 1986). Lacking an understanding of the types and extent of normal maturational changes, both health professionals and clients may tolerate depressive symptoms because they believe them to be a manifestation of aging. Unfortunately, several of the symptoms of clinical depression are compatible with unpleasant, erroneous, but commonly accepted stereotypes of older persons created by the popular press and folklore.

Change is slow. The health care delivery system in the United States is still focused primarily on acute medical and surgical problems and crisis intervention to resolve such problems. For many years preventive health care and mental health services have taken second place in both professional educational programs and the allocation of funding at the local, state, and national levels. Therefore, one of the most common causes of a missed diagnosis is simply selective inattention. Depression is rarely considered as a priority or even a possibility.

In Dreyfus's (1987) study of female outpatients, the incidence of depression among clients during their initial visits to the ambulatory care setting was measured, and the relationship of depressive symptomatology with somatic complaints was correlated. Half of the women in this study had depressive symptoms according to the Beck Depression Inventory. Initial somatic complaints most frequently cited were fatigue, headache, backache, cold or fever, muscle pain, and difficulty sleeping. Four months after the administration of the Beck Depression Inventory and a somatic symptom checklist, Dreyfus conducted a chart review of study subjects. The chart review revealed that depression was not identified as a diagnosis by physicians in any of the study subjects. Therefore, no antidepressants had been prescribed, and no referrals to psychiatrists had been made. The researcher also noted that a significant number of the depressed study subjects did not return for follow-up care. Dreyfus postulated that this lack of appropriate follow-up may have been caused by failure of professionals to respond to depressive symptoms and the loss of energy and motivation that are characteristic of depression. On the basis of her study, Dreyfus suggested that depression inventories be used routinely in the ambulatory care setting. The use of such tools would uncover hidden depression and lead to more appropriate treatment protocols.

Reluctance among older adults to utilize psychiatric services where symptoms might be properly identified further complicates the diagnosis of depression. Because they are unfamiliar with modern mental health approaches, they may avoid such interventions because of the stigma formerly attached to them. Finally, subtle forms of ageism may cause older adults and their problems to be undervalued by health care providers. Thus the older adult may think that if problems are presented, they will be ignored or diminished (St. Pierre et al., 1986).

Theories of the Causes of Depression

The exact cause of depression is unknown, but increasingly the disorder appears to have many causes. Several theories attempt to explain the causes of depression and, depending on the clinician or diagnostician's theoretical leanings, may determine the selection of treatment methods.

Psychosocial Theories

Psychosocial theories focus on the ways in which a person's internal mental life, relationships with others, and life events can lead to depression (Minot, 1986). These theories include psychoanalytical, environmental, psychodynamic, and cognitive explanations for depressive states.

Psychoanalytical theory examines the role of psychic response to loss, anger turned against the self, and regression in the development of depression.

Environmental explanations for depression are based on analyzing the relationship between stressors (major losses, conflicts, or attacks on self-esteem) or inadequacy in the social support system and the expression of depressive characteristics (Minot, 1986).

Psychodynamic theories focus on the development of personality over time and examine the impact of past relationships on the current self. Certain personality styles are assessed for vulnerability to depression (Minot, 1986). Cognitive theory defines depression as the result of habitual reinforcement of negative ideas about oneself, others, and the future. Practitioners of this theory design therapeutic interventions that replace negativistic thinking with positive thoughts and actions (Minot, 1986).

Biochemical Theories

GENETIC THEORIES. Genetic theorists support explanations of depression as a hereditary trait. The work of these researchers is based on studies of twins who have been raised apart (Minot, 1986).

NEUROENDOCRINE THEORIES. Neuroendocrine theorists attribute depression to malfunctioning neurotransmitters in the brain. The activities of dopamine, norepinephrine, seratonin, and epinephrine are being closely scrutinized. Decreases in concentrations of these chemicals occur with aging and may be a major factor in depression among older adults (St. Pierre et al., 1986). Attention is also being directed to patterns of cortisol and thyroid hormone releases because many depressed persons have abnormal responses to thyrotropin-releasing hormone or dexamethasone challenges (Minot, 1986).

Classification of Depression

Depression is classified as a mood disorder. The American Psychiatric Association has established criteria for diagnosing mental health disorders. These standards are listed in the *Diagnostic and Statistical Manual of Mental Disorders,* fourth edition, (DSM-IV). This manual is the standard by which diagnoses are made; the International Classification of Diseases (ICD-9) coding is based on criteria in this document. Therefore the DSM-IV will be used as the major source for identifying types of depression.

Major Depressive Episode
A major depressive episode is defined by the presence of depressed mood and/or loss of interest or pleasure accompanied by four or more of the following symptoms: (1) significant weight loss or gain (5% of body weight in a month) or a change in appetite every day, (2) insomnia or hypersomnia, (3) psychomotor agitation or retardation, (4) fatigue or loss of energy, (5) feelings of worthlessness or inappropriate guilt, (6) diminished ability to think or concentrate, and (7) recurrent thoughts of death or suicidal ideation with or without a plan. These symptoms must have been present for a 2-week period and must represent a change in prior functioning for the disorder to be classified as a major depressive episode. In addition, the symptoms must have been present most of the day for almost every day of the 2-week period. In a major depressive episode, the symptoms are not due to the physical effects of a medical condition or bereavement (unless severe symptoms last for longer than 2 months) (American Psychiatric Association, 1994, p. 327).

Chronic Major Depressive Episode
A depressive episode that has lasted continuously for the past 2 years is identified as chronic major depression (American Psychiatric Association, 1994).

Melancholia
To meet the criteria established for melancholic depression, one of the first two *and* three or more of the other symptoms must be present:

- Loss of interest or pleasure in activities
- Lack of reactivity to usually pleasurable stimuli
- Mood does not improve when something good happens
- Distinct quality of the depressed mood
- Depression that worsens in the morning
- Early morning awakening

- ◆ Psychomotor retardation or agitation
- ◆ Weight loss; anorexia
- ◆ Excessive or inappropriate guilt (American Psychiatric Association, 1994, p. 384)

Seasonal Pattern
A seasonal major depression is defined as a recurrent major depressive disorder that occurs at regular times of the year; for example, begins in the fall or winter and remits in spring. Full remission of symptoms also occurs within a particular 60-day period of the year. Seasonal episodes of mood disturbance must outnumber nonseasonal episodes over the individual's lifetime (American Psychiatric Association, 1994).

Bipolar I Disorder
The client who is in a major depressive episode but who has had one or more manic episodes is diagnosed as a victim of bipolar disorder (American Psychiatric Association, 1994).

Cyclothymia
Cyclothymia is a chronic mood disturbance lasting for at least 2 years that is characterized by numerous hypomanic episodes and periods of depressed mood in which symptoms are not severe enough to meet the criteria for major depressive episode or manic episode (American Psychiatric Association, 1994).

Dysthymia
Dysthymia is a chronic mood disturbance consistently present for at least 2 years in which the client displays a depressed mood. Some of the following symptoms accompany the altered mood: poor appetite or overeating, insomnia or hypersomnia, low energy, low self-esteem, poor concentration, difficulty making decisions, and hopelessness. No evidence of a major depressive episode is evident during the first 2 years of symptom expression (American Psychiatric Association, 1994).

Adjustment Disorder with Depressed Mood
Adjustment disorder is a maladaptive reaction that has persisted for less than 6 months (acute) or 6 months or longer (chronic) and is a reaction to a stressor that can be identified. Onset of the disorder must begin within 3 months of the stressor. The client exhibits symptoms in excess of normal or expected reactions in response to the stressor, or suffers impairment in occupational activities or social interactions. The predominant symptoms are depressed mood, tearfulness, and feelings of hopelessness (American Psychiatric Association, 1994).

Depressive Disorders Not Otherwise Specified
Many other categories of depression exist, but most are a secondary manifestation of another psychiatric disorder such as chronic mental disorder. Depression can also

include a diagnosis of physical illness or be associated with the untoward effects of medications, especially in older people.

Surveys of older adults consistently yield data that indicate a gap between the percentage of older adults who report depressive symptoms and those diagnosed as depressed with the DSM-IV criteria. This gap creates difficulty in accurate estimation of the true number of older adults who are affected by this disease. A study of older adults in North Carolina (Blazer, Hughes, & George, 1987) supported the existence of this disparity in self-reported symptoms and diagnostic criteria. They noted that DSM-IV diagnoses are frequently incongruent with diagnoses assigned by psychiatrists in community populations (Blazer et al., 1987).

Depressive disorders that do not fulfill any of the criteria established previously are classified as depressive disorder, not otherwise specified. These categories of such depressive illness are used by clinicians even though they are not specified by the DSM-IV.

UNCOMPLICATED BEREAVEMENT. Depressed mood that occurs as a result of loss of a loved one is considered a normal expression of grief and bereavement. However, if suicidal ideation, marked functional impairment, psychomotor retardation, or morbid preoccupation with worthlessness occurs, then the client should be reevaluated for major depressive disorder (American Psychiatric Association, 1994).

PSEUDODEMENTIA. Pseudodementia (false confusion) is a depression that mimics dementia. Key differences in the symptoms of the two disorders are used to make a diagnosis. Dementia is usually gradual in onset and marked by an attempt on the part of the client to hide memory loss and remain independent. The client's mood fluctuates, and there may be a history of small strokes or a family pattern of dementia. However, depression in the older adult is usually marked by a relatively abrupt change in behavior. The client's major complaint may be memory loss. Open-ended questions may receive detailed responses whereas direct questions may prompt an "I don't know" response. The depressed client expresses dependency; his or her mood is consistently depressed (Ronsman, 1988).

MASKED DEPRESSION. Masked depression in older adults is used to describe the clinical symptoms commonly observed in depressed older people. About 3% to 4% of older adults suffer from a transient but severe depressive disorder that does not clearly fit any DSM-IV category (Blazer, 1986). This disorder is characterized by minimal sadness, guilt, and self-reproach. The older adult's complaints primarily concern symptoms of cognitive dysfunction, somatic and vegetative symptoms, and atypical pain (Meyers & Alexopoulas, 1988; Mignogna, 1986; Blazer, 1986; Ronsman, 1987). This constellation of symptoms is so consistent in the older adult population that clinicians are urging the creation of a new DSM category. Fogel and Fretwell (1985) have proposed naming the condition either *somatic disorder,* with an as yet unknown biochemical basis, or *depletion syndrome of old age*. In addition to the characteristics previously listed, Fogel and Fretwell would add the following criteria for diagnosis of this illness: onset after age 60, good premorbid psychosocial functioning without a history of overt psychiatric illness, and no evidence of psychosis.

Feeling State in Depression

Statistics and psychiatric diagnoses alone do not convey the significance of depression to individual victims and the family and friends who love them. Numbers cannot tell the story of an older adult who must greet each new dawn barely able or at times totally unable to cope with tasks that were once accomplished without thought or stress. The change may have occurred suddenly with the onset of a mysterious malaise that adds such a burden of fatigue that the effort required to perform simple activities of daily living (ADL) (dressing, eating, grocery shopping) becomes superhuman. Thus meals are skipped, the need for fluid intake is forgotten, clothing is worn soiled, and self-esteem plummets.

The memory becomes unreliable. Facts cannot be recalled at will. Only a portion of yesterday may be remembered, and thoughts come slowly. The fear of losing one's mind and facing institutionalization looms large.

Activities become defined by an internal assessment of the energy that will be required to initiate and sustain involvement. Small and large pleasures are eliminated one by one, resulting in social withdrawal and eventual isolation.

Fatigue is exacerbated by elusiveness of sleep and the knowledge that being unable to sleep and/or waking at odd hours of the night is abnormal. The body is a constant reminder that something is amiss. Severe visceral responses tighten the bowel, create embarrassing flatulence, and cause nausea, stomach pains, dry mouth, and the annoyance of headaches. Muscle aches and pains plague movement. The depressed person feels too ill to participate in sustained activity and begins to envy the energy and accomplishments of others.

For the older adult who has managed more than 6 decades of living, self-esteem is challenged. Feelings of uselessness and being a burden to others may surface. As life becomes constricted and exposure to the world is eliminated, more time is available to ruminate on all the mistakes one has made. Time exists to brood over actions taken that could warrant such punishment.

Daily existence becomes bleak. Locked in a world of little stimuli, the victim cannot determine solutions to problems. Actions seem useless, even if one had the energy to perform them. Life appears doomed, the depressed person is helpless to act, and there seems to be no hope. Suicide may be considered as a solution that makes perfect sense.

The feeling state created by depression is frightening to both victims and professional caregivers. This disorder, more than any other, brings about a death of the soul that may precipitate death of the body.

Assessment

The nurse should ensure that each client has a comprehensive, thorough assessment for both physical and mental disorders. In the older adult, depression can be complicated or caused by a wide variety of factors that have been discussed in this chapter. The potential for misdiagnosis is great, and the subsequent mismanagement based on such a misdiagnosis can be fatal for the client.

The nurse should make certain that the following are included in evaluation of the client for medical disorders:

- ◆ Health history
- ◆ Physical examination
- ◆ Medication history, past and present
- ◆ Blood pressure, sitting and standing
- ◆ Laboratory tests
    Thyroid function studies
    Complete blood count
    Urinalysis
    Serological test for syphilis, if indicated
    DST (dexamethasone suppression test)
- ◆ Electrocardiogram
- ◆ Electroencephalogram
- ◆ Computed tomography
- ◆ Polysomnography

A comprehensive physical examination allows physicians and other members of the multidisciplinary health care team to rule out physical illness and drug-induced depression. Data collected further enable clinicians to identify the presence of biochemical and physiological markers of depression and provide a baseline for decisions about pharmacological and other somatic treatments.

Assessment of the mental health status of the client may be performed by the nurse and should include the following parameters:

- ◆ Collection of a nursing history, including psychosocial assessment
- ◆ Nutritional history (a minimum of 24-hour dietary recall)
- ◆ Family assessment
- ◆ Assessment of ability to perform ADL
- ◆ Mental status examination (see Appendix B)
- ◆ Intensive assessment of client for depressive symptoms (Table 6-3)

Depression Scales

Assessment may be augmented by the use of depression scales and inventories. Commonly used inventories include the Hamilton Rating Scale for Depression (Ham-D), Geriatric Depression Scale (GDS), Zung Self-Rating Depression Scale (SDS), Center for Epidemiologic Studies Depression Scale (CES-D), Inventory of

Table 6-3 Symptoms and Characteristics of Depression in the Older Adult

DSM-IV criterion: daily or nearly daily presence of	Symptoms and characteristics expressed in older adults
Depressed mood	Depressed mood (may be less pronounced in older adults) Irritability Apathy Increased criticism of significant others Expresses feeling of emptiness Crying Flat, monotonous voice Lack of eye contact Flat affect Unkempt appearance Reports feeling sad, if asked Dark physical environment
Markedly diminished interest or pleasure in activities	Social withdrawal Isolation Withdrawal from normal activities Takes no interest or pleasure in activities formerly enjoyed States "I don't want to be with other people" Loss of interest in radio or television Change in sexual interest or pleasure

Weight loss or weight gain	In older adults, usually:
	    Not enjoy eating
	    Lack of appetite
	    Refusal to eat or drink

Insomnia or hypersomnia	Middle of the night insomnia Increase in eary morning awakening Interventions to relieve insomnia in early morning do not seem to help
Psychomotor agitation or retardation observable by others	Lethargy Speaks slowly Actions slow and deliberate Decreased ability to perform ADLs

Continued.

Based on data from the following:

American Psychiatric Association (1994). *Diagnostic and statistical manual* (4th ed.). Washington, DC: Author.

Blazer, D. (1988). Diagnosis and management of the suicidal older adult. *Proceedings of the American Society on Aging Regional Seminar, Mental Health and Aging.* Philadelphia: American Society on Aging.

Burnside, I. (1988). *Nursing and the aged* (3rd ed.). New York: McGraw-Hill.

Dreyfus, J. K. (1987). The prevalence of depression in women in an ambulatory setting. *Nurse Practitioner, 12*(4), 34-50.

Mignogna, M. (1986). Integrity vs. despair: The treatment of depression in the elderly. *Clinical Therapeutics, 8*(3), 248-259.

Minot, S. R. (1986). Depression: What does it mean? *American Journal of Nursing, 86*(3), 14-18.

Weiss, I. K., Nagel, C. L., & Aronson, M. K. (1986). Applicability of depression scales to the old, old person. *Journal of the American Geriatrics Society, 34*(3), 215-218.

Table 6-3   Symptoms and Characteristics of Depression in the Older Adult—cont'd

DSM-IV criterion: daily or nearly daily presence of	Symptoms and characteristics expressed in older adults
	Delayed response to stimuli Expresses envy of the activity levels of others
Fatigue or loss of energy	Extreme fatigue Lassitude Dizziness Falling
Worthlessness, excessive or inappropriate guilt	Worthlessness and guilt may be absent or diminished greatly in older adults compared with younger depressed patients Helplessness—clinging dependency Loss of control—view of events as externally controlled Worries constantly Negativism

Worthlessness, excessive or inappropriate guilt	Low self-esteem
	Expresses feelings like
	   "I'm just a burden on everyone"
	   "I can't do anything anymore"

Diminished ability to think or concentrate	Older adult will describe this as second major concern (somatic complaints are first) Older adult may perceive memory deficits as more severe than those found by professional examiner Inconsistency of memory: good one day, not the next Answers questions with "I don't know" Checks and double-checks things Does not stay focused on topic; responses to questions may ramble or reflect disorganization In contrast, at times responses to questions are remarkably detailed Expresses feelings of confusion Expresses feeling of bewilderment Has difficulty making decisions
Recurrent thoughts of death, suicidal ideation, or suicide attempt	Older adults may *not* overtly express suicidal ideation Morbid preoccupation with death Expression of thoughts that "Life is not worth living," "My family would be better off if I was out of the way"
Somatic or physical complaints, not identified by criterion of DSM-IV	Somatic, physical, or hypochondriacal complaints are often the major initial symptom set expressed by older clients Constipation Dry mouth Stomach pain Nausea Upset stomach Headache Muscle pain Atypical pain

Psychic and Somatic Complaints of the Elderly (IPSCE), and the Beck Depression Inventory (Weiss, Nagel, & Aronson, 1986).

These inventories generally have a scaled response format, and questions require a gradated response to the presence of behaviors expressed in depressive syndrome. Response areas include presence of guilt, sadness, fatigability, pessimism, self-loathing, psychic and motor retardation, anxiety, agitation, and hypochondriasis. Alterations in sleep, appetite, or social interaction; loss of insight; and the potential for self-harm are also assessed. The respondent accrues a total score that is equated with the presence of minimal, mild, moderate, or severe depression. Data collection with these inventories may vary from self-reporting by patients to skilled observation and assignment of scores by a professional health care provider.

After careful examination of these depression scales, Weiss, et al. (1986) suggested that great caution be exercised in the use of these inventories. They noted that none of the scales assess the 2-week persistence of symptoms required by the DSM-III (American Psychiatric Association, 1980) and that each scale omits selected items that are considered critical in assessment of older adults. Among items inconsistently included in the inventories are assessment of somatic complaints, capacity to care for oneself, decreased expression of guilt, presence of feelings of emptiness or helplessness, hypochondriasis, criticism or envy of others, devaluing of lifelong accomplishments, and a history of depressive feelings. These authors also stated that the depression scales commonly in use have not been validated for use in the population above age 60. St. Pierre et al. (1986) also caution clinicians that scales such as the Zung Self-Rating Depression Scale are appropriate for the younger population but do not provide accurate data on the older adult.

Therefore prudence indicates that the clinician should use inventories only as screening tools. Such use would identify clients at high risk for depression and indicate which individuals might require referral for definitive diagnosis. The use of such tools in an ambulatory care setting has been promoted by Dreyfus (1987) as a means of identifying the underlying cause of somatic complaints most often presented in the out-patient settings. She noted that treatments and medications prescribed for the somatic disorders may prove both ineffective and inappropriate without concurrent pharmacological and psychotherapeutic treatment of the underlying depression.

As the population of the United States becomes more racially and ethnically diverse, it is important to develop assessment strategies that accurately identify depression in minority target populations. The use of culturally relevant screening instruments and training of health care professionals to interpret clients' histories in the context of the individual's cultural belief system is essential. For example, in some Asian cultures mental illness is unacceptable, and clients will not seek help with emotional symptoms, nor will medical practitioners from those cultures give their clients mental health diagnoses. Instead, mental health needs will be expressed through somatic complaints. These clients are unlikely to respond in a meaningful way to screening instruments standardized on a white population.

Interventions

The nurse who works to prevent or reduce the effects of depression in older adults may encounter such clients in a variety of settings. He or she will have an array of therapeutic approaches to use in meeting individualized client needs. At times the nurse will have the assistance of colleagues in the decision-making process because she or he has assembled or is a member of a multidisciplinary team. This team may work together to provide services to individuals or delineated population groups. At other times the nurse must act alone, often attempting to provide services with limited personnel, equipment, or cooperation from facility administrators, primary care physicians, or even the clients themselves. Major responsibilities of the nurse in the management of depression are discussed in this section. A sample nursing care plan for a depressed client is provided on pages 135-138.

Feelings about Caring for Depressed Clients

The nurse must carefully examine his or her own psychic strengths and deficits before and during work with depressed clients. The effective nurse is skilled in recognizing his or her own feelings, both those that are good, such as happiness, love, and joy, and those that are threatening, such as anger, hostility, guilt, and fear. If the nurse cannot acknowledge such feelings, his or her acceptance of clients' feelings will be emotionally disruptive and intensely uncomfortable.

Nurses who work with depressed older adults must seek sources of emotional support and nurturing outside the nurse-client interaction. The depressed client will be very self-centered. Until the depressed mood lifts, the client will be unable to provide substantial positive feedback to either professional or family caregivers. Continual exposure to the clinging dependency and negativistic thinking exhibited by the depressed client can lead to rapid burnout. Therefore it is important that nurses create a balanced life outside the clinical setting or they will be emotionally depleted by the needs of clients.

The nurse must be prepared to exercise patience. Progress will be slow. At best, the client's mood will improve after 3 to 4 weeks of therapy with antidepressants. Realistically, nurses and family caregivers must wait patiently for cognitive and behavioral therapies to produce a change in behavior. The time required for behavior change will vary from client to client but will most typically be characterized by advances punctuated by disconcerting setbacks.

Nurses who work with depressed clients must accept the fact that the responsibility for improvement lies with the client and/or client system. The nurse may collaborate with the client, family, and significant others to identify and operationalize therapeutic interventions, but active involvement by the client is a requirement for improvement.

Effective Interpersonal Relationship

Hope is the major commodity that the nurse can offer the depressed client. For the individual locked in a cycle of despair and for whom events seem externally

Nursing Care Plan for an Older Client with Depression

Assessment data	Nursing diagnosis	Goals	Nursing interventions
2/16 **Subjective** "I'm just no good to anyone anymore." "No one would miss me if I was gone." "I just can't seem to get anything done. I just don't care about doing anything." "I don't want to end up being a burden for my son." "I drink a little now and then." **Objective** A fifth of bourbon is sitting on the kitchen counter. An empty bottle is in the trash can. Client has not taken any medications for 1 month. Slow, monotonous speech Flat affect Cluttered row house Client's clothes soiled; hair unkempt Poor dental hygiene	Violence, high risk for: Directed at self related to loneliness	**Short-term** Client will make and keep appointment with mental health clinician for evaluation of depression. **Long-term** Client will demonstrate positive self-esteem by maintaining the household and person. Client will verbalize positive feelings about self.	Using Beck Depression Inventory, screen client for depressive symptoms. Report findings to primary physician. Ask client about suicidal thoughts. If response to above reveals suicidal ideation and a plan, collaborate with physician for immediate hospital admission. In the absence of suicidal ideation, collaborate with the primary physician to refer the client to a mental health clinician for evaluation and diagnosis of depressive symptoms. If client remains in the community, arrange to talk daily to provide telephone reassurance until time of next visit. Schedule home visits by community health nurse two times per week. Identify availability of significant others to check on client between nursing visits.

Continued.

Nursing Care Plan for an Older Client with Depression—cont'd

Assessment data	Nursing diagnosis	Goals	Nursing interventions
Subjective "My husband died in 1964." "I have one son who lives in California. I haven't seen him for 2 years." "My sister used to live next door, but she died last year. She and I were the last two in our family." "My sister used to drive us places. I never learned to drive. Since she died, I have had a hard time getting out." "I don't go to church anymore. I used to go with my sister." "I am afraid to go out. The young kids on this street are into drugs." **Objective** Client has a telephone. Client lives in one side of a Philadelphia twin-row house. A senior center is less than a block from the client's home. Client has no mobility impairment. Client's block of 40 houses has 10 vacant and boarded-up units. One of these is a crack house. Client's church has an active and caring population of older adults.	Social isolation related to lack of support system.	**Short-term** Client will identify persons who can form a support system. **Long-term** Client will regularly participate in church and senior social groups.	Collect history regarding former social activities and friendship networks. Identify persons in these groups who might provide support to client now. Teach client skills for reestablishing social contact if these have been lost. With client's consent, refer her to • Senior center outreach worker for home visit and enrollment in senior center • Minister of her church • Telephone reassurance program at senior center Review client's strategies for self-protection. Refer to local police department for in-home evaluation of door and window locks. Request visits by nursing students for 6 weeks, two times per week. Students will use cognitive and behavior therapies in working with client.

Subjective

"I am not hungry."

"I am just too tired to fix food. It's all I can do to open cans."

"Nothing tastes good."

24-hour dietary recall

Breakfast: "2 pieces of toast, 1 cup of coffee"

Lunch: "Nothing"

Midafternoon snack: "Bowl of chicken noodle soup, 1 cup of coffee"

Dinner: "I wasn't hungry"

Evening snack: "1 glass of buttermilk, 1 glass of water to take Ex-Lax"

Objective

Client now weighs 115 pounds—6 months ago her weight was 127

Skin turgor: Fair

Skin texture: Rough

Pulse: 96

Urinary output: approximately 750 ml/daily

Urine: Strong odor, deep orange in color

Nutrition, altered: Less than body requirements related to lack of desire to eat.

Short-term

Client will eat four small meals per day.

Client will drink 2000 ml of fluid per day.

Long-term

Client will prepare her own meals that provide recommended dietary allowances of all nutrients.

Collaborate with client's physician and a nutritionist to evaluate nutritional and hydration status.

Obtain an order for in-home laboratory work:
Chemistry panel
Urinalysis
Hemoglobin; hematocrit

Report findings to primary physician.

Obtain a nutrient analysis of client's diet from a registered dietitian. Report results and recommendations to primary physician.

Identify source of home-delivered meals for 1 month until client's antidepressants lift mood and she can engage in food preparation.

Identify food and fluid preferences of the client.

Begin diet recommendations and meal plans using preferred foods.

Evaluate economic status and ascertain whether client needs to apply for food stamps.

Continued.

Nursing Care Plan for an Older Client with Depression—cont'd

Assessment data	Nursing diagnosis	Goals	Nursing interventions
			Encourage client to become involved in congregate meals at senior center as depressed mood is relieved.
			Collaborate with client to identify forms of exercise that will aid in increasing bowel motility.
			Instruct client in dietary modifications to reduce constipation: discourage use of laxatives.

controlled, the hope of regaining the power to manage one's own life is a great gift. The nurse must assure the client that help is available, that it will take time, but that improvement will come slowly.

Nurses working with depressed older adults should not assume that all symptoms of social withdrawal are caused by depression. The nurse should determine whether vital assistive devices such as glasses, hearing aids, canes, braces, and walkers are needed or available. It is difficult for clients to interact socially if they cannot see or hear or if they have mobility impairments that prevent them from leaving their rooms or homes.

Establishing an effective relationship with the client takes time. Speech patterns, movements, and thought processes may be markedly slowed. The client initially may not be able to do things at a normal pace. In planning client care, nurses and family caregivers should allow sufficient time to support the client's efforts to perform ADL or to simply be with them. When talking with the client, the nurse should sit and give undivided attention to the interpersonal interaction. Time spent with clients should be used to encourage them to identify feelings, maybe even to feel itself. Some depressed clients will initially report numbness. It is difficult to share feelings with a nurse when one is not consciously feeling anything. Observations on the part of the nurse such as "you look sad" or "I saw you crying yesterday" may indicate to the client that someone cares and may assist in the recognition that feelings are occurring, regardless of whether they can be labeled.

Nurses should assiduously avoid what Burnside describes as the "look and leave syndrome." This undesirable activity occurs when the nurse or family caregiver observes the client crying or visibly upset, is seen by the client making the observation, but walks off without recognition or acknowledgment of the client's distress (Burnside, 1988). Distressing feelings should be addressed directly when they are observed or identified.

Promises made to the client by the nurse should be kept. Socially withdrawn, the client may fear venturing from his or her shell and must exert a great deal of energy to interact with others. Broken trust will discourage the client from making this effort.

Nurses must demonstrate respect for the client. Clients should be asked what they wish to be called, not addressed by their first names without permission. Staff should introduce themselves and describe the nature of their role with the client. If in an institutional setting, the client should be introduced to other clients and personnel. Initially, these introductions may have to be made repeatedly because of memory loss and temporary confusion (Campbell, 1986).

Goals and activities should be planned so that success will be experienced by the client. Successes should build progressively, and greater challenges should be posed as the client successfully achieves initial goals. The nurse should reinforce all expressions of positive thought and performance of positive behavior.

Finally, the nurse should serve as a role model for behaviors. Many depressed older adults have been isolated and have lost socialization skills. They may watch the nurse to obtain clues for appropriate social behaviors, methods of problem solving, and appropriate dress and cosmetics.

The interpersonal relationship between the nurse and client should embrace the client's family. The client's depression can place a severe strain on family relationships. Family members initially supportive of the client may withdraw that support if the client fails to improve. Depression may not be viewed by the family as a legitimate illness like cancer or heart disease but as a personal failing (Parmelee & Katz, 1992). It is important for the nurse to recognize the stress on family members as they seek to meet the needs of the client. The client's family must also manage their own feelings of inadequacy or anger, which may be triggered by a depressed individual who may offer little or no positive feedback. The nurse must work closely with family caregivers as they define the caregiving role, cope with the loss of reciprocity in their relationship with the client, and develop strategies to establish new and positive interactions within the family system.

Interdisciplinary Approach to Client Management
The depressed older adult faces multiple physical and psychological challenges in the resolution of depression. Depression in this group is not a single-cause disorder. Effective management will require the collaboration of the following:

- Nurses
- Clients
- Family members and significant others
- Physicians
- Clergy
- Nutritionists
- Pharmacists
- Activity therapists
- Occupational therapists
- Physical therapists
- Medical social workers
- Lay members of community support groups
- Paraprofessional caregivers
- Representatives of community agencies and resources of the client system
- Volunteers
- Legislators
- Advocates and ombudsmen

Each discipline has a special talent to contribute to the recovery process. Their services should be enlisted as needed in the management of individual clients. Certainly, all groups should be involved in the planning of any overall institutional or community-based program designed to prevent or manage depression.

Somatic Needs and Comfort
The older adult suffering from depression will have a number of somatic complaints. Often he or she will perceive these indispositions to be the major problem, denying

or actively resisting a diagnosis of depression. These somatic symptoms should be addressed promptly to establish trust and a foundation for the psychotherapeutic or somatic therapies that will follow.

Nurses and caregivers must direct their attention to the nutritional status of the client. The client may not have the energy to cut and chew food and may be so preoccupied with internal grief that meals are forgotten. When energy levels are low, meals should be small and offered frequently. A standard-sized plate filled with food may be a barrier to appetite. Initially, foods should be easy to pick up and chew. Hand-held snacks or finger foods may prove to be more effective than full platters. Fluids should be offered frequently to ensure maintenance of hydration. Every effort should be made to make foods colorful, aromatic, and flavorful. Consultations with a dietitian may be helpful for the nurse and/or family caregiver. If dentures have been lost or are not being used because they do not fit properly, the nurse may refer the client to a dentist for evaluation.

Constipation, flatulence, and digestive upset should be aggressively managed. Exercise, stool softeners, and dietary fiber may be used to promote greater comfort for the client.

Sleep disturbances may prove particularly upsetting to the older adult. In the inpatient setting, the staff may wish to schedule time for personalized attention during early morning awakenings. These periods may be used to talk with the client or to give a back rub or a small snack. The nurse may develop strategies for home care clients and caregivers that do not disrupt the caregiver's sleep. Clients should be assured that sleep disturbances will diminish as the depression lifts. Older adults and their caregivers should be taught about the normal changes in sleep patterns that accompany aging. The use of alcohol, sedatives, and hypnotics to induce and sustain sleep should be discouraged.

Complaints of pain by depressed individuals necessitate careful evaluation. Research studies indicate that persons displaying symptoms of major depression report localized pain more frequently and/or report pain to be more intense than do those with minor depression or nondepressives (Parmelee, Katz, & Lawton, 1991; Mansfield & Marx, 1993). Parmelee, et al. (1991, p. 20) report that the relationship of depression to localized pain complaints was strongest when there was a physical disorder to which the pain might logically be attributed. Physicians independently identified one or more physical dysfunctions pertinent to complaints among research subjects, so these complaints of pain could not be dismissed merely as somatizing of anxiety. Thus, the researchers suggest that depressed individuals may be more sensitive to pain and/or more willing to acknowledge it to others. Williamson and Schulz's 1992 research on older adults in community housing adds another dimension to the association between pain and depression. In their research, pain and depression were linked to functional impairment. These scholars suggest that alleviation of pain directed toward increasing functional ability will reduce the severity of depressive symptoms. Similarly, tactics designed to facilitate functional performance and independence, even when such performance is painful, may directly reduce symptoms of depression.

Physical Environment

Often the external physical environment matches the bleakness and gloom of the depressed person. The depressed older adult lives in a darkened room, where shades are drawn, lamps remain turned off, and silence is pervasive. The older depressed adult may be found huddled in bed or in the same chair day after day, staring at the opposite wall. Clutter may present a vivid testimony to the internal surrender of control and/or insufficient energy that can be summoned for ADL. For the older adult living in poverty, environmental decay may be overwhelming. Stained walls, monotone gray or brown colors, crumbling plaster, dingy curtains, inadequate sanitation, intrusive odors, and insects and rodents may cause or deepen despair.

The nurse must promote the creation of an environment that challenges the gloom of depression in both outpatient and inpatient settings. The environment should be made safe for the older adult. Throw rugs, misplaced furniture, electrical cords, and other obstacles should be cleared from walkways. Assistive devices should be provided for clients with limited mobility. Handrails and other aids should be provided if the person is in danger of falling.

Color and pattern should be provided to attract attention and direct thoughts from an ego-centered obsession with personal misery. Straightening up the environment often will reveal attractive surroundings that simply need the occasional introduction of a new object, such as a bright throw pillow, to reduce a feeling of sameness and boredom. Other environments will prove more challenging, especially those inhabited by the poor. Small bouquets of flowers may be the best method for introducing beauty to these surroundings. Often small luxuries such as a cake of scented soap or a box of delicious-smelling powder can boost the spirits of the depressed. Colorful lap robes are another source of pleasure for older adults. They are practical as well, providing needed warmth in rooms that are often chilly.

Lighting is critical to the alleviation of depression. Depressed clients should be actively discouraged from secreting themselves in dark rooms. Darkness deepens the depression. Natural light should be allowed into the environment during the day. At night, sufficient artificial light should be provided to enable clients to read labels on medication bottles, read for pleasure, move around without accident, and prepare food. If confusion or disorientation is present, night lights should be provided during the hours of sleep.

In the inpatient setting, clients should be encouraged to personalize environmental spaces. Photographs, crafts made in occupational therapy, or drawings made by grandchildren will render inpatient spaces less sterile. Personalization of space will also enable staff members to recognize the individuality of the client and serve as a basis for identifying the client's preferences and interests.

Music and art should be introduced into the client setting. Pervasive and continuous silence should be discouraged. Music, radio, and television should be used selectively to encourage the client to reconnect to the larger world in which he or she lives. Singing, dancing, and exercising to music with others allow the client to interact directly with other human beings without bearing full responsibility for conversation or instigation of activities. The power of music, especially hymns, swing, and jazz, brings older adults out of a shell of self-isolation.

Pets should be considered for older adults who are suffering from loneliness and isolation and for whom adequate human support systems are unavailable. Telephones for these clients are a lifeline to the outside world and should be secured. Telephone companies often have special programs for low-income older adults whose resources are insufficient to pay monthly telephone bills.

Rights and Responsibilities of Clients

Nurses should inform clients and family caregivers of their legal rights in relation to treatment and specific therapeutic interventions such as taking medications, permitting room searches, being in seclusion rooms, and receiving electroconvulsive therapy.

Nurses should work with clients and family caregivers in the home to establish clear rules for behavior management. Clear-cut guidelines should be developed regarding the types of behaviors that will necessitate admission to an inpatient treatment setting. Examples of such behaviors include suicidal ideation accompanied by a plan and the means to execute it, noncompliance with medication regimens, refusal to eat or drink, and inability to perform ADL.

Clients must be oriented to their role in the healing process. They must be told that the responsibility for improvement is theirs. Health professionals and caregivers will collaborate in structuring a therapeutic environment, but the client must assume the responsibility for using the services that are offered.

Caution should be used in asking clients about advanced medical directives, which is often required on institutional admission. Severely depressed individuals may be unable to understand the purpose or the process of such documents. Certainly, a client expressing suicidal ideation should not be asked the details of personal decisions about life-sustaining measures. Those decisions can wait until the clinical depression has abated and decision-making skills have returned to normal.

Direction or Participation in Psychotherapy

Psychotherapy and related therapeutic approaches are the treatment of choice for mild and moderate depression in older adults (Blazer, 1986). However, older adults may view psychotherapies with hesitation and suspicion. Many grew up when mental illness carried a stigma and treatment for such illness was inhumane. Therefore it is important for nurses and other health professionals to orient the older adult to psychotherapy. This socialization process should include information on what the client should expect from psychotherapy, clarification of the client's role in the psychotherapeutic process, rules about the way psychotherapy will be conducted, and the rationale behind this method of treatment. Clients should be given an opportunity to clarify their expectations about the treatment process and to express concerns about this mode of therapy. Older adults may not be comfortable with such things as interruption of group members by one another or management of therapeutic silence and may need some orientation to these types of interactions (Thompson & Gallagher, 1986).

Several themes may recur in psychotherapeutic interactions with older clients, including the following (Waller & Griffin, 1984; Mignogna, 1986):

- Grief
- Fighting loneliness
- Fear of death
- Fears of physical illness and disability
- Restitution of loss of loved ones
- Wish to undo some previous life pattern
- Coping with frustration
- Handling stress
- Adjusting to retirement
- Desire for a new start in life

Most older adults with mild to moderate depression will remain in the community. Therefore nurses should be creative in locating and/or establishing therapy or support groups for clients in a wide variety of outpatient settings. The nurse should identify other professionals who can provide one-on-one group therapy. These may include psychologists, occupational therapists, activity therapists, and recreational therapists. In the inpatient, acute care psychiatric setting, the nurse works with many of these professionals in the multidisciplinary team. However, inpatient treatment is brief, often 3 weeks or less. Appropriate therapeutic groups must be located outside the hospital to continue the progress initiated in the inpatient unit. This is critical if the client is taking antidepressants. In the inpatient setting the client's mood may be too depressed to benefit from psychotherapeutic treatment methods. Three weeks after admission, about the time of discharge, the antidepressants will be actively working and the individual may now be ready for psychotherapy. Family therapy may also be warranted if the older adult's symptoms are affecting other family members.

The nurse must plan carefully to ensure a balance between activities and rest. The older adult will benefit from participation in a wide variety of therapy and support groups, but care must be taken not to overprogram the client with activities. The depressed patient will benefit from structure and routine. Thus care should be taken to establish an activity routine that is stable from day to day. The nurse must also consider long-term rehabilitation and plan for a smooth transition from inpatient to outpatient settings. Isolated and lonely older persons may blossom in the hospital where they can interact with others and engage in interesting activities. However, if they return home and no stimulation is available, they will feel more lonely and bereft than before treatment, and depression will return in full force.

Thompson and Gallagher (1986) identified three major types of psychotherapy that are used with older adults. These therapies may be used in one-to-one interactions or in a variety of small therapeutic group settings (Table 6-4).

Table 6-4   Therapeutic Groups for Older Adults with Depression

Type of group	Purpose of group	Example of activities
Behavior Therapy	Aids older adults to identify the relationship between mood changes and life events Enables depressed adults to identify and incorporate pleasurable events into daily living Provides a task-oriented setting for interpersonal interaction	Clients may be asked to perform a series of tasks at each group session. Examples of such tasks are listed below: • Discuss the relationship between pleasant activities and mood. • Identify pleasant activities specific for the individual. • Plan a weekly schedule that includes one pleasant activity each day. • Discuss the value of social activities and friends. • Identify persons who may form a support system. • Examine reasons for not interacting with people who could form a support system. • Call and talk to one person in the support system on the phone. • Invite someone in the support system to share a face-to-face activity.
Cognitive therapy	Promotes the examination of erroneous perceptions of life events Stresses the conversion of negative thoughts to positive ones Provides small-group socialization Provides support from others who are also struggling with life change	Group session focuses on a new topic each session. A minilecture is given on topics related to faulty thought patterns such as automatic thoughts, negative thoughts, overgeneralization, catastrophic thinking, dichotomous thinking, alternative explanations, and reality testing. At each session the client is also given an assignment to perform such as the following: • Keep a record of dysfunctional thoughts. Relate these to present mood. • Choose one negative thought. Convert this to a positive thought.
Music therapy	Focuses thoughts and feelings on activities unrelated to internal despair Allows for interpersonal interaction without bearing total responsibility for the interactions Allows alternate forms for expression of feelings	Have client select music that best fits depressed feeling tone. Discuss selection. Use music of differing tempos to elevate mood. Encourage clients to express their feelings nonverbally by coordinating movements to music. Encourage singing with others as a nonthreatening form of social interaction.

Table 6-4 **Therapeutic Groups for Older Adults with Depression—cont'd**

Type of group	Purpose of group	Example of activities
Reminiscing	Promotes a review of past life experiences to identify successful coping strategies	Use photos of family members or events to stimulate discussions. Select topics such as childbearing, job seeking, and childrearing; have older adult describe the management of these life experiences. Focus on areas of life such as school experiences, play activities, participation in church, celebration of holidays as discussion points for group members to share their own experiences. Identify positive coping skills.
Exercise	Stimulates movement and discourages passivity Stimulates biochemical processes in the brain that reduce stress Provides a task-oriented medium for social interaction Promotes muscle tone and gastrointestinal motility	Twenty-minute sessions of low-impact aerobics for senior adults Outdoor activities such as walking, cycling, and swimming Stress management exercises (e.g., guided imagery, responsive relaxation) Dancing
Poetry	Promotes expression of feelings in words	Older adults select poems that express the inner moods they are feeling; the poetry is then read and discussed with other group members. Writing of poems is encouraged and is often a good device for the expression of bottled-up feelings.

Table 6-4 **Therapeutic Groups for Older Adults with Depression—cont'd**

Type of group	Purpose of group	Example of activities
Assertiveness training	Assists older adults to identify how to get what they want from others Promotes identification of the impact of verbal and nonverbal behavior on others	Describe passive and assertive feelings. Identify body language associated with passive behavior; with assertive behavior. Life situations are presented, and role playing is used to practice a variety of new behaviors. Role playing is enhanced by the use of props or simple costumes. Situations may include saying no to someone who is pressuring them to do something they really do not wish to do. An example would be an adult child asking the older adult to babysit for toddler grandchildren. Situations may include confrontations with workmen who have performed jobs poorly, refusal of monetary solicitations, and making specific requests to others for aid and assistance.
Cooking	Promotes and maintains physical health Provides for socialization with others through task-oriented activities Enhances coping skills and mastery of ADL	Cooking groups focus on the preparation of low-cost, easy to prepare, nutritious meals. Segments may include introduction of Healthy Hearts program sponsored by American Heart Association. Emphasis is on preparing and storing meals that can be eaten over time because older adults often do not have energy to cook three meals a day. If possible, field trips can be planned to markets to teach the selection of low-fat, low-sodium products.

Table 6-4 Therapeutic Groups for Older Adults with Depression—cont'd

Type of group	Purpose of group	Example of activities
Caregiver support	Same as above	Caregivers of older depressed adults and caregivers who are themselves depressed will benefit from participating in a caregiver group. The group can have both topical presentations on client management issues and a discussion period for sharing and ventilating feelings. Topics for discussion may include loss of freedom, role reversal, shared living, integrating the dependent adult into the family, respite care, financial management, and management of old and new psychic pain.
Chronic illness adaptation	Provides information regarding management of specific chronic diseases Same as above support groups Enhances coping skills and mastery	Older depressed adults with chronic illnesses such as diabetes, chronic obstructive pulmonary disease, heart disease, or cancer will benefit from inclusion in groups that discuss management of disorders, use of assistive devices and community resources to aid in maintenance of health.
Widow/widower support	Provides acceptable outlet for expression of grief and loss Provides socialization Introduces a variety of strategies for coping with life changes	Research suggests that older adults benefit from inclusion of both sexes in a survivor support group. Problems and feelings of bereaved older adults tend to be more similar than dissimilar. Topics for discussion include management of loneliness, socialization as a single person, assumption of tasks and responsibilities of deceased spouse, and adaptation of a new lifestyle.

Based on data from Thompson & Gallagher (1986) and Burnside (1988) and on interviews with Ana Y. Askew, OTR, Supervisor of Occupational Therapy, Blue Ridge Hospital; Department of Behavioral Medicine and Psychiatry, University of Virginia, Charlottesville, and Gary Bilsky, RN, Nurse Manager, Geropsychiatric Unit, Albert Einstein Hospital, Philadelphia.

INSIGHT THERAPY. Insight therapy uses techniques for dealing with posttraumatic stress and is a brief psychodynamic technique. The goal of therapy is to assist the older adult to identify life events and situations that have been painful in the past and to correlate feelings and reactions to these events with the current situation that may have triggered a depression. Psychoanalytical techniques are not useful with older adults because of the length of time and cost that may be involved in such therapy.

COGNITIVE THERAPY. Cognitive therapy is based on the theory that depression is caused by how the client interprets events rather than on the events themselves. The goal of therapy is to help the older adult identify and alter dysfunctional patterns of thinking. Attention is given to control of negative thoughts, errors in thinking, and overreactions to perceptions.

BEHAVIOR THERAPY. Behavior therapy is based on the premise that depression occurs when the patient experiences a negative balance between unpleasant and pleasurable events. The goal of therapy is to help the older adult to identify pleasurable events and then use that knowledge to decrease life events and experiences that contribute to depressed mood.

Provision for Continuity of Care

Mental health services are fragmented in most communities. Therefore, the nurse may need to assist clients and family members in identifying and using appropriate community resources. Most older adults will remain in their own homes. The majority will have chronic medical conditions in addition to their depressive illness. Nurses can assist in the following tasks:

- ◆ Coordination of mental health care and services provided by the primary physician
- ◆ Identification of outpatient treatment resources (support groups, activity programs, friendly visitors, home health services, and outpatient mental health centers)
- ◆ Planning for mental health follow-up such as evaluation of blood levels of antidepressants and decreases in depressive symptomatology
- ◆ Establishment of a reasonable network for the client to use for outpatient→inpatient→outpatient treatment. Nurses should help the client, family, and/or significant others to identify contact people in the treatment cycle who can assist in gaining access to the health care delivery services needed at any given time.

Somatic Therapies

Older adults diagnosed with recurrent moderate or severe depressive symptoms may be treated with medications, electroconvulsive therapy, and/or sleep deprivation therapy.

Pharmacological intervention most often includes the use of antidepressants.

However, some older adults with treatment-resistant depression may receive lithium in combination with the tricyclic antidepressants (Meyers & Alexopoulas, 1988). Psychostimulants may be ordered for selected older adults who display apathy (Goff & Jenike, 1986), and antipsychotics may be used for those who experience delusions or hallucinations with depression (Mignogna, 1986). Management of these medications is discussed extensively in Chapter 5.

Nursing management of medications includes administration of medications, assessment of efficacy, management of side effects, and promotion of compliance. Compliance is easy to ensure in the inpatient setting, where health care personnel have control. However, the nurse working with the client in an outpatient setting may have to deal with noncompliance as a major issue. Promotion of compliance will include some of the following strategies:

1. Teach the client and caregivers that results of antidepressants will not be felt for 2 to 3 weeks after the initiation of therapy.
2. Teach the client and caregiver to identify and manage side effects.
3. Determine the client's literacy level and understanding of written materials related to medication usage.
4. Evaluate all medications used by the client and identify any potential drug interaction. In the home, examine all medications, prescription and nonprescription. It is not unusual for clients to forget to mention to the physician treating depression that several medications are being taken for medical illnesses.
5. Because primary physicians may not be familiar with geriatric pharmacology and/or antidepressant medication, evaluate treatment regimens that they prescribe. Evaluate initial dosages to determine that they begin at one third to one half the dose rates given to younger adults (Goff & Jenike, 1986; Mignogna, 1986). Determine that the frequency of administration orders makes sense. One severely depressed client in the community setting had a prescription that read "Ludiomil, prn at hour of sleep for depression."
6. Evaluate the client's ability to pay for the medication and to travel to and from the pharmacy to pick it up. Assess the availability of support persons to perform these tasks if the client is unable to do so.
7. Teach the client the importance of returning to the physician to have blood levels of medication evaluated. Check on availability of transportation to medical centers or physician's office for follow-up. If mobility is a problem, check with local home health agencies to determine whether laboratory work can be done in the home.
8. If the client takes many medications, discuss combining medications or simplifying regimens to reduce the likelihood of pill swallower's syndrome. Evaluate the client's and caregiver's ability to identify each medicine, their understanding of the action of the medicine, and knowledge of side effects that should be reported to the physician. Make sure the client can see well enough to read medication labels.

9. If monoamine oxidase inhibitors are used, assess the client's and caregiver's understanding of dietary restrictions. Older clients who have difficulty with shopping and food preparation will depend on others (such as Meals on Wheels or Congregate Meals) for meals. They may not be able to follow dietary guidelines essential for the proper use of these medications. The physician may not have been able to obtain this information in the inpatient setting.

10. The nurse should ascertain whether all physicians being seen by the client are aware of the order for an antidepressant and whether consistent information is being given by each physician regarding the use of the medication. If the primary physician minimizes the need for the medication and the psychiatrist emphasizes its importance, the client will become confused. Noncompliance will become a real possibility, depending on which professional he or she trusts the most.

Nursing actions in relation to the implementation of electroconvulsive therapy (ECT) include teaching the client about the procedure, preparing the client for the procedure, accompanying him or her during the procedure, and providing nursing care in the immediate postprocedure period. ECT is effective in 50% of older adults who are nonresponsive to medications and in up to 80% of those with endogenous symptoms (Goff & Jenike, 1986). The nurse must be alert and warn the physician if the patient develops symptoms or disorders that contraindicate ECT treatment, such as severe hypertension, increased intracranial pressure, myocardial infarction, or suspected cerebrovascular accident (Mignogna, 1986). Nurses should also be alert to the client's need for reorientation after ECT as a result of temporary memory loss. Caregivers who bring older adults for outpatient ECT should be reminded to monitor client activities for several hours after they return home because forgetfulness or confusion may occur.

Prevention of Depression through Education

Management of depression in older adults is a 24-hour-a-day, 365-day-a-year job. Depression occurs in every city, town, and neighborhood in our country. No nurse can manage the problem alone, but through the art of multiplying himself or herself can marshal an army of interested and committed comrades. Multiplication occurs as a result of educating others—potential clients, clients, family caregivers, paraprofessionals, professionals, and legislators. No nurse can be in all places at all times. The educated consumer and/or professional colleague can implement needed therapeutic interventions in the nurse's absence if taught to do so.

Effective educational programs should be based on prevention. Comprehensive education related to depression in older adults should address prevention of depression (primary prevention), early treatment and diagnosis (secondary prevention), and rehabilitation of the chronically depressed (tertiary prevention). Suggested prevention topics are listed in Table 6-5.

Educational programs may be developed and provided directly by the nurse or

Table 6-5   Topics for Health Education to Prevent Depression in Older Adults

Type of prevention	*Suggested topics for health education*
Primary	Maintenance of physical health
	Diet
	Exercise
	Smoking cessation
	Patterns of sleep and rest
	Routine health examinations through adulthood
	Preventive immunization
	Stress management
	Relaxation techniques
	Breathing exercises
	Positive self-talk
	Use of humor to combat depression
	Assertiveness training
	Guided imagery
	Visualization
	Preparation for retirement
	Development of leisure skills
	Integration of part-time employment with retirement benefits
	Continuing educational opportunities
	Establishing non–work related support systems
	Managing on a reduced income
	For women: Independent management skills
	Financial management
	Simple household maintenance
	Hiring and managing repairmen
	Simple car maintenance
	Engaging in social activities without a spouse
	For men: Independent management skills
	Food shopping
	Meal planning and preparation
	Laundry management
	Cleaning
	Social networking
	Health care management
	Strategies for dealing with changes associated with normal aging
	Causes of depression in older adults
	Bereavement as a normal life crisis
	Roles and functions of individual health care disciplines
	For young adults: Effective communication with older adults
	For older adults: Effective communication with younger adults
	Community resources available for social activities
	Financing health care: Medicare and other programs

Table 6-5   Topics for Health Education to Prevent Depression in Older Adults—cont'd

Type of prevention	*Suggested topics for health education*
Secondary	Physical changes not characteristic of normal aging
	Management of loss
	Strategies for managing chronic illness to minimize disability (these should be disease specific)
	Signs and symptoms of depression
	Screening client populations for depression
	Using mental health services
	Treatment techniques used in depression
	Medication management
	Roles and responsibilities
	Family caregivers
	Professional caregivers
	Identifying, establishing, and running support groups
	Management of older depressed adults in a variety of settings
	Home
	Board-and-care homes
	Day care programs
	Inpatient psychiatric unit
	Outpatient mental health clinic
	Senior center
	Prevention of suicide
	Intervention during bereavement
Tertiary	Community resources for long-term follow-up care
	Management of older depressed adults in
	Long-term care facilities
	State mental hospitals
	Dealing with depression in the terminally ill
	Assisting the survivor of a significant other who has committed suicide
	Dealing with placement of a loved one in an institution

by other individuals identified by the nurse. Older adults themselves should not be overlooked as teachers. They have much to offer paraprofessional and professional caregivers and are extremely effective with their own peer groups.

Training of health care professionals should be one facet of a comprehensive educational effort. Physicians and nurses should be taught to replace shallow, cursory mental status exams with meaningful assessments of the parameters of depression. All too frequently the data supplied on health histories to document mental status is limited to the description that the client is A&Ox3 (alert and oriented to time, place, and person). This type of information is useful in describing lethargic or comatose individuals but is less helpful in identifying the presence or level of depression. Even severely depressed individuals can be alert to time, place, and person. Standardized, objective depression screening instruments such as the Geriatric Depression Scale and Beck Depression Inventory should replace imprecise and subjective measures of mental status.

Nurses and caregivers, professional and nonprofessional, often encounter clients with extremely stressful and complex life situations. Teachers of caregivers should caution these providers of care to refrain from projecting their own feelings into the client's situation. If their own feelings in the client's situation would be depression and loss of hope, such feelings in the client may be accepted as an understandable and normal reaction to stressors. Thus, clinical depression will cease to be perceived as an abnormality to be aggressively treated and will instead become a normal albeit uncomfortable condition to be endured.

Education for caregivers should sensitize both professional and lay health care providers to the effects of depression on a client's ability to process information and comply with health care regimens. Depressed clients will process information more slowly, become more easily confused, have a shorter attention span, possess less psychic and physical energy, and have more decisional conflict than nondepressed individuals. Consequently, caregivers should allow more time for teaching and/or performance of self-care when working with depressed older adults than they would when working with nondepressed persons. Periods of instruction should be kept short and focused on a single objective. Repetition of information or performance of skills during single educational sessions and over time is essential. Positive reinforcement and praise are critical for enabling the depressed individual, struggling with low self-esteem and uncertainty, to master self-care and behavior modification.

Education for health care consumers may be provided on a one-to-one basis, in small groups, or in crowded auditoriums. The message of prevention can be spread to large numbers of clients through written materials such as columns in newspapers and newsletters, pamphlets, and books. Finally, in this audiovisual age, television and videotapes should not be overlooked as appropriate media for education. The responsible nurse will take every opportunity in every setting of practice to teach others.

Older adults are very receptive to both informal and formal educational programs. Educational activities are a good substitute for work lost through retirement. Learning may fill time, stimulate interest, foster socialization, enhance coping, and promote self-esteem (Pfeiffer, 1985).

Outreach

Health care professionals must be aggressive in case finding and outreach to identify older adults with depression. Special efforts should be directed toward the needs of minority populations, many of whom have limited access to health care services (NIH, 1992).

Lobbying

Nurses, individually or through professional health care organizations and senior adult groups, should propose authorization and funding of mental health programs and associated support services that are affordable and accessible.

Funding for Program Development

In this era of tight government funding and budget cutbacks, the nurse may wish to explore alternate avenues for funding of programs. Some of these may include charitable foundations, business corporations, private trusts, voluntary mental health agencies, churches, and private fund-raising activities like balls, raffles, and direct donations.

Research

Nurses should direct attention toward research that improves outpatient treatment of depression, utilizing ancillary and volunteer workers to alleviate or prevent depression, and identifying educational strategies that will effectively reach older adults with prevention information.

Evaluation

Nurses involved in establishing individual care plans develop specific goals and client outcomes at the outset of treatment. The same strategy should be used in the creation of programs designed to alleviate depression. Both individual care and care to larger groups should be evaluated to ascertain whether goals have been met and client outcomes achieved.

❖ *Suicide*

Suicide is a final, irreversible solution to despair. It is the worst outcome of depression. Expression of suicidal ideation triggers anxiety in health care professionals, who zealously institute suicide precautions, occasionally excluding the human contacts needed in favor of rigorous checking protocols. Completed suicide attempts evoke remorse and guilt in family, friends, and professionals involved with the victim.

Significance of the Problem

Older adults are disproportionately represented among suicide victims. Although comprising only 11% of the total population, they account for 25% of completed attempts (Meyers & Alexopoulas, 1988). Suicide attempts are less frequent among older adults than among persons at other stages of the life cycle, but the ratio of suicide attempts to completed suicide drops from 20:1 in those below age 40 to 4:1 after the age of 60 (Blazer, 1988). A study by Manton, Blazer, and Woodbury (1987) noted a rapid rise in suicide rates among nonwhite men that contrasts with the usual clinical focus on older white men as the individuals at highest risk. Manton et al. noted that the overall percentage of suicide deaths associated with advanced age increased between 1969 and 1980. Furthermore, the percentage of deaths expected from suicide after age 70 increased 10% for white men and 44% for nonwhite men during this period. Finally, there is an age-related increase in the rate of suicide in elderly individuals of Asian extraction in the United States (Richardson, Lowenstein, & Weissberg, 1989).

Profile of Risk

Older adults identified as being at risk for suicide are those who are widowed or divorced, retired, living alone or in isolation, in poor physical health, suffering from chronic pain or discomfort, suffering bereavement because of real or perceived losses, abusers of alcohol or drugs, and from a family with a history of suicide (Blazer, 1988; Neville & Barnes, 1985).

Individuals who are older, male, isolated, clinically ill, delusionally depressed, or intoxicated run the highest risk for the successful completion of a suicide attempt (Neville & Barnes, 1985). In the inpatient setting the client at greatest risk is the one who has made an attempt before hospitalization, is not immobilized by depression, and has not discussed suicide plans with staff (Campbell, 1986).

A delusionally depressed person is five times more likely to commit suicide than a nondelusional one. The delusional client views the world as a dark and gloomy place. Because he or she may not want to leave loved ones alone in such a place, this client should be considered at high risk for homicide-suicide if there are dependents such as older spouses or parents for whom they care (Neville & Barnes, 1985).

Bereavement may also be a risk factor for suicide. The risk of suicide in a bereaved spouse is the highest in the first day or two after the spouse's death and remains relatively high for a year. Anniversaries of the death and other anniversaries of significant dates in the couple's life together (for example, birthdays and wedding anniversaries) may trigger a suicide attempt in those with suicidal ideation (Richardson et al., 1989).

Assessment

Suicidal Ideation

Suicide, rather than a topic to be avoided, is one that must be addressed head on with clients. Blazer (1986) suggested a graduated series of questions to be used to explore this topic.

- Have you ever thought life is not worth living? If answer is yes, then
- Have you ever considered harming yourself? If answer is yes, then
- Do you have plans for harming yourself? (If an older adult describes a plan, the risk increases.)
- Have you ever begun to act on that plan?
- Have you ever made a suicide attempt?

If the older adult responds affirmatively to these final questions and provides details of a plan, the risk of his or her carrying out a successful suicide escalates dramatically.

Lethality

In the presence of suicidal ideation, assessment of lethality will influence decisions about the amount of protection a client needs. Such an assessment will determine whether the client should be placed in a protected inpatient environment or can be maintained in the community.

Methods of self-destruction with high lethality include firearms, jumping, hanging, drowning, carbon monoxide poisoning, consumption of barbiturates or aspirin, car accidents, and extreme exposure to cold. Methods considered to be of low lethality include wrist cutting, breathing house gas, consumption of nonprescription drugs excluding aspirin and acetaminophen, and consumption of tranquilizers (Neville & Barnes, 1985).

The presence of a plan with high lethality plus access to the materials for implementation places the client's life in jeopardy and indicates a need for inpatient supervision.

Balance between Despair and Coping

In both inpatient and outpatient management of suicide, professionals must direct attention to the despair and pain experienced by the client. The client's own perception of the situation should be elicited. Does the client express only despair about the future or are there faint glimmers of hope? The nurse should explore the client's history of coping with past life stressors and disappointments. Are there successful strategies that can be drawn on? The presence or absence of support systems such as family, friends, and clergy should be evaluated. Can support systems be used on behalf of the client? Does the client feel alone or actually live alone most of the time? If actually alone, are periods of time without the presence of others sufficient for execution of a suicide plan?

Alcohol or Substance Abuse

Suicide is seen as an impulsive act (Blazer, 1988). Substance abuse affects perceptions, ability to reason, and judgment. Suicidal ideation in combination with substance abuse creates a lethal couple. Therapeutic intervention in the inpatient setting may be indicated if lethality and plan are not very low level or if strict supervision by community caregivers is not possible.

Interventions

Antisuicide Contract

The ideal suicide contract states: "No matter what happens, I will not kill myself, accidentally or on purpose, at any time" (Neville & Barnes, 1985, p. 16). Clients may try to set conditions on making such a statement. The nurse should consistently negotiate to move the client toward the unconditional contract. The nurse should negotiate for the least lethal, most prolife agreement. At a minimum, the client's promise to contact a professional or significant other before acting on feelings to terminate life should be obtained (Blazer, 1988; Neville & Barnes, 1985).

Time Periods Noted for Suicide

Weekends and holidays may pose a special risk for individuals who are considering self-destruction (Neville & Barnes, 1985). Mental health centers, senior centers, and other support facilities or socialization activities may be closed, thus depriving the individual of human contact and access to perspective on problems.

A common belief transmitted to generations of health care workers is to carefully watch depressed clients as the depressive symptoms lift. At this point, the person has enough energy to act on suicidal ideation. This caveat remains true today. However, health care workers must also direct attention to the 6- to 12-month period after inpatient hospitalization. Fawcell et al. (1987) studied 954 depressed clients who were being treated in five academic medical centers. They found that the highest frequency of suicides occurred in the period after successful treatment and discharge from the inpatient psychiatric setting. Similar trends in successful suicide attempts have been identified by other researchers. Fawcell et al. postulated that this accelerated suicide rate is due to withdrawal of inpatient support systems and failure to replace them with appropriate long-term follow-up care.

Protected Environment

Clients whose suicidal ideation is well developed should be protected from their own impulses by prudent precautions. Family members, trying to manage the client on an outpatient basis, should be taught to assess suicidal ideation and to identify symptoms or actions that indicate the need for immediate transfer to inpatient settings. Medications for both medical and psychiatric conditions should be monitored carefully, and pill counting may be instituted. Prescriptions may require tight control and should be written for limited amounts. Medications may have to be dispensed to the patient by family caregivers. Implements identified as a part of a suicide plan should be removed from the environment. Additionally, family members should consistently evaluate the client's mood and activities. Periods of great calm coupled with giving away prized possessions, writing wills, or making statements such as "Soon you won't have to worry about me" should trigger alarm and indicate a need for further professional follow-up.

Control of the environment can be intensified in the inpatient psychiatric setting. Medications are dispensed by staff members, who must watch to see that they are swallowed. If concern exists that the client will overdose by hoarding oral medications, they may be administered in liquid or injectable form. Suicide observation schedules may be instituted with criteria set for behaviors that require restraints, such as one-to-one restriction, 5- to 10-minute observations, 15-minute observations, 30-minute observations, or daily evaluation of risk (Bydlon-Brown & Billman, 1988).

Dugan (1987) cautions professionals not to become so involved with observation and checkoffs that the client's pain is not addressed. Nurses must acknowledge and recognize despair. Dugan entreats professionals to take time to sit with the client and honor mechanisms of catharsis like tears, ranting, raving, verbalizing, and circular grieving that leads to repetition of the same themes for days or weeks until the painful emotion is exorcised.

Appropriate Response to Suicidal Telephone Call

Nurses and other health professionals may receive a suicide call that must be managed carefully to promote a positive outcome. Neville and Barnes (1985) discuss several strategies that are effective in dealing with such a call. Strategies suggested by the authors follow.

1. The fact that the person has called is a positive sign. It indicates that ambivalence exists and that the person has not yet made a final decision. Keep the caller talking. Time may allow the professional to tip the scale in favor of life.
2. Remember that the caller is in control. Do not pressure the person to give name or address. Do not confront, argue with, or antagonize the caller. Do not use hostility or sarcasm. Any of these actions may cause the caller to disconnect.
3. Avoid reflection of feelings. Instead, use a direct problem-solving approach. Example:
   Caller: "I lost my job. I don't know where to get another."
   Counselor: (This) "Have you applied for any other?" *(Not this)* "You must be feeling upset about losing your job." (Neville & Barnes, 1985, p. 16)
4. Conduct assessment of suicide ideation, lethality, and coping abilities.
5. Attempt to negotiate a suicide contract.
6. Verbally acknowledge the extreme emotional pain of the caller.
7. Encourage ventilation of feelings. Accept feelings as expressed; do not place value judgments on them or use confrontative communication approaches.
8. Assist the caller to explore other things he or she could do instead of killing him or herself.
9. Verbally give positive recognition and reinforcement to all positive thoughts, feelings, or actions described by the caller.
10. Remind the caller that you are there, that you are listening, and that you care.

The nurse should avoid disrupting the call to consult with colleagues. A tablet should be kept by the phone to use in writing notes to convey information or to request help. Written records of the phone call should be kept for other professionals who may work with the caller during subsequent phone calls or in face-to-face interactions. Referrals made as a result of the suicide call should also be documented.

Carefully Planned or Benign Suicide

Older adults may not verbally express suicidal ideation, but such ideation may be extraordinarily sophisticated, as evidenced by one successful suicide for every four unsuccessful attempts. For many older adults, suicide may not be an impulsive act but a carefully considered decision based on quality of life issues. The daily newspaper abounds with stories of older spouses who perform "mercy killings" to terminate the life of a loved one whose life has lost quality and meaning. Some of these mercy killings are active homicide; others are assisted suicide.

Passive forms of terminating life are gaining acceptability in our society through the use of no-codes and the execution of living wills. However, the United States, unlike Japan, where suicide may be an honorable act, has not given support to active forms of suicide. Health professionals discuss clients who have hoarded drugs that were used to end their lives when pain became unbearable or when their physical condition rendered them dependent on others for basic needs and ADL. Organizations such as the Hemlock Society advocate euthanasia as a matter of public policy.

Ethical debates regarding active euthanasia have been stimulated by the right-to-die crusade of Jack Kevorkian, a pathologist from Michigan. Kevorkian has been dubbed Dr. Death for advocating and participating in assisted suicides for terminally ill clients. The publicity surrounding his involvement in an increasing number of deaths has prompted changes in Michigan law, which initially did not prohibit assisted suicide. Kevorkian's activities have been condemned by organized medicine, which highlights the extreme vulnerability of the terminally ill to destructive impulses precipitated by severe pain and/or depression. Kevorkian's opponents note that both depression and chronic pain, often the underlying causes of suicide in older adults, are treatable conditions. Therefore, Kevorkian's activities are viewed not as acts of mercy but as acts of murder (Colburn, 1993).

The controversy surrounding assisted suicide has initiated further examination of active euthanasia as a value. Ballot initiatives have been proposed to allow participation by medical practitioners in euthanasia. Such initiatives have begun to spell out the conditions of participation by health professionals in acts of mercy killing. These conditions often include evaluation of the client by a number of practitioners to assure that they are competent to make requests for assistance in terminating life. So far, these right-to-die ballot initiatives have been defeated. However, both professional and consumer groups continue to discuss and shape legislative proposals for the future.

The nurse must be alert to passive or benign forms of suicide frequently found among older adults. Death may occur as a result of a fall, wandering in front of a car, a fatal car crash, or malnutrition. Two clients from one caseload illustrate such benign suicides as shown on p. 161.

Follow-up Support for Survivors of a Suicide Victim

The nurse must work closely with survivors of a successful suicide victim. Spouses, midlife caregivers, and grandchildren of older adults need support as they seek to understand the meaning of a self-precipitated death. In addition to the normal stresses of bereavement, these survivors must struggle with pronounced feelings of guilt. Nurses should refer survivors of a suicide victim to community support groups.

Case Study **Benign Suicide Based on a Quality of Life Issue**

An older adult client was married for years to a man who had leukemia. During the process of treatment for leukemia, he received a number of blood transfusions and from one of these contracted acquired immunodeficiency syndrome (AIDS). The client contracted AIDS from her husband. When the client's husband died, she was left with limited financial resources. Azidothymidine (AZT) has been prescribed for her treatment but is very expensive. In her case, she must either allow a lien to be placed against her home or sell it to buy the medication that would prolong her life. The patient has made the decision to forgo treatment with AZT because she wishes to leave tangible assets to her children.

Case Study **Benign Suicide Precipitated by Family Indifference**

I made a home visit to follow up on a 76-year-old man who had recently been discharged from the hospital for treatment of a mild stroke. I was greeted at the door by a young adult who informed me that "my mother's husband's father is upstairs." In response to a query about how the client was doing, the young woman replied, "I don't know. I never go up there. He wets the bed and is disgusting." When I entered the client's upstairs bedroom, I found a home health aide completing a bath. The home health aide expressed concern about the client, whom she viewed as a nice old man and whose condition she described as having deteriorated progressively over the past 2 weeks. The home health aide reported that when the man was discharged from the hospital, he was oriented and able to assist with self-care activities. The day of my visit, he was lethargic and unresponsive. His skin turgor was poor with tenting, and the home health aide reported no known intake or output. The client obviously was suffering from severe dehydration. I placed a phone call to his daughter-in-law and elicited the following story. Until 3 weeks before the visit, the client was an active man and assumed responsibility for household chores, including meal preparation. His stroke was mild but left him with slight mobility impairment and some loss of bowel and bladder control, which he viewed as distressing. He required some in-home care. After discharge, heated arguments between the daughter-in-law and her husband occurred about who would take care of the client. This was a second marriage; the daughter-in-law refused to stay home and care for the client. Therefore the man's son assumed responsibility for his care but could only perform caregiving activities late at night when he was home from work. The client initially expressed concern that he was so much trouble to his son and expressed embarrassment that his son had to handle the results of his incontinence. The daughter-in-law and her daughter ceased to visit his room. The client then turned his face to the wall and began to refuse all food and fluids. At the conclusion of my home visit, he was admitted to an inpatient facility, where he subsequently died.

Intervention during bereavement may prevent the family pattern of suicide from being repeated as survivors reach advanced age.

Recognition of Issues of Control

Nurses must recognize that regardless of how much concern is displayed or how much vigilance is exercised, some clients successfully commit suicide. The choice—life or death—is ultimately in the client's hands. Health care professionals, family, and friends cannot assume responsibility for another's life, no matter how much they may wish to do so. They are not to blame when suicide occurs. Staff members who work with suicidal patients must realize the anxiety provoked by these clients and would do well to seek peer support when working with suicidal clients. Family members dealing with suicidal clients can benefit from involvement in suicide support groups and should be referred to them.

❖ *Bereavement*

Bereavement is a time in life that is dreaded but inevitable. It is a time of transition, marked by keeping the essence of what went before and using it as the foundation for creating a new and different life. It is a time of intense personal pain that when accepted and lived, leads to growth and change. Normal bereavement cannot be accelerated; it occurs at its own pace and in its own time. The bereavement period may be defined and sanctioned by cultural mores that establish rituals and activities to organize the overt expression of grief. However, the real process of grief and bereavement usually extends well beyond the time socially authorized and sanctioned. It is during the day-by-day evolution of the grieving process that the nurse must collaborate with the client for a successful outcome. Nursing intervention will be most necessary in the days and weeks after the casseroles have all been eaten, the flowers have faded, and the frenzied activities accompanying the funeral have ended.

Bereavement may be characterized by many of the symptoms present in depressive disorders. The most prevalent physical symptoms include insomnia, weight loss, and lack of energy. Survivors generally identify their emotional reaction to the loss as normal, even if some of the physical and psychic manifestations are unpleasant or frightening. Expressions of worthlessness, marked retardation of activity, functional impairment, and suicidal ideation are not usual expressions of normal grief and should alert the nurse to the need for evaluation of the client for major depression. Older adults involved in the normal bereavement process generally respond well to supportive interventions such as one-to-one contacts, involvement in support groups, activity therapy, and psychotherapy. Medications are not generally required in the management of normal bereavement. When sedatives or tranquilizers are given, they may block normal, necessary expressions of grief and ultimately delay the bereavement process or trigger dysfunctional grieving.

Significance of the Problem

Bereavement is part of the life of the older adult. It is estimated that 80,000 to 100,000 widows and widowers suffer from true depression nationwide (Burnside, 1988). The first year after loss of a spouse is commonly viewed as a time during which morbidity and mortality increase (Richter, 1984). Thus the period of bereavement is of special concern to health care professionals.

By the year 2000 there will be two women aged 65 and older for every man over 65 years of age in the United States (Brock & Sullivan, 1985). The bereaved are most likely to be widows. Among those 65 to 75 years of age, widows outnumber widowers 6:1; for those over 75, the female to male ratio is 5:1. Thus a society of widows exists within our country (Kalish, 1985).

Brock and Sullivan (1985) focused on the special difficulties of American widows. They note that women have not planned for and are poorly prepared for the crisis of widowhood, even though they will in all probability face it. They noted that many years will be lived as a widow and that because of the disproportion of the sexes in late life, the prospect of remarriage is slim. They identified widows at highest risk for dysfunctional bereavement as those whose identity had been defined solely by the role of wife and mother and who were financially dependent on their husbands. Successful bereavement outcomes were experienced by women who had adequate income coupled with the ability to manage finances, those who had been employed, those who had gained skills in social interactions, and those who were immersed in a close-knit, sex-segregated world of kin, neighbors, and friends after the spouse's death.

In a 2-year study of gender differences in bereavement, Lund, Caserta, and Diamond (1986) found that both sexes of older adults appear to share similar experiences in respect to major aspects of grief resolution and psychosocial adjustment. Lund et al. further reported that 70% of the study population, regardless of sex, reported loneliness to be the greatest single difficulty after the death of a spouse. Twenty percent of subjects reported difficulty in managing responsibilities that had formerly been allocated to the deceased spouse. Men reported problems with meal preparation, cleaning, and grocery shopping, whereas women struggled with yard work, home repairs, car repairs, and balancing checkbooks. Lund et al. (1986) found that bereavement is a long-term experience that does not end at 2 years. At the end of the study period, subjects still exhibited signs of avoidance, disbelief, anger, and difficulty making a transition to new roles and responsibilities. They also noted a consistent tendency in the older adult to report simultaneous occurrence of competing and conflicting behaviors during bereavement. The older adults reported feeling mild depression, shock, anger, and confusion while simultaneously feeling confident about self and emerging coping skills.

Breckenridge, Gallagher, Thompson, and Peterson (1986) found no difference in depressive symptoms (sadness, tearfulness, dissatisfaction with self, insomnia, weight loss, and poor appetite) reported by bereaved elders who expected spousal death and those for whom death was sudden. However, these researchers noted that the bereavement process for older adults who lost a spouse as a result of a lengthy chronic illness was more difficult and turbulent than that of the bereaved spouse confronted with a sudden, unanticipated death.

Although the greatest attention has been focused on spousal loss, the health care professional must not overlook bereavement triggered by the death of adult children, grandchildren, siblings, and friends of the older adult. These deaths may occur in rapid succession and leave the older client enmeshed in constant bereavement or progressing through a series of bereavements. In addition, the death of a beloved pet and companion may trigger expressions of grief and loss in the isolated, older adult. Grief, loss, and bereavement can also occur as a response to loss of something tangible or intangible that is highly regarded. Such a loss may be a personal object, a social role, or a physical attribute.

Goals of the Bereavement Period

The survivor must accomplish four major goals during the bereavement period:

- ◆ Acceptance of the reality that death (loss) has occurred
- ◆ Acceptance of the fact that grief is emotionally and physically painful
- ◆ Adjustment to an environment that no longer includes the deceased
- ◆ Withdrawal of emotional energy invested in the deceased and subsequent reinvestment of that energy in new persons, objects, or activities.

Assessment

Symptoms that occur during the bereavement process may be divided into four major categories: (1) physical expression of grief, (2) cognitive expression of grief, (3) affective expression of grief, and (4) behavioral expressions of grief; these are described by Kalish (1985).

Characteristics of Bereavement

The characteristics of bereavement are considered normal and should abate over time. The older adult may tend to replace some of the affective symptoms (for example, sadness) with somatic complaints, just as in other types of depression. The older adult is also more likely to demonstrate self-isolation and hostility toward friends and family (Richter, 1984).

Physical Expressions of Grief
The bodily sensations of grief are these:

- ◆ Pangs—waves of somatic distress that last for 20 minutes to a hour at a time. These are characterized by choking with shortness of breath, need for sighing, empty feeling in abdomen, lack of muscular power, and tension or mental pain. Pangs may begin a few hours after the death and last approximately 2 weeks.

- Numbness—lacking feeling or having what is felt to be appropriate feeling.
- Depersonalization.
- Dry mouth.
- Hypersensitivity to noise.

Cognitive Expressions of Grief

Cognitive aspects of grief are these:

- Disbelief
- Confusion
- Preoccupation with thoughts of the deceased
- Encounters with the deceased in ways that make the person seem to be living
- Tendency to review repeatedly all of the events leading up to the death. This may include trying to find some meaning or significance in the death.

Affective Expressions of Grief

Feelings of grief may include the following:

- Sadness, sorrow, depression (mild to moderate).
- Relief-especially if deceased was ill for an extended time.
- Anger and guilt-anger may be accompanied by a sense of abandonment and separation anxiety. Expressions of anger may elicit guilt because the survivor feels that it is inappropriate to be angry at someone who has died. Anger may also be displaced by blaming the deceased for not trying hard enough and blaming God or health care professionals. Guilt may be expressed by concern that the survivor should have or could have prevented the death by taking different actions. Guilt may occur when benefits are received as a result of the decedent's death, such as monetary gain and acquisition of personal possessions or property. Finally, guilt may be engendered by survival itself.
- Denial-expressed by refusing to believe in the reality of the death. Plans that include the decedent are still made. The environment and possessions are kept exactly as the decedent left them, and the term "we" is used when talking about the present or future.

Behavioral Expressions of Grief

Obvious behavioral expressions of grief are these:

- Depressed appetite
- Sleep disturbances (insomnia or sudden awakening)
- Visiting places or carrying reminders of the decreased or studiously avoiding doing so
- Social withdrawal
- Crying
- Dreams of the deceased, both pleasant and unpleasant

- ◆ Frequent sighing
- ◆ Absentminded behavior
- ◆ Inability to concentrate
- ◆ Restless overactivity
- ◆ Treasuring objects that belonged to the deceased
- ◆ Searching-perception that others look like the deceased or repetitive recall of the decreased triggered by both present and past events

Interventions

The nurse should distinguish between normal and abnormal grieving. If marked or morbid preoccupation with self-reproach or guilt, marked retardation of activity, or suicidal ideation are present, or if characteristics of normal early bereavement do not progressively abate or are excessive (such as the appearance of delusions), the client should be referred for evaluation for major depressive illness. In management of end-stage physically ill clients, the nurse should also be alert to anticipatory bereavement or anticipatory grief that has gone awry. If caregivers and family members enter a period of bereavement before the death of the client and that mourning period is successful, the client may be abandoned before death actually occurs. Such an untoward event may occur in the very old and institutionalized (Kalish, 1985).

The nurse should allow the client to express feelings and emotions and to verbally review the life and death of the deceased by listening, acknowledging, and supporting feelings. The nurse should suggest involvement of the bereaved in community support groups such as those for widows and widowers and cognitive or behavioral therapy groups.

The nurse should provide information for the clients and family on community resources that can assist with adjustments in lifestyle. These may include senior centers, adult day care programs, church groups, financial planners, women in transition organizations, and university for seniors programs.

The client and family members should be helped to distinguish normal from abnormal feelings. Often the painful emotions and physical expressions of grief lead survivors to fear that they are losing their minds. For the older adult, the fear of losing one's mind may lead to fear of loss of independence. This fear may precipitate alcohol or drug abuse to blunt the physical and psychological discomfort of grieving. Clients should be assured that bereavement symptoms are a normal part of grieving and that they will abate with time. The nurse can help clients to explore options and alternatives and support problem solving as new lifestyle situations arise. Successes and accomplishments in lifestyle changes of the survivor should be celebrated with positive feedback, both verbal and nonverbal; hugs are not forbidden.

If the nurse identifies caregivers who are managing end-stage illness of loved ones before the terminal event, referral to a hospice program should be explored. Family members will then receive bereavement support services after death. In some locations, bereavement counseling may be available even if the family was not a client of the hospice before the decedent's death.

If the survivor is socially isolated, the nurse should consult the client about referral to telephone or friendly visitor programs. Follow-up should be continued for at least a year, with special attention to making contacts or providing that they be made with the survivor on holidays, wedding anniversaries, and on the anniversary date of the decedent's death.

The nurse should encourage the client to manage somatic symptoms with attention to basic bodily needs such as adequate nutrition and rest. Somatic symptoms that cause physical illness or exacerbation of chronic conditions should be referred to the physician for further diagnosis and treatment.

Nurses should assist survivors to identify sources of emotional support and identify ways of requesting such support. Many older adults do not want to bother anyone and will not seek the human consolation that is needed during bereavement. Social support must be supplied if major depression is to be prevented. Social support may be found among family members, friends, clergy, and mental health centers.

Nurses who work with the bereaved on a consistent basis, such as in a hospice program or who must use increased emotional reserves to deal with one special client, should seek peer support for themselves.

❖ *Summary*

Depression is a significant problem for older adults. Fortunately, only a small percentage of clients develop a severe depressive episode that requires inpatient psychiatric treatment. Mild and moderate depression will be endemic in over half of the older adults in long-term care facilities; these individuals should be identified. However, the majority of older adults will not be seen by the nurse in acute care units or in extended care facilities. These individuals will reside in their own homes or be seen in community settings. In this noninstitutionalized population, over one third will experience periods of mild to moderate depression. Some older adults will experience these symptoms in association with physical illness or as an untoward reaction to medications. Relief will be provided for these clients when the underlying medical condition is treated or when the offending medication is withdrawn. For the majority of the remaining clients, the depressive episodes will be an adjustment to loss and bereavement or a response to loneliness and isolation.

Suicide is a final and dramatic testimony to despair. This act is perceived by the client as the final solution for hopelessness. Suicide is linked with severe depressive episodes and occurs more frequently when drug or alcohol abuse is present. Suicidal ideation may not be verbalized by older clients; thus, family, friends, and health care professionals may be quite surprised when confronted by a death efficiently executed. Older adults commit suicide at a rate disproportionate to their representation in the population. For every four suicide attempts, one is completed. Suicides among older adults can be impulsive, but an alarming number are carefully planned and are the result of quality of life decisions. Finally, suicide tends to be underreported among older adults because benign forms of suicide, frequently seen by health professionals and described by family caregivers, are not a part of current epidemiological tabulation.

Bereavement and associated adjustment reactions are normal responses to loss and grief. These reactions are accompanied by some of the symptoms of mild or moderate depression and selected expressions of grief unique to the psychic assimilation of painful loss. The bereavement period appears to paralyze the survivor temporarily. In reality, successful bereavement is not a time of stagnation but a time of transition from an old pattern of living to a new one. During normal bereavement, depressive symptoms abate as lifestyle adjustments are accomplished.

The nurse's primary task in the management of depression, suicide, and bereavement is prevention. Nurses should promote educational programs that provide clients with skills to manage life transitions and crises. Since many life crises are predictable and certain, strategies can be implemented as early as midlife to reduce the negative impact of change in later years.

When the development of depressive symptoms cannot be prevented or when these symptoms are a normal reaction to a life event, the nurse must act to contain the depression in the mild to moderate range. Early identification and treatment of depressive episodes is critical. In the less severe stages of depression, older adults respond well to interventions that involve socialization, such as activity therapy and participation in small task-oriented or support groups. For older adults afflicted with more severe depression or suicidal ideation, aggressive treatment must be supported by the nurse. Somatic therapies such as antidepressant drug treatment and electroconvulsive therapy may be appropriate and linked effectively to psychotherapeutic interventions.

In controlling depression and the related manifestations of bereavement or suicide, nurses collaborate with clients, family caregivers, and other professional discipliness to enable the client to access appropriate services. Nurses also coordinate existing programs to form a continuum of services for clients in their care. When treatment and support services are not available, nurses participate with members of other disciplines to develop appropriate community programs. Ultimately, the responsibility for relief from depressive episodes must be assigned to the client because active involvement in treatment methods is essential for cure to occur. The nurse simply serves as a facilitator.

❖ *References*

American Psychiatric Association. (1980). *Diagnostic and statistical manual* (3rd ed.). Washington, DC: Author.

American Psychiatric Association. (1994). *Diagnostic and statistical manual* (4th ed.). Washington, DC: Author.

Black J and Matassarin-Jacobs E. (1993). Luckman and Sorenson's *Medical-surgical nursing: A psychophysiologic approach* (4th ed.). Philadelphia: Saunders.

Blazer, D. (1986). Depression: Paradoxically, a cause for hope. *Generations, 10*(3), 21-23.

Blazer, D. (1988). *Diagnosis and management of the suicidal older adult.* Proceedings of the American Society on Aging Regional Seminar, Mental Health and Aging. Philadelphia: American Society on Aging.

Blazer, D., Hughes, D. C., & George, L. K. (1987). The epidemiology of depression in an elderly community population. *The Gerontologist, 27*(3), 281-287.

Breckenridge, J. N., Gallagher, D., Thompson, L. W., & Peterson, J. (1986). Characteristic depressive symptoms of bereaved elders. *Journal of Gerontology, 41*(2), 163-168.

Brock, A. M., & Sullivan, P. O. (1985). From wife to widow: Role transition in the elderly. *Journal of Psychosocial Nursing, 23*(12), 6-12.

Burnside, I. (1988). *Nursing and the aged* (3rd ed.). New York: McGraw-Hill.

Bydlon-Brown, B., & Billman, R. (1988). At risk for suicide. *American Journal of Nursing, 88*(10), 1358-1361.

Campbell, L. (1986). Acute care in the hospital. *American Journal of Nursing, 86*(3), 288-291.

Colburn, D. (1993, September 14). Assisted suicide. *Washington Post Health.* p. 7.

Copel, L. C. (1988). Loneliness. *Journal of Psychosocial Nursing, 26*(1), 14-19.

de la Cruz, L. (1986). On loneliness and the elderly. *Journal of Gerontological Nursing, 12*(11), 24-27.

Dreyfus, J. K. (1987). The prevalence of depression in women in an ambulatory setting. *Nurse Practitioner, 12*(4), 34-50.

Dugan, D. O. (1987). Death and dying: Emotional, spiritual, and ethical support for patients and families. *Journal of Psychosocial Nursing, 25*(7), 21-29.

Fawcell, J., Scheftner, W., Clark, D., Hedeker, D., Gibbons, R., & Coryell, W. (1987). Clinical predictors of suicide in patients with major affective disorders. *American Journal of Psychiatry, 144*(1), 35-40.

Ferry, M. E., Lamy, P. P., & Becker, L. A. (1985). Physician's knowledge of prescribing for the elderly. *Journal of the American Geriatrics Society, 33*(9), 616-625.

Field, W. E. (1985). Physical causes of depression. *Journal of Psychosocial Nursing, 23*(10), 7-11.

Fogel, B. S., & Fretwell, M. D. (1985). Reclassification of depression in the medically ill elderly. *Journal of the American Geriatrics Society, 33*(6), 446-448.

Gallagher, D., Rose, J., Rivera, P., Lovett, S., & Thompson, L. (1989). Prevalence of depression in family caregivers. *The Gerontologist, 29*(4), 449-456.

Garrett, J. E. (1987). Multiple losses in older adults. *Journal of Gerontological Nursing, 13*(8), 8-12.

Gift, A., & McCrone, S. (1993). Depression in patients with COPD. *Heart and Lung, 22*(4), 289-297.

Goff, D. C., & Jenike, M. A. (1986). Treatment-resistant depression in the elderly. *Journal of the American Geriatrics Society, 34*(1), 63-70.

Goldsmith, J., Jackson, D., Kramer, M., Brenner, B., Stiles, D., Tweed, D., Holzer, D., & MacKenzie, E. (1986). Strategies for investigating effects of residential context. *Research on Aging, 8*(4), 609-631.

Groom, D. (1993). Elder care: A diagnostic model for failure to thrive. *Journal of Gerontological Nursing, 19*(6), 12-16.

Kalish, R. A. (1985). *Death, grief, and caring relationships*. Monterey, CA: Brooks/Cole.

Kennedy, G., Kelman, H., & Thomas, C. (1990). The emergence of depressive symptoms in late life: The importance of declining health and increasing disability. *Journal of Community Health, 15*(2), 93-104.

Krause, D. (1986). Stress and sex differences in depressive symptoms among older adults. *Journal of Gerontology, 41*(6), 727-731.

Loebl, S., & Spratto, G. R. (1986). *The nurses drug handbook*. New York: Wiley and Sons.

Lund, D. A., Caserta, M. S., & Diamond, M. F. (1986). Gender differences through two years of bereavement among the elderly. *The Gerontologist, 26*(3), 314-319.

Mansfield, J., & Marx, M. (1993). Pain and depression in the nursing home: Corroborating results. *Journal of Gerontology, 48*(2), p96-p97.

Manton, K. G., Blazer, D. G., & Woodbury, M. A. (1987). Suicide in middle age and later life: Sex and race specific time table and cohort analysis. *Journal of Gerontology, 42*(2), 219-227.

Matteson, M. A., & McConnell, E. S. (1988). *Gerontological nursing: Concepts and practice.* Philadelphia: Saunders.

Meyers, B. S., & Alexopoulas, G. S. (1988). Geriatric depression. *Medical Clinics of North America, 72*(4), 847-863.

Mignogna, M. (1986). Integrity versus despair: The treatment of depression in the elderly. *Clinical Therapeutics, 8*(3), 248-259.

Minot, S. R. (1986). Depression: What does it mean? *American Journal of Nursing, 86*(3), 284-288.

Neville, D., & Barnes, S. (1985). The suicidal phone call. *Journal of Psychosocial Nursing, 23*(8), 14-18.

NIH Consensus Panel. (1992). Diagnosis and treatment of depression in late life. *Journal of the American Medical Association, 268*(8), 1018-1024.

Osato, E., Stone, J., Phillips, S., & Winne, D. (1993). Clinical manifestations: Failure to thrive in the elderly. *Journal of Gerontological Nursing, 19*(8), 28-34.

Parmelee, P., & Katz, I. (1992). "Caregiving" to depressed persons: A relevant concept? *The Gerontologist, 32*(4), 436-437.

Parmelee, P., Katz, I., & Lawton, M. (1991). The relation of pain to depression among institutionalized aged. *Journal of Gerontology, 46*(1), p15-p21.

Parmelee, P., Katz, I., & Lawton, M. (1992). Incidence of depression in long-term care settings. *Journal of Gerontology, 47*(6), m189-m196.

Pfeiffer, E. (1985). Some basic principles of working with older patients. *Journal of the American Geriatrics Society, 33*(1), 44-47.

Richardson, R., Lowenstein, S., & Weissberg, M. (1989). Coping with the suicidal elderly: A physician's guide. *Geriatrics, 44*(9), 43-51.

Richter, J. M. (1984). Crisis of mate loss in the elderly. *Advances in Nursing Science, 6*(4), 45-54.

Ronsman, K. M. (1987). Therapy for depression. *Journal of Gerontological Nursing, 13*(12), 18-25.

Ronsman, K. M. (1988). Pseudodementia. *Geriatric Nursing, 9*(1), 50-52.

Ryan, M., & Patterson, J. (1987). Loneliness in the elderly. *Journal of Gerontological Nursing, 13*(5), 6-12.

St. Pierre, J., Craven, R., & Bruno, P. (1986). Late life depression: A guide for assessment. *Journal of Gerontological Nursing, 12*(7) 5-10.

Thompson, L., & Gallagher, D. (1986). Psychotherapy for late life depression. *Generations, 10*(3), 38-41.

Waller, M., & Griffin, M. (1984). Group therapy for depressed elders. *Geriatric Nursing, 5*(7), 309-311.

Weiss, I. K., Nagel, C. L., & Aronson, M. K. (1986). Applicability of depression scales to the old, old person. *Journal of the American Geriatrics Society, 34*(3), 215-218.

Williamson, G., & Schultz, R. (1992). Pain, activity restriction, and symptoms of depression among community residing elderly adults. *Journal of Gerontology, 47*(6), 367-372.

Chapter 7

❖ *Delirium, Dementia, and Other Cognitive Disorders*

Anne Langston Lind*

It is generally accepted that there are some changes in intellectual functions in older persons just as there is some loss in physical abilities with aging. Normal aging, however, does not include intellectual impairment, depression, confusion, hallucinations, or delusions. These symptoms are due to disease and indicate the need for diagnosis and treatment. Intellectual impairment in the older person may be due to conditions that can be cured, conditions that can be improved with treatment, or conditions that have a relentless downhill course (National Institute on Aging Task Force, 1980).

The *Diagnostic and Statistical Manual of Mental Disorders* (DSM-IV) of the American Psychiatric Association (1994) groups conditions previously identified as organic mental disorders into delirium, dementia, and amnestic and other cognitive disorders; mental disorders due to a general medical condition; and substance-related disorders (p. 123). Impaired cognition is the primary characteristic of dementia, delirium, and amnestic disorder, but Detwiler (1993) emphasizes that other disorders may also be characterized by impaired cognition. These disorders have the common feature of disturbed behavior because of disease or dysfunction of the brain, either transient or permanent.

* With appreciation to Mira Kirk Nelson for her contribution to this chapter.

Cognitive disorders are a heterogeneous group; therefore no single description can characterize them all. The differences in clinical presentation reflect differences in the localization, mode of onset, progression, duration, and nature of the underlying pathophysiological process.

The organic factor responsible for these disorders may be a primary disease of the brain or a systemic illness that affects the brain. Use of or withdrawal of a psychoactive substance also can cause these disorders. Another cause can be the use of a toxic agent that is either currently disturbing brain function or has had some long-lasting effect on the brain.

This chapter will discuss some of the major types of cognitive impairment that are organically based and explore the primary degenerative dementias, including Alzheimer's disease, Parkinson's disease, Huntington's disease, Pick's disease, and Creutzfeldt-Jakob disease. In addition, vascular dementia (multi-infarct dementia), transient ischemic attack, and delirium will be examined. A discussion of the nursing process used with these organically based disorders will conclude the chapter.

❖ *Dementia*

Dementia is a broad category of disorders related to particular neurological diseases that characteristically appear in older age. These conditions are characterized by loss of intellectual ability and are severe enough to interfere significantly with usual activities of daily living, work, or social relationships. Memory, judgment, and abstract thought are impaired, but the level of consciousness is not affected as it is in delirium. Dementia may be temporary or permanent and is the result of a disease or an abnormal condition in which an underlying causative factor is sought. If the client is diagnosed and treated promptly, the dementia may clear without any long-term effects. The conditions of approximately 25% to 35% of individuals complaining of memory problems have a treatable cause. In some cases such as primary degenerative dementia of the Alzheimer's type, no specific causative organic factor may be found (American Psychiatric Association, 1994; Cohen & Eisdorfer, 1986a).

Diagnosis

Early diagnosis of dementia is crucial. If the disease or condition is treatable, the problem may be reversed if detected soon enough. If the dementia is irreversible and due to Alzheimer's disease or a related disorder, early diagnosis leads to early intervention and treatment. Early diagnosis allows patients to be in the best position to deal with the impact of dementia on their futures. If an accurate diagnosis is delayed, the consequences may cause many problems, such as emotional distress, family upheaval, and even physical harm to the patient or others. Because there is no specific diagnostic test for dementia, the physician must rely on careful assessment of history, physical examination, laboratory and neurological tests, and observation by health care professionals, family, and friends of the client (Souder, 1992). Scales used to assess cognitive functioning are the Brief Cognitive Rating Scale, Global Deterioration Scale, Clinical Dementia Rating, and Alzheimer's Disease Assessment Scale (Abraham & Neundorfer, 1990).

One of the primary features of dementia is deterioration of intellectual abilities of sufficient severity to interfere with social or occupational functioning. Memory loss is usually the first sign of dementia, and deterioration often continues until the memory is no longer testable. Another feature of primary importance to the disorder is loss of impulse control (Chiverton, 1990). See Box 7-1 for the diagnostic criteria for dementia of the Alzheimer's type.

Impaired abstract thinking is indicated by reduced capacity for generalization, differentiation, logical reasoning, and concept formation. Events that occurred many years ago tend to be remembered better than events that occurred more recently, although this pattern of loss is variable. Impaired judgment is often an early sign of the disorder and may cause great concern among family members and associates, especially if they do not understand the nature of the underlying disorder. Control of aggressive and sexual impulses is reduced, and the capacity for empathic understanding of significant others gradually deteriorates. A previously caring and responsive person often becomes extremely self-centered and oblivious to the needs of others. The change in the client's personality can be very distressing to family members (Weiner and Svetlik, 1991).

Lucas, Steele, and Bognanni (1986) described mood disturbances common in patients with dementia syndromes. A patient may suffer from emotional lability, which is characterized by periods of crying or laughing for minutes to hours without any explanation but usually associated with environmental stimuli. The emotional lability may appear as sadness, irritability, combativeness, or inappropriate elation. Scales that assess mood and behavior include the Geriatric Depression Scale and the Dementia Mood Assessment (Abraham & Neundorfer, 1990).

Pseudobulbar palsy, a mood disturbance, is a pathological expression of emotion associated with bilateral lesions in the corticobulbar tracts in the cerebral hemisphere or in the brain stem. It is characterized by an uncontrollable expression of emotion, usually crying. When presented with some particular stimulus the patient will start to cry for a period of seconds to minutes. The crying is unrelated to the patient's current level of feeling. When questioned, the patient does not know why he is crying and feels embarrassed that he is not able to control it.

Another mood disorder sometimes associated with dementia is mania. People who are manic have an abnormal elevation of mood and are often mistaken for good-humored, outgoing people who are annoying with their incessant activity, energy, and enthusiasm. In mild cases manic behavior may be seen as meddlesome interference in the affairs of others. In more severe cases the client may be provoked into violent and destructive behavior.

Delusions and hallucinations are present at times in dementia syndrome. Delusions are false beliefs such as fear of poisoning or persecution; hallucinations are sensory experiences occurring most frequently in the auditory or visual spheres. Abnormal behaviors may occur, as clients often act on the content of the belief or

---

Box 7-1 **Diagnostic Criteria for Dementia of the Alzheimer's Type**

A. The development of multiple cognitive deficits manifested by both
   1. memory impairment (impaired ability to learn new information or to recall previously learned information)
   2. one (or more) of the following cognitive disturbances:
      a. aphasia (language disturbance)
      b. apraxia (impaired ability to carry out motor activities despite intact motor function)
      c. agnosia (failure to recognize or identify objects despite intact sensory function)
      d. disturbance in executive functioning (i.e., planning, organizing, sequencing, abstracting)

B. The cognitive deficits in Criteria A1 and A2 each cause significant impairment in social or occupational functioning and represent a significant decline from a previous level of functioning.

C. The course is characterized by gradual onset and continuing cognitive decline.

D. The cognitive deficits in Criteria A1 and A2 are not due to any of the following:
   1. other central nervous system conditions that cause progressive deficits in memory and cognition (e.g., cerebrovascular disease, Parkinson's disease, Huntington's disease, subdural hematoma, normal-pressure hydrocephalus, brain tumor)
   2. systemic conditions that are known to cause dementia (e.g., hypothyroidism, vitamin B_{12} or folic acid deficiency, niacin deficiency, hypercalcemia, neurosyphilis, HIV infection)
   3. substance-induced conditions

E. The deficits do not occur exclusively during the course of a delirium.

F. The disturbance is not better accounted for by another Axis I disorder (e.g., Major Depressive Disorder, Schizophrenia).

From American Psychiatric Association (1994). *Diagnostic and Statistical Manual of Mental Disorders* (4th ed.) pp. 142-143. Washington, DC: author; with permission.

---

sensory experience. Hallucinations and delusions must be described and documented accurately to include frequency, duration, content, and the client's behavior and reaction to these abnormal experiences. Delirium is a common cause of hallucinations and delusions.

Illusions are common in patients with dementia syndromes. Illusions are misrepresentations of sensory perceptions that are triggered by actual environmental stimuli, whereas hallucinations have no source in fact. Accurate observation and documentation will distinguish between a visual illusion and a visual hallucination and can determine the correct intervention strategy (Lucas et al., 1986).

Reversible Causes

The reversible causes of dementia are listed in Box 7-2. Many of these disorders can be cured and others can be substantially alleviated. Some common causes of impaired cognitive function are therapeutic drug intoxication, depression, and metabolic or infectious disorders (Weiner, Tintner, & Goodkin, 1991).

Drug-related problems are one of the most common causes of cognitive impairment. If these problems are detected early and corrected, the disturbances can usually be corrected. Medication can cause either dementia or delirium. A variety of medications have been implicated, including digitalis, diuretics, analgesics, sedatives, oral antidiabetics, anti-inflammatory agents, and psychopharmacological drugs. Diuretics used in the treatment of high blood pressure may cause an electrolyte imbalance and hence cognitive problems. Drugs such as digitalis, hormone preparations such as thyroid, and insulin are commonly taken over many years. Long-term use of medications can lead to problems in later life, since side effects can damage cognitive abilities in some persons (Cohen & Eisdorfer, 1986a; National Institute on Aging Task Force, 1980).

Depression is the most common mental health problem among older adults. Although the common symptoms of depression are similar to those in younger persons, older patients may deny depressed mood and instead have multiple somatic complaints, hypochondriasis, or pain. Depression in older people may be accompanied by a mild to profound reversible dementia. Severe cases of this type of dementia make it extremely difficult to distinguish depression from a progressive degenerative dementia, and misdiagnosis is not uncommon (National Institute on Aging Task Force, 1980).

Depression can cause significant cognitive impairment, especially in the older adult. Much of the research on cognitive assessment for dementia has focused on methods of differentiating between depression and primary degenerative dementias. Research indicates that depression and dementia coexist in approximately 25% of cognitively impaired older adults. Differentiating those with depression alone from persons with coexisting depression and dementia is extremely difficult (Office of Technology Assessment Task Force, 1988). Depression is discussed more fully in Chapter 6.

According to Cohen and Eisdorfer (1986a, 1986b), infectious disorders are frequent causes of dementia. An illness accompanied by fever, regardless of cause, may precipitate problems in memory and thinking in persons of any age. Older persons with even modest infections may become confused and lethargic, eat sparingly, and find little pleasure in social activities. This may cause the person to ignore requests to do many things, to refuse to answer questions, and to give the false

Box 7-2 **Causes of Potentially Reversible Dementia**

Psychiatric
    Depression
    Schizophrenia
    Ganser's syndrome
    Malingering
    Toxic
    Drugs (prescription or street)
    Alcohol
    Chemical poisoning (arsenic, mercury, lead, lithium, and other metals;
        organic compounds and solvents)
Metabolic
    Azotemia and renal failure (diuretics, dehydration, obstruction, hypoka-
        lemia)
    Hyponatremia (diuretics, excess ADH, salt wasting, water intoxication)
    Volume depletion
    Hypoglycemia or hyperglycemia
    Hepatic encephalopathy
    Hypothyroidism or hyperthyroidism
    Hyperparathyroidism
    Cushing's syndrome
    Wilson's disease
    Acute intermittent porphyria
    Infection and/or fever (in elders, pneumonia, urinary tract infection)
    Anoxia
    Anemia
    Congestive heart failure
    Chronic obstructive pulmonary disease
    Vitamin deficiencies (B_{12}, folic acid, thiamine, niacin)
    Brain disorders
    Stroke
    Trauma (subdural hematoma, post-concussion syndrome)
    AIDS and opportunistic infections
    Other infections (neurosyphilis, chronic meningitis, brain abscess, pro-
        gressive multifocal leukoencephalopathy)
    Neoplasm (primary or metastatic)
    Cerebral vasculitis
    Normal pressure hydrocephalus
    Multiple sclerosis

Adapted from Weiner MF, Tintner RJ, & Goodkin K. (1991). Differential diagnosis. In MF Weiner (Ed.). *The dementias: Diagnosing and management* (pp. 77-106). Washington DC: The American Psychiatric Press; with permission.

appearance of progressive dementia. Acquired immunodeficiency syndrome (AIDS) has a direct effect upon the central nervous system because of invasion of the central nervous system by the virus and subsequent infections of the central nervous system and other organ systems. AIDS dementia complex, a very serious complication, is a severe dementia in more than half of affected patients, and it has a survival prognosis of 1 to 6 months (Goodkin, 1991).

Many physical disorders are the result of disturbances in the body's metabolism, the chemical reactions by which the materials necessary for life are synthesized, utilized, and broken down for excretion or reuse. Disruption of metabolism can be caused by many things such as a shortage of enzymes and minerals, dehydration, or poor diet. A person with thyroid problems may feel run-down, have difficulty concentrating, and become forgetful. A disturbance in the body's electrolytes such as sodium and potassium may result from dehydration, excessive fluid consumption, or kidney problems. A change in mental state may be caused by too much or too little sodium or potassium.

Malnutrition will eventually lead to significant metabolic changes that are often first observed as memory loss or other cognitive problems. Vitamin deficiencies are common in older persons, and it is estimated that at least 10% of all persons over the age of 65 are deficient in vitamin A, vitamin C, thiamine, and riboflavin.

Visual and hearing losses have a significant impact on the ability of an individual to understand and to answer questions. Older persons with sensory impairments may appear unable to answer questions, which significantly reduces their ability to communicate effectively.

Social isolation and sensory deprivation are major causes of confusion. Deprivation of human touch, activity, and excitement is experienced by many older persons who live alone and has a potent effect on their behavior. Without rewarding relationships the mind may become dull, forgetful, or confused. Living apart from other people may create a major problem for older persons suffering social and sensory deprivation (Cohen & Eisdorfer, 1986a).

Irreversible Causes

Not all of the disorders leading to intellectual loss are reversible. When reversible causes of dementia have been ruled out, the differential diagnosis between Alzheimer's disease, cerebrovascular diseases, and other brain diseases that cause dementia may be easy or quite difficult. Cerebrovascular diseases involve problems in the circulation of blood to the brain. Small strokes may occur in persons with irreversible dementias. These strokes and a reduction in flow of blood to parts of the brain lead to memory loss (Cohen & Eisdorfer, 1986a).

Primary Degenerative Dementias

Alzheimer's disease is the most prevalent of all irreversible dementias. Other irreversible dementias include some forms of Parkinson's disease, Huntington's disease, Pick's disease, and Creutzfeldt-Jakob disease.

Alzheimer's Disease

Alzheimer's disease is a progressive disorder of the central nervous system with an average duration of 5 to 8 years from onset to death. Like other dementing illnesses, it is an irreversible, insidious, life-threatening disorder that involves a progressive loss in cognitive ability, self-care skills, and adaptation that ultimately leads to the death of the afflicted individual (Kermis, 1986). At this time there are no known drugs or other treatments that can stop or reverse the progress of Alzheimer's disease (Cohen & Eisdorfer, 1986a). The Alzheimer's Association (see Appendix G) has described Alzheimer's disease as the fourth leading cause of adult deaths, with 4 million Americans afflicted by this devastating, expensive disease (Alzheimer's Disease and Related Disorders Association, 1992). Studies of risk factors associated with Alzheimer's disease have shown positive associations with a family history of dementia, familial Down's syndrome, increased maternal age at birth, and a history of head trauma (Amadeuci, Falcini, & Lippi, 1992).

Alzheimer's disease was first described in 1907 by Alois Alzheimer (1864-1915), a neuropathologist in Tübingen, Germany, who detailed its characteristic neurological changes in the brain of a 51-year-old woman with the disease. Her symptoms began with memory loss, disorientation, depression, hallucinations, and profound dementia. She died 4½ years after onset of the disease. In a postmortem examination brain atrophy and distortions in the cortical neurofibrils were found. These distortions were later named Alzheimer's tangles and are sometimes called Alzheimer-type changes (Burnside, 1988).

The course of Alzheimer's disease usually begins after age 70 and progresses downward. Between 2% and 4% of the population over age 65 is assumed to have Alzheimer's disease. This prevalence increases steadily with age, and the disease is believed to affect 20% to 30% of the population who reach age 85. It is believed that Alzheimer's disease accounts for 50% to 70% of all older patients diagnosed as demented. Dementia of the Alzheimer's type is believed to be the fourth or fifth leading cause of death in persons over age 65, accounting for 90,000 to 100,000 deaths per year in this age group (Kermis, 1986).

Dementia of the Alzheimer's type is found more frequently in women than in men, and there appears to be a familial predisposition to the disease. Genetic predisposition to the disease has not been definitively proved, but studies have identified structural and biochemical similarities between Alzheimer's disease and Down's syndrome. If they survive, Down's syndrome patients eventually develop Alzheimer's disease (Kermis, 1986).

Alzheimer's disease is difficult to diagnose, especially in its early stages when it resembles many other disorders. A definite diagnosis of Alzheimer's disease can be made only on autopsy or biopsy of brain tissue, where the distinctive neurological changes in the brain can be noted. The main characteristics include neurofibrillary tangles, neuritic plaques, and granulovacuolar bodies.

Neurofibrillary tangles are made up of insoluble protein in nerve cells of the brain. Neuritic plaques occurring outside of damaged brain nerve cells consist of beta-amyloid protein mixed with branches of dying nerve cells. A pattern in the death of nerve cells has been related to the symptoms of abnormal behavior presented by the victims of the disease. The first area of the brain to be affected is the hippocampus, which stores recent memories. As the parietal lobes are affected, long-term memory is lost, which may be associated with depression. Finally, destruction of the neurons of the cortex causes hallucinations, severe thinking disorders, seizures, and the inability to walk, talk, or swallow (Williams, 1986; Brownlee, 1991).

STAGES. Three stages of Alzheimer's disease have been identified by Williams (1986). The first stage covers approximately 2 to 4 years. This stage is characterized by loss of memory, time and spatial disorientation, affect changes, increased paranoia and depression, and mistakes in judgment. The second stage may extend over 2 to 20 years. The dementia progresses with memory defects, including forgetfulness of recent and remote events, and complete disorientation with lessening of the person's ability to comprehend. The third stage is terminal; clients usually do not live longer than a year after reaching this stage. It is characterized by marked irritability, insertion of wrong words in speaking (paraphasia), and common seizures. The individual eventually becomes emaciated, helpless, and bedridden. The most frequent cause of death is pneumonia, with other infections, malnutrition, and dehydration as contributing factors (Kermis, 1986; Williams, 1986).

Another method of identifying the stages of Alzheimer's disease is outlined in the Global Deterioration Scale, which classifies the symptoms into seven levels of cognitive functionings (Reisberg, Ferris, deLeon, & Crook, 1982). See Table 7-1 for the Global Deterioration Scale and accompanying changes in the person with primary degenerative dementia.

RESEARCH. Structural changes in the brain are the result, not the cause, of Alzheimer's disease. The great challenge is to discover what causes the degeneration. At present, research concentrates on several major hypotheses.

The *acetylcholine model* is based on the hypothesis that some of the cognitive defects in Alzheimer's disease are the direct result of a reduction in the acetylcholine-mediated transmission of nerve impulses (Burnside, 1988). Acetylcholine is a neurotransmitter important in learning and memory. For several years intensive research efforts have focused on the study of drugs that might increase the amount of neurotransmitter acetylcholine, which is deficient in a brain affected by Alzheimer's disease. As acetylcholine does not enter the brain when taken directly, it can be introduced only through substances such as lecithin and choline. When taken orally, these substances are broken down in the body to form acetylcholine, which enters the brain. Tacrine (1, 2, 3, 4 - tetrahydroacridine) administered in combination with lecithin was found to improve results of tests of cognitive abilities but not activities of daily living. This symptomatic improvement occurred in patients with mild to moderate Alzheimer's disease. Liver dysfunction has been reported in some patients receiving tacrine treatment (Adem, 1992; Eagger, Levy, & Sahakian, 1992).

The *genetic model* is based on the possibility of a faulty gene or genes. Perhaps some factor in a person's genetic makeup renders him or her particularly vulnerable

Table 7-1 Global Deterioration Scale Compared with a normal individual of the same age and sex, rate the subject's level of cognitive functioning

Level	Cognitive functioning
1 No cognitive decline	No subjective complaints of memory deficit. No memory deficit evident on clinical interview.
2 Very mild cognitive decline	Subjective complaints of memory deficit, most frequently in following areas: (a) forgetting location of objects; (b) forgetting familiar names. No objective evidence of memory deficit on clinical interview or in employment or social situations. Appropriate concern with respect to symptomatology.
3 Mild cognitive decline	Earliest clear-cut deficits. Manifestations in more than one of the following areas: (a) patient may have gotten lost when traveling to an unfamiliar location; (b) co-workers become aware of patient's relatively poor performance; (c) word and name finding deficit become evident to intimates; (d) patient may read a passage or a book and retain relatively little material; (e) patient may demonstrate decreased facility in remembering names upon introduction to new people; (f) patient may have lost or misplaced an object of value; (g) concentration deficit may be evident on clinical testing. Objective evidence of memory deficit obtained only with an intensive interview conducted by a trained geriatric psychiatrist. Decreased performance in demanding employment and social settings. Denial begins to become manifest in patient. Mild to moderate anxiety accompanies symptoms.
4 Moderate cognitive decline	Clear-cut deficit on careful clinical interview. Deficit manifest in the following areas: (a) decreased knowledge of current and recent events; (b) may exhibit some deficit in memory of personal history; (c) concentration deficit elicited on serial subtractions; (d) decreased ability to travel, handle finances, etc. Frequently no deficit in following areas: (a) orientation to time and person; (b) recognition of familiar persons and faces; (c) ability to travel to familiar locations. Inability to perform complex tasks. Denial is dominant defense mechanism. Flattening of affect and withdrawal from challenging situations occur.

Adapted from Reisberg, B., Ferris, S. H., de Leon M. J., and Crook, T. (1982). The global deterioration scale for assessment of primary degenerative dementia. *American Journal of Psychiatry, 139*(9), 1136-1139; with permission.

Table 7-1　Global Deterioration Scale Compared with a normal individual of the same age and sex, rate the subject's level of cognitive functioning—cont'd

Level	Cognitive functioning
5　Moderately severe cognitive decline	Patient can no longer survive without some assistance. Patient is unable during interview to recall a major relevant aspect of his or her current life, e.g., an address or telephone number of many years, the names of close family members (such as grand-children), the name of the high school or college from which he or she graduated. Frequently some disorientation to time (date, day of week, season, etc.) or to place. An educated person may have difficulty counting back from 40 by 4s or from 20 by 2s. Persons at this stage retain knowledge of many major facts regarding themselves and others. They invariably know their own names and generally know their spouse's and children's names. They require no assistance with toileting and eating but may have some difficulty choosing the proper clothing to wear and may occasionally clothe themselves improperly (e.g., put shoes on the wrong feet).
6　Severe cognitive decline	May occasionally forget the name of the spouse upon whom they are entirely dependent for survival. Will be largely unaware of all recent events and experiences in their lives. Retain some knowledge of their past lives but this is very sketchy. Generally unaware of their surroundings, the year, the season, etc. May have difficulty counting from 10, both backward and, sometimes forward. Will require some assistance with activities of daily living, e.g., may become incontinent, will require travel assistance but occasionally will display ability to familiar locations. Diurnal rhythm frequently disturbed. Almost always recall their own name. Frequently continue to be able to distinguish familiar from unfamiliar persons in their environment. Personality and emotional changes occur. These are quite variable and include: (a) delusional behavior, e.g., patients may accuse their spouse of being an impostor; may talk to imaginary figures in the environment, or to their own reflection in the mirror; (b) obsessive symptoms, e.g., person may continually repeat simple cleaning activities; (c) anxiety symptoms, agitation, and even previously nonexistent violent behavior may occur; (d) cognitive abulia, i.e., loss of willpower because an

Continued.

Table 7-1 Global Deterioration Scale Compared with a normal individual of the same age and sex, rate the subject's level of cognitive functioning—cont'd

Level	Cognitive functioning
	individual cannot carry a thought long enough to determine a purposeful course of action.
7 Very severe cognitive decline	All verbal abilities are lost. Frequently there is no speech at all—only grunting. Incontinent of urine; requires assistance toileting and feeding. Loose basic psycho-motor skills, e.g., ability to walk. The brain appears to no longer be able to tell the body what to do. Generalized and cortical neurological signs and symptoms are frequently present.

to an environmental factor. In some families 10 or more members representing four or five generations have developed a dementia of the Alzheimer's type (Burnside, 1988). Chromosomes 19 and 21 have been linked to Alzheimer's disease. Chromosome 21 contains the gene that makes beta-amyloid protein, the major substance in neuritic plaques. Amyloid precursor protein, found in normal brain tissue, has an undefined function. A genetic defect allows production of beta-amyloid, producing neurological damage that may be proven to be strongly connected to Alzheimer's disease (Brownlee, 1991; Weiner, Tintner, & Goodkin, 1991).

The *toxin model* is described by some researchers who believe that the salts of aluminum may contribute to the development of Alzheimer's disease. These salts may be found in drinking water and may be added to food and drugs such as processed cheeses, antacids, and buffered acids. Aluminum salts may also be released from aluminum cans and utensils. An irreversible dementia has been seen in persons who have undergone kidney dialyses with dialysis solutions containing aluminum. Several investigators have reported higher concentrations of aluminum in the brains of Alzheimer's clients than in those of healthy older persons without dementia. (Burnside, 1988; Cohen & Eisdorfer, 1986a). People with exposure to airborne particles of aluminum have shown a higher than average occurrence of Alzheimer's disease. The abundance of aluminum in the earth and the body's mechanisms to protect people from retaining ingested aluminum have raised doubts that Alzheimer's disease is directly related to aluminum (Brownlee, 1991).

The *abnormal protein model* is named for the abnormal protein structures in the brain of the Alzheimer's client. The brain manufactures many proteins used to build internal structures within the nerve cell. Unusual twisted filaments discovered in the neurofibrillary tangles of brains of Alzheimer victims prompted research to determine how protein metabolism is disrupted. Exactly how these abnormal filaments are formed is still unknown. Some evidence suggests that an anomalous protein may be produced in the brain of the Alzheimer's client and that the presence of this atypical protein leads to the formation of abnormal filaments. Tangles in the neurons containing broken-down cellular tissue allow transport of acetylcholine (Brownlee, 1991; Burnside, 1988).

The *infectious agent model* arose from early suggestions that Alzheimer's disease was caused by a slow-growing virus. Current research suggests that if this disease is caused by an infectious agent, it is accompanied by a particular genetic makeup, a concurrent immune disorder, or a prior exposure to a toxin in the environment. However, there is no evidence that Alzheimer's disease can be transmitted from human to human (Burnside, 1988; Cohen & Eisdorfer, 1986a).

The scientific community is optimistic that intensified research efforts and new technological advances will someday lead to the discovery of what causes Alzheimer's disease and related disorders (Cohen & Eisdorfer, 1986a).

Parkinson's Disease

Since its description by James Parkinson in 1917, Parkinson's disease has become recognized as second only to stroke as the most common neurological disorder in older adults (Matteson, 1988; McDowell, 1986).

As many as 1 million to 1.5 million people in the United States are afflicted by Parkinson's disease, and approximately 40,000 to 50,000 new cases are identified annually. It has been identified in all races and is found worldwide. Age of onset is usually between 55 and 60, although it can occur earlier or later, even into the 80s. The disease strikes men and women equally (Matteson, 1988; McDowell, 1986). There are similarities in symptoms, pathology, and neurotransmitter function between Parkinson's disease and Alzheimer's disease. Research has not clearly defined this relationship (Weiner, Tintner, & Goodkin, 1991).

Parkinson's disease is predominantly a motor disorder characterized by slowness and weakness of voluntary movement, cogwheel rigidity, and tremor. The term *parkinsonism* is often used to describe movement disorders with such symptoms whether or not Parkinson's disease is actually present.

Usually there is no clear point of disease onset. The most common initial symptom is tremor, usually starting on one side of the body, most often in an upper extremity. The tremor often spreads to involve both sides. The person generally tends to slow down and to experience difficulty in performing daily activities.

Slowness of voluntary movment may become so severe that the person is unable to initiate movements. Increased difficulty in walking becomes evident, with more short, quick steps and difficulty in resuming walking after stopping. The client may shuffle his feet when he walks. Older persons have poor balance and may fall often. They may have trouble getting in and out of bed, turning in bed, and bathing themselves. They may have trouble dressing themselves and using eating utensils to cut their food. Handwriting may become illegible. Affected individuals have an expressionless face, with muffled or monotonous speech, excessive salivation, and limited ocular mobility. Although some clients with Parkinson's disease have no mental disturbances, others are disoriented, confused, depressed, delusional, and hallucinatory (Kermis, 1986; Matteson, 1988; McDowell, 1986).

It is important for clients with Parkinson's disease to remain as physically, socially, and intellectually active as possible. Exercise programs and increased activity are important in maintaining optimal performance. Patients should be encouraged to remain as independent as possible and to continue daily activities without assistance regardless of the time required to accomplish these tasks. It may become necessary for the family to force social activity, since the client may easily become less interested in such activities; however, once the client participates, he or she usually finds these activities interesting and enjoyable. The person will rarely initiate a social activity, especially if there is some evidence of declining intellectual capacity. The disease can progress to the point of complete dependency (McDowell, 1986).

Dopamine in the form of levodopa, the treatment of choice for Parkinson's disease, frequently produces side effects similar to those characteristic of dementing illnesses. According to McDowell (1986), one of the side effects is the development of marked postural instability. Clients report that after several years of treatment their balance has become poor, and they frequently fall forward or backward while getting in or out of chairs. Occasionally they fall for no reason, and injuries are common. The exact cause of this postural instability is not clear. Loss of postural reflexes, common with Parkinson's disease, seems to become more marked as the disease progresses under treatment with levodopa.

Huntington's Disease

Huntington's disease, formerly called Huntington's chorea, is characterized by uncontrollable writhing movements, called choreiform movements. The disease begins with disturbances of gait and slurred speech and progresses to neurological and intellectual deterioration. These symptoms can be mistaken for alcoholism by observers because the victims resemble intoxicated persons in their movement and speech (Kermis, 1986). The extrapyramidal and subcortical areas of the brain and nervous system are affected, producing jerky movements accompanied by memory loss, paranoia, irritability, and impaired impulse control (Matteson, 1988). Symptomatic treatment may be by haloperidol (Haldol), baclofen (Lioresal), or bromo-scriptine (Parlodel) (Weiner, Tintner, & Goodkin, 1991).

Huntington's disease is an autosomal dominant disorder with full penetrance; that is, when the defective gene is inherited, there is a 100% probability that the disorder will occur. Many times there is no family history indicated because of either the social stigma attached to the disease or the premature death of parents for unknown reasons.

Huntington's disease usually begins between the ages of 25 and 45, with an average duration of 15 years. It is a fairly rare disorder, occurring two to seven times in every population of 100,000 in the United States, and represents less than 5% of the dementias. The outcome is fatal, usually from heart failure or pulmonary complications caused by asphyxiation or aspiration of food (Kermis, 1986; Matteson, 1988; Wills, 1986).

Pick's Disease

Matteson (1988) states that the onset, course, and clinical presentation of Pick's disease are very similar to those of Alzheimer's disease and are often categorically linked and treated in the same manner. There are some subtle differences between the two diseases, and it is important to have some knowledge of a condition that is almost exclusively associated with aging. This condition occurs more frequently in women than in men, usually after age 70. The onset of the disease is slow and progresses until death with an average duration of 4 years.

A major difference between Alzheimer's disease and Pick's disease is in the pathological process. Alzheimer's disease is characterized by diffuse involvement of higher brain structures, whereas Pick's disease is characterized by extreme atrophy of localized cortical areas. The frontal and temporal lobes narrow and the number of neurons in the affected areas decreases. As a result, the senile plaques, neurofibrillary tangles, and granulovacuolar degeneration characteristic of Alzheimer's disease rarely appear with Pick's disease.

Symptoms of progressive impairment of cognition, memory, and orientation are similar to those of Alzheimer's disease. Language disorders are common, and depression and apathy may also accompany the disease. Inappropriate actions and major personality changes occur in early stages of the disease. Because there is no known cure, treatment is aimed at management of the symptoms. Working with family caregivers and modifying the home environment are important in the early stages; institutionalization may be necessary in the later stages (Kuhlman, DeBoer & Wilson, 1992; Matteson, 1988).

Creutzfeldt-Jakob Disease

Creutzfeldt-Jakob disease, or subacute spongiform encephalopathy, is a noninflammatory viral dementia. It is a rare disease, with approximately one case for every million people, and death occurs within 9 months to a year after the onset of symptoms. The average age of onset is usually between 50 and 60 years, but the age range is from 21 to 79 (Kermis, 1986).

The disease is a rapidly progressive, diffuse disorder of the nervous system involving severe neurological impairment with marked dysfunction. The histopathology of the brain disorder is similar to that seen in Alzheimer's disease. Concurrent symptoms include impaired cognition, myoclonus, ataxia, muscle wasting, extrapyramidal movements (choreoathetoid movements, tremor), early blindness, hallucinations, and illusions. These symptoms and the rapid onset of dementia characterize Creutzfeldt-Jakob syndrome. There is no known treatment to stop the progression of the disease (Kermis, 1986; Matteson, 1988; Souder, 1992).

Vascular Dementia (Multi-Infarct Dementia)

Multi-infarct dementia, the second most common dementia, is a vascular disorder characterized by multiple large and small cerebral infarctions. This disorder is classified as vascular dementia in the DSM-IV (American Psychiatric Association, 1994). Approximately 25% of all dementia cases are vascular, and hypertension and diabetes are closely associated with this disease. Other factors contributing to the disease include obesity, smoking, peripheral vascular disease, arrhythmias, myocardial infarction, and transient ischemic attacks. The usual age of onset is 55 to 70 (Souder, 1992).

Multi-infarct dementia occurs earlier than the primary degenerative dementias and appears to follow no familial patterns. It is more common in men than women, which is the opposite of the degenerative dementias. The progression is highly variable, depending on the occurrence of new lesions in brain tissue. Some of the features of multi-infarct dementia include pseudo-bulbar palsy with emotional lability, dysarthria, dysphasia, and convulsive seizures. The client usually has a history of hypertension and exhibits abrupt ischemic episodes that lead to weakness, slowness, hyperreflexia, and extensor plantar responses. Fluctuation in level of cognition and stages of confusion or delirium are common. The personality is for the most part left intact, although explosive or unstable emotions often occur. Disturbances in memory, abstract thinking, judgment, and impulse control are also common. Clients with multi-infarct dementia are often unaware of these mental barriers. These behavioral difficulties must be noticed and dealt with by staff persons; otherwise, they will hamper any attempts at successful rehabilitation (Kermis, 1986; Raskind & Storrie, 1981).

Treatment is primarily preventive by controlling hypertension, diabetes, and intravascular clotting. Treatment of depression by appropriate medications is an important part of therapy (Weiner et al., 1991).

Transient Ischemic Attack

A transient ischemic attack (TIA), sometimes called a little stroke, is characterized by transient focal neurological signs and symptoms that occur suddenly and last usually less than an hour and never more than 24 hours. In about 90% of persons with TIA, this syndrome is caused by a microembolism to the brain from atherosclerotic plaques in the aortocranial arteries. In the remainder, it is caused by mural thrombi, valvular diseases of the heart, vegetations on the heart valve, polycythemia, or other blood-clotting disorders (Harrell, 1988).

The specific symptoms of a TIA vary according to which vessel is involved, the degree of obstruction of the vessel, and the collateral blood supply. If the anterior (carotid) system is involved, the person may experience ipsilateral blindness, monocular blurring, gradual obscuration of vision, flashes of light, and headaches. If the posterior (vertebrobasilar) system is involved, symptoms may include tinnitus, vertigo, simultaneous bilateral sensory and motor symptoms, diplopia, facial weakness, ataxia, and falling without losing consciousness.

Older persons who have a TIA may ignore an attack as the symptoms completely resolve. However, they should be seen by a physician to prevent a possibly disabling stroke in the future (Harrell, 1988).

❖ Delirium

Delirium is an organic brain disorder involving widespread cerebral dysfunction in which memory, thinking, and perception are simultaneously impaired. Delirium

---

Box 7-3 **Diagnostic Features of Delirium**

Vital Feature: Disturbance of consciousness with altered cognition not caused by dementia. Evidence of relationship to physiological results of a medical condition, substance use, medication, toxin, or a combination of these.

    A. Lessened clarity of awareness of environment.
        Reduced ability to maintain attention (resulting communication impairment).

    B. Change in cognition: memory impairment, disorientation, language disturbances, perceptual disturbances.
        Often associated with disturbances in sleep-wake cycle.
        Rapidly shifting emotional disturbances.
        Escalation of disturbed behavior at night.

    C. Occurs rapidly, in hours or days. Fluctuates during day.

Adapted from American Psychiatric Association (1994). *Diagnostic and Statistical Manual of Mental Disorders* (4th ed.). pp. 124-133. Washington, DC: Authors; with permission.

---

may be differentiated from dementia by its acute onset with reversible causes, whereas dementia usually is a chronic irreversible cerebral dysfunction (Foreman, 1986). According to Wills (1986), the distinguishing features of delirium are altered consciousness, inability to sustain attention, and a fluctuating clinical course.

Matteson (1988) states that the essential features associated with delirium are disturbances in attention, disorganized thinking, disorientation, disturbance of short-term memory, clouded sensorium, perceptual disturbances, and changes in psychomotor activity. The DSM-IV diagnostic features of delirium are listed in Box 7-3.

Delirium is a common condition, with an estimated one third to one half of hospitalized older clients becoming delirious at some time during their hospitalization (Wills, 1986). Although delirium may occur at any age, older persons seem more likely to develop the symptoms than younger persons. Delirium has a sudden onset, often starting at night. Its duration is relatively brief, although it usually lasts longer in an older person (Gomez & Gomez, 1987).

Causes

Delirium is generally caused by a widespread disturbance of brain metabolism and is a temporary and reversible disorder if treated early. Some of the causes are infections, fluid and electrolyte imbalance, cardiovascular disease, cerebrovascular disease, central nervous system disease, metabolic disorders, malnutrition, trauma, sensory deprivation, exposure to extremes in temperature, and exogenous toxins such as alcohol and medications.

According to Gomez and Gomez (1987), delirium in older persons may be caused by nearly all illnesses and chemical agents, including drugs and alcohol. Intoxication from drugs prescribed for a medical condition is probably the most frequent single cause of delirium. The central cholinergic system, necessary for memory, learning, attention, and wakefulness, is affected by aging, and this problem is aggravated by the use of anticholinergic medications. Delirium is most likely when several anticholinergic drugs are prescribed concurrently. Therefore polypharmacy, especially with anticholinergic medications, should be avoided as much as possible, and the nurse attending the older patient should be aware of these dangers.

A major factor contributing to delirium is a reversal of the sleep-wake cycle; patients sleep during the day and are awake at night. Sensory deprivation caused by loss or diminution of hearing and sight can cause confusion and impaired cognition. Older people use visual and auditory cues to orient themselves in the dark. If these cues are abolished, the result can lead to anxiousness and disorientation. Other contributing factors include head trauma; burns; hepatic, renal, or pulmonary failure; and hip and other injuries (Gomez & Gomez, 1987).

Treatment

If clinically possible, all drugs should be withdrawn for a few days. Medications often can be reduced in dosage or discontinued altogether without a significant change in the patient's physiological status. This is possible because of the tendency to add new drugs without removing old ones. Aggressive and successful therapy of the primary medical or surgical problem is important. In addition, measures directed at correction of anemia, nutritional deficiencies, electrolyte imbalance, and dehydration should be undertaken.

Therapeutic goals include a reduction in agitation and confusion with an improvement in sleep. Most deliriums will improve with treatment of the underlying disease or with removal of the noxious agent. Without a correct diagnosis and complete treatment, there is a potential for slow recovery and perhaps permanent brain damage (Wills, 1986).

❖ Nursing Process

According to Hall (1988a), altered thought processes is a common nursing diagnosis of older clients. Confusion, disorientation, and/or misinterpretation of the environment may develop in older clients and be severe enough to impair performance in basic activities of daily living.

Stress resulting from relocation, sleep deprivation, interruption of normal routine, sensory deficits, and/or physical stressors may alter behavior. Altered thought processes may be caused by physiological changes that alter the character or metabolism of the cerebral cortex. These changes include tumors, cerebral trauma, diminished oxygenation, and progressive degeneration. In addition, chronic or acute mental illness or lifelong developmental disabilities may contribute to altered thought processes.

An older person with the deficits in mental status seen in dementia may appear intact initially because of compensation mechanisms. These mechanisms, including preservation of social graces, can initially fool nurses by covering up existing dementia symptoms. In the case of delirium the existence and progression of cognitive impairment must be identified before the underlying conditions can be treated. Mental status changes must be confirmed to provide appropriate and adequate nursing care, whether it be acute care, long-term care, or care in the community. Assessment procedures can reveal the degree of cognitive impairment and implement individualized nursing care strategies (Gomez & Gomez, 1987; Linderborn, 1988; Abraham & Neundorfer, 1990).

Assessment

Assessing clients with altered thought processes can be problematic. The client with concerns about memory loss or other troublesome behavior is usually brought to the attention of the primary health care provider (nurse practitioner or physician). Behavior must be validated to establish the diagnosis. A comprehensive history and a physical assessment, including a mental status examination, should be completed for individuals suspected of having an organic mental disorder. In addition, a thorough documentation of current functional abilities and behavioral symptoms should be included. As with symptoms of physiological problems, it is important to analyze the behavioral symptoms. Often clients are unable to share reliable information about their psychosocial and health history or to provide a thorough drug inventory. The nurse must validate information received from the client with information from family members who may be reluctant to discuss the client's problems. The nurse should interview the client and/or family members to determine the following:

- ◆ *Onset of the behavior.* Sudden onset in terms of hours or days as opposed to insidious gradual onset over months may help differentiate between delirium and dementia. Progression of behaviors is also determined.
- ◆ *Timing of the behavior* (time of day or night when the behavior is present or when it becomes worse). Note intermittent or constant patterns and duration of the behavior in question. Timing may help in differentiating between delirium and dementia and in planning individualized nursing care.
- ◆ *Whether the behavior seems to be related to any precipitating factors.* What seems to make the behavior improve or to make the behavior worse? This information may assist the nurse in understanding the client's lifestyle and coping ability and in planning nursing interventions.
- ◆ *How the client's and the caregiver's activities of daily living have been affected by the behavioral symptoms.*

◆ *What the behavioral symptoms mean to the client and to the caregiver.* These last two questions assist in understanding a variety of factors, such as lifestyle, individual and family coping, and perception of the behavior by the client and the caregiver.

After a thorough history of the patient has been completed, a physical assessment should be done to determine fit with diagnostic criteria and to discover coexistent physiological illnesses (Souder, 1992). The physical assessment should include chest x-ray examination, electroencephalogram, electrocardiogram, urinalysis, SMA 12/60, T_3 and T_4 thyroid studies, CBC, VDRL, serum creatinine, electrolytes, B_{12}, serum folate, and either a computed tomography scan, a positron emission tomography scan, or a nuclear magnetic resonance imaging (Burnside, 1988; Cohen & Eisdorfer, 1986a). These tests assist in discovering possible organic causes for the alteration in thought processes.

Mental status should be assessed in memory, abstract thinking, judgment, mood or affect, orientation, attention or concentration, level of consciousness (wakefulness or sleepiness), communication or language abilities, and personality changes, such as suspiciousness or loss of impulse control. Assessment of mental status by screening tests such as the Mini-Mental State Examination may be helpful. Depression may be diagnosed as dementia and should be differentiated in assessment of mental status (Souder, 1992).

Burnside (1988) recommends that when dementia is suspected, the nurse should look for the following:

◆ Medications not taken correctly
◆ Previously balanced checkbook no longer balanced
◆ Deterioration in personal appearance, such as clothes not fastened correctly, clothes on backward, or clothes not the client's own
◆ Food spilled frequently
◆ Altered sleep patterns
◆ Wandering behavior not recognized by the client
◆ Beginning deterioration in manner or social graces

Assessment of sensory status should be included, especially that of hearing and vision, as deficits in these senses profoundly affect the way a person perceives and interprets the environment. Studies have shown that confusion may result from deficits of vision (Ninos & Makohon, 1985).

Nursing Diagnoses

One or several nursing diagnoses will emerge after completion of the assessment. Some of the possible nursing diagnoses applicable to those with organic mental disorders are shown in Box 7-4. (See the complete list of NANDA diagnostic categories in Appendix F.) It is important to identify and plan for all diagnoses present. Because of the myriad possible nursing diagnoses for clients with organic

---

Box 7-4 **Sample Nursing Diagnoses for Organic Mental Disorders**

1. Thought processes, altered
2. Communication, impaired verbal
3. Self-care deficit, bathing/hygiene
4. Self-care deficit, dressing/grooming
5. Self-care deficit, toileting
6. Health maintenance, altered
7. Family processes, altered
8. Home maintenance management, impaired
9. Nutrition, altered: less than bodily requirements
10. Knowledge deficit
11. Physical mobility, impaired
12. Injury, high risk for
13. Sensory-perceptual alterations
14. Sleep pattern disturbance
15. Activity intolerance
16. Violence, high risk for: directed at self/others
17. Role performance, altered
18. Caregiver role strain
19. Coping, ineffective individual
20. Powerlessness

Adapted from North American Nursing Diagnosis Association (1992). *NANDA Nursing Diagnoses: Definition and Classification 1992-1993*. Philadelphia: Author; with permission.

---

mental disorders, discussion of nursing care in this chapter will focus on altered thought processes.

Planning

After making a diagnosis of altered thought processes, the nurse should determine the client's ability to manage environmental stimuli, level of function, and concomitant medical conditions. In planning care the nurse should evaluate the client's coping mechanisms and past interests to provide meaningful activities and positive interactions with others. Nursing interventions are based on defining behavioral symptoms, determining cause(s), and eliminating causes whenever possible. Altered thought processes are often misdiagnosed by nurses because of the baffling behavioral nature of the defining characteristics, the broad scope of behavioral symptoms, and the wide range of causes. Since there is a broad range of causes, it is impossible to develop a single care plan for altered thought processes. However, Hall (1988a) outlines key components of every plan:

- ◆ Providing for client safety
- ◆ Intervening to eliminate the cause(s) whenever possible
- ◆ Eliminating overwhelming environmental, intrapersonal, or interpersonal stressors
- ◆ Providing structure and routine to provide pattern and meaning
- ◆ Developing interpersonal relationships that promote trust
- ◆ Evaluating interventions

Intervention

A majority of clients are cared for at home by family members or other caregivers, which limits the role of the nurse. It is important for the nurse to assess the family and caregivers for any significant health problems in addition to their state of chronic grief in reaction to the client's condition. As the family becomes part clients and part members of the caregiving team, it is important to assess their understanding of the client's diagnosis and care as well as their own health and social needs. Assisting family members with support, information about resources, and referrals is an important component in the care of the client with an organic mental disorder. Local and national chapters of the Alzheimer's Association offer many sources of assistance for family members when the victim is cared for at home or in a long-term care facility (Souder, 1992).

If the client is institutionalized, it is important for the family to continue to provide care through visiting, social activities, and performing individualized tasks. The effect of having Alzheimer's disease in a family member manifests itself in many ways. One person may try to compensate for the increasing deficits of the client. Family members may become frustrated, angry, sad, and depressed. The need to deal with the common defense mechanisms of denial and projection often used by the client demands innovative approaches. Progress of the disease resulting in incontinence of the client together with physical and emotional exhaustion of the primary caregiver may determine the timing and need for nursing home placement. Such a placement does not, however, relieve the caregivers of responsibility for their loved one, because they continue to provide care and emotional support, but not on a 24-hour daily basis (Weiner & Svetlik, 1991). *The 36-Hour Day* (Mace & Rabins, 1991) is an excellent guide for family members of dementia patients.

In a long-term care facility, care is provided primarily by nursing assistants. The nursing assistants may have received little training in care of the client with behavioral problems. In this setting the nurse assumes supervisory, supportive, and evaluative roles. Therefore it is important for the nurse to have a conceptual framework to use in planning care, educating staff, counseling family, and evaluating outcomes based on predetermined criteria. See Chapter 11.

Hall's Conceptual Model for Planning Care
Conceptual models provide a means of organizing and guiding research and practice in the field of nursing. A model developed by Hall known as *progressively lowered stress*

threshold (PLST) uses psychological theories of stress, coping, and adaptation in addition to behavioral and physiological research on Alzheimer's disease and related disorders (Hall & Buckwalter, 1987).

In this model Hall (1988a) categorized the symptoms of dementing illnesses into three groups: cognitive, or intellectual, losses; affective, or personality, losses; and conative, or planning, losses—all of which result in functional decline. A fourth group of dysfunctional behaviors was noted to occur with increasing regularity as the disease progresses. The behaviors included night awakening, agitation, late-day confusion, fearfulness, panic, agitated wandering, sudden withdrawal from activities, and catastrophic episodes. Several symptoms must be present to establish the diagnosis of altered thought processes.

Adults with dementia exhibit three main types of behavior: baseline, anxious, and dysfunctional. Although these types occur throughout the course of the disease, the proportions of each behavior type change with the progression of the disease. Baseline, or normative, behavior is a generally calm state, incorporating cognitive, affective, and conative losses. It is characterized by two elements: (1) the person is socially accessible and able to communicate needs and to respond to communications from others, and (2) the person is cognitively accessible and oriented to the environment. These clients are able to function within the limits of their neurological deficits. As the disease progresses, baseline behaviors are diminished and replaced by more anxious and dysfunctional behaviors (Hall, 1988a; Hall & Buckwalter, 1987).

Anxious behavior occurs when the demented individual feels stress. The patient avoids eye contact and seeks to avoid offending stimuli. The caregiver is still able to make or maintain contact with the patient. If the stress level continues or increases, dysfunctional or catastrophic behavior (cognitively and socially inaccessible) follows. In a dysfunctional state the patient is unable to communicate effectively or use environmental stimuli in an appropriate manner. Dysfunctional or catastrophic behaviors are viewed as stress-related and indicate a progressive lowering of the stress threshold. These behaviors cause excessive disability and further limit the client's ability to function and interact with the environment (Hall & Buckwalter, 1987). Dawson, Kline, Wianco, and Wells (1986, p. 299) define excessive disability as a "reversible deficit that is more disabling than the primary disability, existing when the magnitude of the disturbance in functioning is greater than might be accounted for by basic physical illness or cerebral pathology." Thus the client with a dementing illness who has prolonged periods of high stress will develop additional functional impairment and losses that clear when the stressors are removed (Hall & Buckwalter, 1987).

Stressors

Hall's model outlines five groups of stressors that produce excessive disability in the patient with altered thought processes: (1) fatigue; (2) change of environment, routine, or caregiver; (3) overwhelming and/or competing stimuli; (4) demands that exceed capacity to function; and (5) physical stressors such as acute illness, discomfort, and/or medication reactions. The nursing care plan should alleviate these stressors by recognizing anxious or agitated client behavior as an indication that further intervention is needed (Hall, 1988a). Wandering, a common symptom of Alzheimer's disease, may be the person's means of coping with the disease. Hall (1988c) developed a behavioral assessment tool to evaluate patients for cognitive decline and/or the need for a low-stimulus environment (see Appendix D).

FATIGUE. Family members should anticipate the first visits to be emotional or difficult and understand that they can discuss this with the staff. They should be encouraged to schedule visits in small groups within the client's consistent schedule. Clients tire rapidly from performing basic daily functions and frequently require rests or naps. If clients sleep several times during the day, their ability to sleep at night may be minimized.

Resting in a recliner with the head extended or spending quiet time in the room for 40 minutes at 10 AM and 90 minutes at 2 PM will usually refresh the client without promoting night wakening. Activities and visitors should not be scheduled at that time. If the client is up frequently at night, it may be necessary to decrease the rest periods during the day. If the client arises at night, do not turn on the lights because this cues the person that it is morning. Use photosensitive night lights for consistent low-level illumination at night (Hall, 1988a, 1988b). Sleep deprivation adds to an already existing cognitive dysfunction. If the client has trouble sleeping, a back rub, a warm glass of milk, or a soothing conversation may permit relaxation and subsequent sleep.

Fatigue can also be avoided by organizing shorter group activities for the client. Depending on the progression of the disease, the client may only be able to tolerate group activities in the morning with rest or quiet activities in the afternoon (Hall, 1988a, 1988b). The client should be well rested before going out. Family members should be counseled to provide time for the client to rest before and after traveling.

CHANGE OF ENVIRONMENT, CAREGIVER, OR ROUTINE. According to Burnside (1988), it is important to assess the environment of the client with altered thought processes. The physical environment should be safe, promote freedom, and stimulate without overloading. For example, a client moved suddenly into a darkened room may experience increased confusion and agitation.

Hall (1988a) found that altered ability to plan, initiate, and carry through voluntary activities is devastating to clients with altered thought processes. They will become frustrated at trying to initiate or complete simple tasks and may refuse to attempt any activity they feel they cannot complete. To compensate for this, many clients develop a consistent routine with very little variation. For some clients it may be necessary for the caregiver to develop a schedule that is posted in the room for the client to follow daily without variation. A change in the environment, such as holiday decorations, should be limited to specific areas so that the client's environment remains relatively stable. Any change in routine or environment forces the client to rethink all activities, and any increased disability should be noted by caregivers. It is critical to provide support to patients that will help them to continue to maximize their own self-care or activities of daily living as long as possible (Heacock, Walton, Beck, & Mercer, 1991; Niemoller, 1990).

Consistent staffing of caregivers is very important to minimize interruption of the thinking process of the client (Hall, 1988a). The availability of pets and children to provide touch, affection, spontaneity, and interest seems to help clients (Burnside, 1988). The nurse should evaluate the client's ability to tolerate change both before and after any scheduled activity. If the client becomes upset or shows any intolerance of the activity, plans should be made for a less complex activity or a rest period (Hall, 1988a, 1988b).

MISLEADING, OVERWHELMING, OR COMPETING STIMULI.   Clients with altered thought processes have limited ability to receive and interpret stimuli, particularly high noise levels, multiple activities, and crowds of people. DeBoer & Wilson (1988) state that to reduce environmental stimuli, only necessary procedures should be performed. While working with the client, move slowly, speak clearly, and provide information deliberately. Patience and direct, literal phrasing enhance understanding. The client should have time to process the communication and to reply. Directions should be simple and direct, without unneeded choices (Lee, 1991; Williams, Doyle, Feeney, Lenihan, & Salisbury, 1991).

Frequent misinterpretation of visual stimuli, such as television or pictures of people or animals, is common for clients with advanced altered thought processes. A person speaking over a public address system may be interpreted as someone in the attic. These misinterpretations are labeled as pseudohallucinations. As the caregiver learns of these misinterpretations, determination and elimination of the source are necessary. Clients tend to choose comfortable levels of stimuli. Some facilities have smaller, self-contained units for Alzheimer's disease clients that minimize competing stimuli while allowing areas for rest or small group activities. Patients should not eat in large group dining areas but should be allowed additional quiet time with one or two other clients while eating. Encourage the family to bring favorite snacks and food for the client's pleasure (Dawson et al., 1986; Hall, 1988b).

It is important that the facility approximate the home environments of the group it serves. Avoid overdecorating, which will be uncomfortable for the clients. The total environment should be evaluated for level of auditory and visual stimuli. The atmosphere of the Alzheimer's unit should be routine, orderly, safe and simple (ROSS) (Williams, Doyle, Feeney, Lenihan, & Salisbury, 1991). Music therapy is being evaluated with institutionalized Alzheimer's patients and may be used effectively with them. Further study of the Music Therapy Assessment Tool (MTAT) is needed (Glynn, 1992).

DEMANDS TO ACHIEVE THAT EXCEED FUNCTIONAL CAPACITY.   In clients with altered thought processes, language loss hampers attempts to read and speak. Some families and staff feel they must test the client daily to observe how much memory is lost. Questions they cannot answer and being told they are wrong frustrate the client.

Reality orientation may promote agitation but can be meaningful to clients if the goals are realistic (Hall, 1988a).

Rader, Doan, and Schwab (1985) state that reality orientation is not appropriate for all cognitively impaired persons. If the client has only mild confusion and is asking for reality information, then reality orientation may be valuable. However, if memory loss is severe, reality orientation will probably fail. With these clients reality orientation seems only to deepen anxiety and exaggerate separation from what they love and trust. According to Detwiler (1993), reality orientation is a nursing approach generally helpful to clients with cognitive impairments. Systematic reality orientation should include time, place, and person. Involvement in a caring group is an important factor in causing a positive behavioral change. Personal and physical contact is found to have a positive impact on group members. Clients who receive reality orientation seem to be happier and more involved with other people even if the level of confusion does not change significantly. Hall (1988a, 1988b) advises avoiding reality orientation unless the client requests it or safety is threatened. However, discussion of a pastime, holiday, or other concrete item may promote comfort and some understanding of the environment. With clients where reality orientation is not effective, Feil (1992) recommends validation therapy for confused older persons in various stages of disorientation.

PHYSICAL STRESSORS. The mental condition of the client with altered thought processes will worsen with pain, discomfort, acute illness, or other physiological alterations. Caffeine is one of the most commonly used physical stressors, and its use should be eliminated. Other common stressors are pain from any source, impacted bowels, full bladder, infections, influenza, and medication reactions and interactions. Dysfunctional behavior resulting from physical stressors is also known as acute confusional syndrome or delirium. Clients exhibiting stress-related behavior should receive a physical assessment to determine presence of any serious illness (Hall, 1988a).

Safety

Safety is a very important area in planning care for clients with altered thought processes. As the disease progresses, clients are unable to consider their own safety needs and risks. Older persons who wander present numerous safety problems and are a challenge to all persons caring for them whether at home or in an institution (Hall, 1988a).

Falls are another safety problem for these clients. Obstacles, slippery floors, and inadequate lighting should be eliminated from the environment. The family and the facility staff should discuss realistically the potential for falls. The agreement reached on use of restraints and safety measures should be recorded for future use (Hall, 1988a).

Other safety measures should include an awareness of hazardous objects that should be used with supervision, such as razors, canes, and electrical devices. Testing of water temperatures before bathing and food and beverage temperatures before eating are necessary interventions. Caregivers should be careful not to leave anything at the bedside that might harm the client. Substances that might be ingested, such as toiletries, cleaning solutions, and plants, should be monitored carefully. All staff should be trained in hazards to assure a safe environment for the clients (Hall, 1988a; Matteson, 1988).

Wandering

Wandering is leaving the nursing unit, facility, or a designated area without approval of the caregiver. Clients who have problems with wandering or elopement must be identified and plans must be made to minimize these risks. Plans can include locating the client's room near an area where additional supervision can be provided. Clothes can be labeled, and photographs of clients can be kept on file to be used in looking for any lost residents. Special alarm systems should be installed to alert staff when elopement occurs (Burnside, 1988; Hall, 1988a).

Wandering can be misunderstood and frustrating to a nursing staff, who may think of wandering as an aimless activity holding many hazards for the client (Heim, 1986). According to Burnside (1988), wandering can be both a psychosocial problem (meddling in others' belongings during wandering time) and a physical care problem. Wandering can be the result of restlessness and activity seeking. A client may unknowingly wander from home or off the grounds of an institution with the intention of running an errand or exploring the surroundings. A client in an advanced stage of dementia may wander because of disorientation or inability to sustain intentions. The client cannot remember what he or she started out to do. Heim (1986) states that clients may have underlying reasons for wandering, such as boredom, tension, hunger, pain, or need for warmth. There also may be deteriorative diseases of the central nervous system or cardiac decompensation.

Hall (1988b) classifies wandering agendas as (1) purposeless, including tactile or environmentally cued searching, or (2) purposeful, including recreational, reminiscent or fantasy, and agitated wandering. Wandering or pacing by an active client with Alzheimer's disease helps to maintain mobility and avoids the hostile and combative behavior resulting from physical restraint (Williams, et al., 1991).

Tactile wanderers are clients nearing the end of the ambulatory dementia phase. Characteristics include the use of their hands to explore the environment. As they feel their way through doorways and along halls, they remain calm as they appear to elope by accident. These clients have often lost the ability to communicate. Nursing interventions include guiding clients away from hallways and doors, supervising their walking, and redirecting them to other tactile objects.

Environmentally cued wanderers are usually in the mid to late ambulatory dementia phase. They appear calm and tend to follow cues within the environment. A chair may cue them to sit, a window invites them to look out, hallways entice them to keep walking, and a door may ask to be walked through. These clients elope on a regular basis and may appear to be searching for something. Nursing interventions include assessing the environment for cues to wander. Doors may be disguised with wall coverings and may be fitted with special closures that prohibit opening by clients. Chairs can be provided as cues for the client to stop. A barrier may be created by applying a brightly colored tape to the floor. Diversionary activities are useful for keeping the client's attention.

Recreational wanderers may be in the confused or ambulatory dementia phase of the illness. The wandering is purposeful, occurs regularly, and appears to serve a need for exercise. The client may have a history of an active lifestyle. The nurse should plan for a staff member to take the client for a walk on a regular basis at the same time of day and over the same route. Walking affords an excellent opportunity for a one-to-one interaction with the client.

Reminiscent or *fantasy wanderers* are usually calm and in the ambulatory dementia phase of the illness. Their desire to elope stems from a delusion or fantasy based on something in their past, such as going to work, going to see parents, or doing chores. The client may announce the intention of leaving the facility to go home. The nurse should remind the client that these actions are not necessary and redirect his or her attention to other actions.

Agitated wanderers are upset and may exhibit stress-related dysfunctional behavior. The client will be preoccupied with leaving the facility and may have packed a bag to leave. Staff will find that the client is cognitively and socially inaccessible and will be unable to reason with him or her. Staff is open to assault by the client who attempts to maintain control of the situation. Immediate interventions are necessary. The nurse should not confront the client while trying to defuse the situation. Tell the client about fears and concerns the staff have if the actions are carried out. Offer suggestions of alternatives or diversions to delay the action. This will allow the client time to regain composure, and the staff will generally be able to control the situation. Remove any offending stressors. If the client leaves, accompany or follow with enticements to return to the facility as quickly as possible, assuring safety and security. Tranquilizing medications may be necessary. The staff should assess and evaluate the situation for prevention of further episodes of agitated wandering (Hall, 1988b).

Wandering at night or by moonlight poses additional problems and concerns for the client and staff. Limiting the client's area of movement to one that can adequately be monitored is essential. It is important to adapt to the individual needs of each client by determining the cause if possible and incorporating appropriate interventions into the plan of care (Berky, 1991).

Rader et al. (1985) suggest alternative methods to quiet the restlessness accompanying dementia. They believe that wandering and confusion often stem from feelings of loneliness and separation. These feelings could be alleviated by a behavior agenda that includes verbal and nonverbal planning and actions to fulfill the client's social, emotional, and physical needs. Many clients have fear engendered by separation from the people and environment with which the person was previously most connected and comfortable. Efforts must be made to help the client recapture these feelings of safety and belonging. Many clients will have an intense desire to be needed. Staff can satisfy that need by finding activities through which the client can be of service. These activities could include pushing another's wheelchair, folding linens, or other such activity. By ignoring the needs of the client, staff contribute to wandering and agitation, which can precipitate combative behavior. Clients confined to wheelchairs may also wander. Rather than repeatedly pushing or pulling the client and chair to a safe area, the caregiver may elicit the cooperation of the client by holding the hand and asking the client to take a walk with the chair (Tucker, 1991).

Other methods for management of wandering include chemical and physical restraints; however, these present inherent problems. Use of sedatives by older people often adds to their confusion and increases their mental deficits. Use of restraints may result in severe physical and emotional problems for the clients because of enforced immobility. The only alternative is to let the client wander, but most homes and institutions do not have a safe enough environment to allow this (Young, Muir-Nash, & Ninos, 1988).

Evaluation

Evaluation of nursing care plans for clients with altered thought processes should be based on the degree to which the stated goals or expected outcomes were accomplished. Nursing care plans can be modified as needed according to the results of evaluation and changes in the clients' condition. Matteson (1988) states that evaluation is based on the success with which older clients are able to maintain function and the attainment of social supports for both clients and families.

Using Hall's PLST model, care can be evaluated using behavioral indicators that change with increased stress. These behavioral indicators include the amount of food ingested, client weight, functional level, social level, and presence of stress-related behaviors. Although new literature is continually being published concerning care of clients with altered thought processes, continued nursing research is needed to validate assessment instruments, techniques, and interventions (Hall, 1988a).

❖ Summary

There are some changes in intellectual functions with aging; however, normal aging does not include intellectual impairment, depression, confusion, hallucinations, or delusions. These symptoms are caused by disease and indicate the need for diagnosis and treatment. Intellectual impairment may be due to conditions that can be cured, conditions that can be improved with treatment, or conditions that have a relentless downhill course.

Early diagnosis of the cause of mental impairment is essential. If the condition is treatable, the problem may be reversed on early detection. If the condition is irreversible, early diagnosis provides a baseline for intervention.

Dementia is a type of mental impairment that affects memory, abstract thinking, judgment, reasoning, language, and personality. The symptoms of dementia are severe enough to interfere with activities of daily living, work, and social relationships.

Some of the primary degenerative dementias are Alzheimer's disease, Parkinson's disease, Huntington's disease, Pick's disease, and Creutzfeldt-Jakob disease. Alzheimer's disease is insidious, life-threatening, and the most prevalent of the irreversible dementias.

Other types of dementia include vascular dementia (multi-infarct dementia) and transient ischemic attacks (TIA). Multi-infarct dementia is a vascular disorder in which there are multiple large and small cerebral infarctions; it is the second most common cause of dementia. Transient ischemic attacks are sometimes called little strokes, and the specific symptoms depend on which vessel is involved, the degree of obstruction to that vessel, and the collateral blood supply. Older persons tend to ignore these attacks, which can result in a disabling stroke.

Delirium is a condition involving widespread cerebral dysfunction. Memory, thinking, and perception are simultaneously impaired. Delirium is usually differentiated from dementia by its acute onset with reversible causes; dementia usually is a chronic irreversible cerebral dysfunction.

A thorough comprehensive assessment is critical for planning individualized nursing care. The PLST model provides a means of organizing nursing care for clients with dementing illnesses. The nursing care plan should include alleviation of the five groups of stressors that produce anxious or agitated client behavior. Nursing care plans should provide safety measures for all clients, with special precautions for those who wander.

Evaluation of the nursing care plan is based on the accomplishment of expected outcomes. Interventions can be modified as needed according to evaluative data. Continuing nursing research in the care of clients with organic mental disorders is needed to improve assessment instruments and interventions.

Case Study **Alzheimer's Disease**

Mrs. Jones is a 76-year-old retired department store salesperson who has resided with her daughter and her daughter's family for the past 8 years. She has been a widow for the past 10 years. She began having memory problems before her retirement about 11 years ago at age 65. She began to forget names of her customers, to lose things, and to have problems driving.

Mrs. Jones has one daughter with whom she lives, two brothers who live in another state, and one close friend who lives nearby. She no longer knows the names of her brothers, her friend, her three grandchildren, her son-in-law, or her daughter. She has wandered from home two or three times in the past year. She has not seen a physician in about 2 years. The only medications she takes are doxepin (Sinequan), 150 mg at bedtime, and acetaminophen (Tylenol) for pain as needed.

The daughter has employed a woman to care for Mrs. Jones during the day while she works; however, the cost of care has exhausted all the financial resources left to Mrs. Jones by her deceased husband. The daughter has decided that since she must continue to work, she will place her mother in a nursing home nearby.

On Mrs. Jones's admittance to the nursing home, the following nursing care plan was prepared.

Nursing Care Plan for a Client with Alzheimer's Disease

Assessment data	Nursing diagnosis	Goals	Nursing interventions
2/1 **Subjective** Daughter: "Over the past few months, Mother has lost all of her memory and does not know my name or that of my husband or children. She is almost like another person. She becomes confused if her daily routine is changed. She is unable to plan her day or any events."	Thought processes, altered related to organic impairment	**Short-term** Client will be comfortable (not fearful or frustrated). Client will maintain as much independence as possible within disease process. Client will be safe and free from injury.	Avoid reality testing and reality orientation unless requested by the client or safety is threatened. Use reminiscence and validation to increase self-esteem. Use one-to-one or small group activities.
Objective Daughter: Tearful when discussing mother. Affect sad and anxious. Client: Not oriented to person, place or time. Appearance: Walks well; eye contact limited.	Sensory-perceptual alterations related to environmental changes and sensory overload	**Short-term** Client will not be overstimulated, withdrawn, or agitated. Client will not attempt to wander because of anxiety or fear. Client will be able to function in a set routine without needing to plan.	On admission assess client's ability to tolerate activities and stimuli. Try to match stimulus level to that of resident's home. Introduce new stimuli slowly. Confine to room for 48 hours. Use yellow tape on floor in front of door to create a boundary.

Continued.

Adapted from the following:
Harvis, K. A. (1990). Care plan approach to dementia. *Geriatric Nursing, 11*(2), 76-80.
Lee, V. K. (1991). Language changes and Alzheimer's disease: A literature review. *Journal of Gerontological Nursing 17*(1), 16-20.
North American Nursing Diagnosis Association (1992), *NANDA nursing diagnoses: Definitions and Classification, 1992-1993.* Philadelphia: Author.
Van Ort, S. and Phillips, L. (1992), Feeding nursing home residents with Alzheimer's disease. *Geriatric Nursing, 13*(5), 249-253.

Nursing Care Plan for a Client with Alzheimer's Disease

Assessment data	Nursing diagnosis	Goals	Nursing interventions
Affect: Pleasant, smiles occasionally. Mood: Anxious at times; silly at times. Memory: Immediate and remote memory severely impaired. Abstract thinking: Absent. Attitude: Sociable. MSQ score = 9 errors (severe). Attention span: Easily distracted. Thought content: Cognitively impaired. Thought processes: Jumps from topic to topic; illogical and unable to complete sentences at times. Insight: Absent.			Avoid misleading stimuli (pictures of people, animals, etc.). Family pictures are helpful. Decrease or eliminate if possible the use of a public address system. Avoid use of TV and use easy listening music instead. If client is confused or agitated, decrease stimuli and simplify routine. Develop a schedule that the client can follow daily. Post schedule in room and on nursing care plan. Do not vary from schedule.
Subjective Daughter: "Mother cannot initiate dressing and becomes mixed up but will finish dressing if someone helps her start."	Self-care deficit: bathing/hygiene Self-care deficit: dressing/grooming Self-care deficit: toileting related to cognitive impairment from disease process	**Short-term** Client will maintain as much independence as possible in self-care. Client will remain continent; incontinence will be managed. Skin integrity will be maintained. Maintain bowel habits	Assist in bathing, dressing, and grooming. Allow client to do as much as possible for herself at her own pace. Provide a regular schedule of bathroom visits, but at least after meals and at bedtime. Assist in cleaning and wearing glasses daily. Lay out clothing; minimize simple choices if the client is unable to respond or becomes frustrated.

Subjective
Daughter:
"Mother has wandered away from home two or three times in the past year."

Injury, high risk for related to altered cerebral function

Client will not injure herself or others.

Supervise client while she bathes, eats, and participates in activities.
Keep all hot or sharp objects safely out of reach.
Monitor all medications, lotions, and other dangerous materials.
Monitor stairways, doors, and door alarms carefully.
Schedule exercises individually or in small groups.
If client becomes agitated, remove to a quiet area.
Orient family to safety policies and procedures so they understand that staff will not be able to prevent all wandering.
If wandering occurs, assess the possible reasons.
Avoid physical restraints.

Subjective
Daughter:
"Mother gets up from the table before she finishes eating. She likes most foods."

Nutrition, altered: less than body requirements related to inability to feed self and focus on meals

Long-term
Client's weight will be maintained.

Simplify mealtimes with fewer utensils and food choices.
If client is unable to use utensils, provide finger foods.
Do not force client to make choices when she has difficulty with decisions but provide as many choices as she can handle.
Have family bring favorite snacks and food.
Provide quiet environment.
Offer liquids between meals.
Weigh weekly; note changes.

Continued.

Nursing Care Plan for a Client with Alzheimer's Disease—cont'd

Assessment data	Nursing diagnosis	Goals	Nursing interventions
Subjective "I can't find my lackerby. Ask her; she must know it all."	Communication, impaired verbal related to organic changes in brain.	Establish and maintain effective communication.	Remain calm. Keep sentences short and simple. Allow time to respond. Use illustrations for communication. Do not argue. Offer to look for "lost" items.
Objective Pulling clothing out of drawers and piling it on her bed. Anxious expression. Holding her purse under her arm.			
Subjective "No one cares about me. They just want my money. Daughter "I have tried to do my best, but I don't know what to do. I feel guilty and tired all the time."	Family processes, altered related to roles and relationships, separation from family member.	Maintain family relationships. Provide support to family members.	Refer family to Alzheimer support groups. Provide reading materials about Alzheimer's disease. Explain relationship of behaviors to process of dementia. Provide reassurance to patient: touch, hugs. Remind of daughter's visit, but do not argue or contradict.
Objective Daughter: Anxious expression. Visits daily. Client: Crying when talking about family. Points to pictures of daughter's family and says she wishes she knew who they are.			

❖ *References*

Abraham, I. L., & Neundorfer, M. M. (1990). Alzheimer's: A decade of progress, a future of nursing challenges. *Geriatric Nursing, 11*(3), 116-119.

Adem, A. (1992). Putative mechanisms of action of tacrine in Alzheimer's disease. *Acta Neurologica Scandanavica, 85* (Suppl. 139), 69-74.

Alzheimer's Disease and Related Disorders Association, Inc. (1992). Statistical data on Alzheimer's disease (INQ 230Z). Chicago: Author.

Amadeuci, L., Falcini, M., & Lippi, A. (1992). Descriptive epidemiology risk factors for Alzheimer's disease. *Acta Neurologica Scandanavica, 85* (Suppl. 139), 21-25.

American Psychiatric Association. (1994). *Diagnostic and statistical manual of mental disorders* (4th ed.). Washington, DC: Author.

Berky, P. S. (1991). Alzheimer's by moonlight. *Geriatric Nursing, 12*(6), 292-293.

Brownlee, S. (August 12, 1991). Alzheimer's: Is there hope? *U.S. News & World Report, 111*(7), 40-49.

Burnside, I. M. (1988). Dementia and delirium. In I. M. Burnside (Ed.). *Nursing and the aged: A self-care approach* (3rd. ed., pp. 733-767). New York: McGraw-Hill.

Chiverton, P. (1990). Dementia is not a diagnosis. *Geriatric Nursing, 11*(1), 24-25.

Cohen, D., & Eisdorfer, C. (1986a). *The loss of self.* New York: New American Library.

Cohen, D., & Eisdorfer, C. (1986b). Dementing disorders. In E. Calkins, P. J. Davis, & A. B. Ford (Eds.). *The practice of geriatrics* (pp. 194-205). Philadelphia: Saunders.

Dawson, P., Kline, K., Wianco, D., & Wells, D. (1986). Preventing excess disability in patients with Alzheimer's disease. *Geriatric Nursing, 7*(6), 299-301.

Detwiler, C. S. (1993). Organic mental disorders. In B. S. Johnson (Ed.). *Psychiatric-mental health nursing: Adaptation and growth* (pp. 629-643). Philadelphia: J. B. Lippincott.

Eagger, S. A., Levy, R., & Sahakian, B. J. (1992). Tacrine in Alzheimer's disease. *Acta Neurologica Scandanavica, 85* (Suppl. 139), 75-80.

Feil, N. (1992). Validation therapy. *Geriatric Nursing, 13*(3), 129-133.

Foreman, M. D. (1986). Acute confusional states in hospitalized elderly: A research dilemma. *Nursing Research, 35*(1), 34-38.

Glynn, N. J. (1992). Music therapy assessment tool. *Journal of Gerontological Nursing, 18* (1), 3-9.

Gomez, G. E., & Gomez, E. A. (1987). Delerium. *Geriatric Nursing, 8*(6), 330-332.

Goodkin, K. (1991). Differential diagnosis. In M. Weiner (Ed.). *The dementias: Diagnosis and management* (pp. 77-106). Washington, DC: American Psychiatric Press.

Hall, G. R. (1988a). Alterations in thought process. *Journal of Gerontological Nursing, 14*(3), 30-37.

Hall, G. R. (1988b, September). Assessing and managing the Alzheimer's patient. Paper presented at the preconference seminar of the National Gerontological Nursing Association, New Orleans.

Hall, G. R. (1988c). Behavioral assessment for low stimulus care plan. Unpublished manuscript, University of Iowa, Iowa City.

Hall, G. R., & Buckwalter, K. C. (1987). Progressively lowered stress threshold: A conceptual model for care of adults with Alzheimer's disease. *Archives of Psychiatric Nursing, 1*(6), 399-406.

Harrell, J. S. (1988). Age-related changes in the cardiovascular system. In M. A. Matteson & E. S. McConnell (Eds.). *Gerontological nursing concepts and practice* (pp. 194-217). Philadelphia: Saunders.

Harvis, K. A. (1990). Care plan approach to dementia. *Geriatric Nursing, 11*(2), 76-80.

Heacock, P., Walton, C., Beck, C., & Mercer, S. (1991). Caring for the cognitively impaired. *Journal of Gerontological Nursing, 17*(3), 22-25.

Heim, K. M. (1986). Wandering behavior. *Journal of Gerontological Nursing, 12*(11), 4-7.

Kermis, M. D. (1986). *Mental health in late life: The adaptive process.* Boston: Jones & Bartlett.

Kuhlman, G., DeBoer, G., & Wilson, H. S. (1992). Applying the nursing process for clients with organic mental syndromes and disorders. In H. S. Wilson & C. R. Kneisl (Eds.). *Psychiatric Nursing* (4th ed., pp. 184-213). Redwood City, CA.: Addison-Wesley.

Lee, V. K. (1991). Language changes and Alzheimer's disease: A literature review. *Journal of Gerontological Nursing, 17*(1), 16-20.

Linderborn, K. M. (1988). The need to assess dementia. *Journal of Gerontological Nursing, 14*(1), 35-39.

Lucas, M. J., Steele, C., & Bognanni, A. (1986). Recognition of psychiatric symptoms in dementia. *Journal of Gerontological Nursing, 12*(1), 11-15.

Mace, N., & Rabins, P. (1991). *The 36-hour day: A family guide to coping with persons with Alzheimer's disease, related dementing illnesses, and memory loss in later life* (revised edition). Baltimore: Johns Hopkins Press.

Matteson, M. A. (1988). Age-related changes in the neurological system. In M. A. Matteson & E. S. McConnell (Eds.). *Gerontological nursing concepts and practice* (pp. 248-263). Philadelphia: Saunders.

McDowell, F. H. (1986). Other neurologic diseases of the elderly. In E. Calkins, P. J. Davis, & A. B. Ford (Eds.). *The practice of geriatrics* (pp. 225-239). Philadelphia: Saunders.

National Institute on Aging Task Force. (1980). Senility reconsidered: Treatment possibilities for mental impairment in the elderly. *Journal of the American Medical Association, 244*(3), 259-263.

Niemoller, J. (1990). Change of pace for Alzheimer's patients. *Geriatric Nursing, 11*(2), 86-87.

Ninos, M., & Makohon, R. (1985). Functional assessment of the patient. *Geriatric Nursing, 6*(3), 139-142.

North American Nursing Diagnosis Association. (1992). *NANDA nursing diagnoses: Definitions and classification 1992-1993.* Philadelphia: Author.

Office of Technology Assessment Task Force. (1988). Confronting Alzheimer's disease and other dementias. New York: Lippincott.

Rader, J., Doan, J., & Schwab, M. (1985). How to decrease wandering, a form of agenda behavior. *Geriatric Nursing, 6*(4), 196-199.

Raskind, M. A., & Storrie, M. C. (1981). The organic mental disorders. In E. W. Busse & D. G. Blazer (Eds.). *Handbook of geriatric psychiatry* (pp. 305-328). New York: Van Nostrand Reinhold.

Reisberg, B., Ferris, S. H., deLeon, M. J., & Crook, T. (1982). The global deterioration scale for assessment of primary degenerative dementia. *American Journal of Psychiatry, 139*(9), 1136-1139.

Souder, E. (1992). Diagnosing dementia. *Journal of Gerontological Nursing, 18*(2), 5-11.

Tucker, N. J. (1991). Wheelchair walking. *Geriatric Nursing, 12*(1), 37.

Van Ort, S., & Philips, L. (1992). Feeding nursing home residents with Alzheimer's disease. *Geriatric Nursing, 13*(5), 249-253.

Weiner, M. F., & Svetlik, D. (1991). Dealing with family caregivers. In M. F. Weiner (Ed.).

The dementias: Diagnosis and management (pp. 185-199). Washington, DC: American Psychiatric Press.

Weiner, M. F., Tintner, R. J., & Goodkin, K. (1991). Differential diagnosis. In M. F. Weiner (Ed.). *The dementias: Diagnosis and management* (pp. 77-106). Washington, DC: American Psychiatric Press.

Williams, L. (1986). Alzheimer's: The need for caring. *Journal of Gerontological Nursing, 12*(2), 21-28.

Williams, M. P., Doyle, G. C., Feeney, E., Lenihan, P., & Salisbury, S. (1991). Alzheimer's unit by design. *Geriatric Nursing, 12*(1), 34-36.

Wills, R. (1986). Cognitive changes of normal aging and the dementias. In D. L. Carnevali & M. Patrick (Eds.). *Nursing management for the elderly* (2nd ed., pp. 241-256). Philadelphia: Lippincott.

Young, S. H., Muir-Nash, J., & Ninos, M. (1988). Managing nocturnal wandering behavior. *Journal of Gerontological Nursing, 14*(5), 6-12.

## Chapter 8

❖ *Schizophrenia, Paranoid, Anxiety, and Somatoform Disorders*

Brenda Riley

The functional psychiatric problems most frequently found in the aged are obsessive-compulsive disorders (a type of anxiety disorder), paranoia (a type of paranoid disorder), and depression. This chapter will focus on schizophrenia, paranoid disorders, anxiety disorders, and somatoform disorders. Depression in older adults is discussed in Chapter 6.

❖ *Schizophrenia*

Schizophrenia is a functional psychosis, a thought disorder characterized by altered concepts of reality, such as delusions and hallucinations. Other symptoms characteristic of an individual diagnosed as having schizophrenia include illogical thinking and speech, loose associations, inappropriate affect, disorganized psychomotor behavior, decreased ability to function in work and social activities, and poor hygiene.

The American Psychiatric Association (1994) has stated that the onset of schizophrenia usually occurs during early adulthood. Older schizophrenics generally have had long-standing problems and have been taking antipsychotic medications for years. Exacerbations of the illness may occur in later years as the stresses of aging increase. The person may become more withdrawn or paranoid. Thus, acute symptoms decrease and residual symptoms are more common as the schizophrenic ages. Winokur, Pfohl, and Tsuang (1987) found that older schizophrenics were most likely to have problems with affect, orientation, memory, and amount of verbal communication. However, Whanger and Meyers (1984) state that as the person ages, hallucinations often become less frequent and delusions may disappear. It is not unusual for schizophrenics to improve with age.

Strauss (1987) writes that it is rare for schizophrenia to develop in old age. The geriatric schizophrenic has most likely suffered from the illness for many years. Many schizophrenics have been cared for by their families in the home for years and have rarely or never been hospitalized. When parents or siblings die, the older schizophrenic is often left alone. Unable to manage at home, some become institutionalized; others become street people.

There are a number of theories about the causes of schizophrenia: family communication, sociocultural, psychological, and biological. It has been noted that the disorder is more prevalent in some families than in others (American Psychiatric Association, 1994; Butler, Lewis & Sunderland, 1991). Emphasis is currently being placed on genetic links in schizophrenics: "The first-degree biological relatives of individuals with schizophrenia have a risk for schizophrenia that is about 10 times greater than that of the general population" (American Psychiatric Association, 1994, p. 283).

Diagnostic Categories

There are five major diagnostic categories of schizophrenia used in diagnosing older adults as well as other age groups: (1) disorganized type, (2) catatonic type, (3) paranoid type, (4) undifferentiated type, and (5) residual type.

Disorganized Type

The disorganized schizophrenic may have disorganized speech and behavior and have an inappropriate or flat affect. Delusions are not organized around a coherent theme. The person may demonstrate grimacing and odd mannerisms (American Psychiatric Association, 1994). Hebephrenic schizophrenics, a subtype, were often housed in the back wards of large state mental hospitals until the mid-twentieth century. Many hebephrenics were older and had been hospitalized for years.

Catatonic Type

Clients who are diagnosed as having catatonic schizophrenia may be stuporous or they may demonstrate excitement and display purposeless motor activity. Catatonic stupor may include motoric immobility or an inappropriate position (waxy flexibility). One older resident of a nursing home would sit in a gerichair all day, stare into space, not speak, and hold first one arm and then the other straight up in the air for long intervals. She was nonambulatory but would eat certain foods without a word when fed. Extreme negativism and mutism may be seen (American Psychiatric Association, 1994).

Paranoid Type

Paranoid schizophrenia is more prevalent than either catatonic or disorganized schizophrenia and tends to begin later in life. The person with this diagnosis may have little impairment in cognition (American Psychiatric Association, 1994). Delusions are a dominant feature and are usually persecutory or grandiose in nature. The paranoid person is generally unable to trust others, and hostility is a common characteristic of this diagnosis. Hallucinations related to the delusions may also be present.

PARAPHRENIA. Paraphrenia is late-onset persecutory delusions. This term is not included in the diagnoses listed by the American Psychiatric Association (1994). The symptoms of paraphrenia are often difficult to differentiate from those of chronic schizophrenia, dementia, and delirium (Hall & Buckwalter, 1989). However, paraphrenia occurs when paranoid symptoms are manifest without symptoms of organic dementia or severe cognitive and affective impairment (Roth, 1987). Delusions and hallucinations are poorly systematized, and the deterioration of schizophrenia is not present. Paraphrenia is more common in women than in men (Hall & Buckwalter, 1989), and visual or hearing impairments may be a factor (Butler et al., 1991). Genetic, epidemiological, and developmental factors are being studied to determine the causes of paraphrenia (Hall & Buckwalter, 1989). A study by Naguib, McCuffin, Levy, Festenstein, and Alonso (1987) indicated that paraphrenics may be genetically different from schizophrenics. Paraphrenics are often physically and socially isolated.

The 80-year-old with paraphrenia may suddenly begin to believe that friends and neighbors of 40 years are stealing items such as jewelry or yard tools from him or her. Others begin to believe that their children or grandchildren have begun stealing cars, dishes, and other valued objects from them.

Undifferentiated Type

The undifferentiated type includes symptoms that are not as obvious or as easily discriminated as those in the three types previously discussed. The person having this diagnosis has psychotic symptoms such as delusions and hallucinations and may also demonstrate disorganized speech that may make it difficult to understand what the client is saying. (American Psychiatric Association, 1994).

Residual Type

The person who is classified as schizophrenic, residual type, has had at least one previous schizophrenic episode. Psychotic symptoms such as delusions and hallucinations may not be obvious; however, symptoms such as flat affect, eccentric behavior, or odd beliefs are present (American Psychiatric Association, 1994).

Nursing Care

The following discussion will describe nursing interventions that are appropriate for the various types of schizophrenia. Nursing interventions for behaviors that occur with schizophrenics and with clients who have other diagnoses will be included.

When caring for the schizophrenic of any age, it is important to remember that progress may be slow and the goal may be remission rather than cure. However, observing relief of symptoms and increased quality of life for the older patient and the family can be rewarding for the caregiver. Since one of the major tools for providing care for the schizophrenic is the interactive process between the client and the caregiver, it is desirable that the caregiver be able to do a self-analysis related to the therapeutic process to determine the effect of the interaction on the client and the illness. Ongoing self-evaluation is necessary to determine which interventions are effective and which are not. This process is personal and dynamic; therefore, in a health care facility it is important that provisions be made for continuity of care by assigning the same caregivers to the client whenever possible.

Characteristics important in any relationship become even more so when working with a schizophrenic person. Since distrust is a common problem, honesty on the part of the caregiver is essential. It is necessary to move into the relationship at the client's pace, usually slowly, with a matter-of-fact, kind but firm attitude that is not too friendly. This approach allows trust to build, whereas an overly friendly attitude may be frightening and motivate the client to maintain distance rather than to form a relationship.

The client's verbal communication may be symbolic or illogical. Over time the meaning may become clear. The nurse may respond to symbolic or illogical statements by saying, "I don't understand what you mean" or "By that statement do you mean . . .?" Nonverbal communication should be noted as well, since it may clarify the meaning of words. Winokur et al. (1987) observed that speech may decrease in the older schizophrenic. Special effort is required to understand verbal and nonverbal communication in this population.

When clients are severely withdrawn, it is necessary for the nurse to help them meet basic biological needs such as food and fluid. The caregiver may have to encourage the client to eat at mealtime and to offer fluids throughout the day. Assistance with activities of daily living such as bathing, dressing, toileting, and oral care may be necessary (Stuart & Sundeen, 1995).

Some withdrawn clients may be mute or talk sparingly. The nurse should let such persons know that they will be listened to when they decide to talk. To encourage verbalization, the nurse should ask questions that are not intimidating. Mute clients are often well aware of their surroundings. The nurse should address the client with respect and convey the expectation that the client will talk when ready. Older clients may have more problems with orientation and memory than the newly diagnosed schizophrenic (Winokur et al., 1987). Reality orientation is important with this group.

During the initial assessment interview the nurse should listen to the client's description of delusions and hallucinations but avoid encouraging continued description in future interactions. Frequent questioning regarding these symptoms may promote sick behavior rather than healthy coping skills. The nurse should not attempt to disprove delusions or hallucinations. Generally, as anxiety decreases and the person becomes more comfortable, the delusions and hallucinations will decrease. A goal related to these symptoms is to decrease anxiety. Some clients are never able to give up their delusions and hallucinations. They are advised by caregivers not to discuss them with others, so that they will be accepted in the community (Stuart & Sundeen, 1995). Buckwalter (1992) discusses phantom seeing and hearing, which are experienced by many older persons. The cause of these problems seems to be lack of sensory input. The phantom sights and sounds can be startling to the individual. Consistent attentive staff and adequate meaningful sensory stimulation help to decrease phantom experiences. Hearing and sight impairments should be treated whenever possible.

Since schizophrenics may be out of touch with reality and living in a world of their own, they may be uninterested in hygiene and forget to bathe, shave, comb their hair, and brush their teeth. Telling them that it is time for these activities often promotes compliance. At other times it may be necessary to assist the client with maintaining hygiene.

Touch can be therapeutic; however, the schizophrenic who does not trust may find invasion of personal space and physical contact threatening. Therefore, the nurse should allow the client to set the limits on touching. If the client touches the caregiver, then it is usually acceptable for the caregiver to touch the client.

Physical activity such as walking provides a relief from anxiety and aids in sleep. Also, walking with someone is a nonthreatening way to share an experience that may help build a therapeutic relationship.

The environment should be safe, pleasant, and not too stimulating. It should be designed to promote the goals of treatment and to have seating areas as well as areas for games or group activities. Each client should follow a daily schedule based on individual needs.

Catatonic and paranoid schizophrenic clients demonstrate anger. The nurse must understand that the anger is a reaction to internal as well as external environmental factors. Therefore anger may be expressed in relation to thought disorders such as delusions and hallucinations. Anger may also be related to a perceived threat from someone in the external environment. It is important that the nurse not personalize the anger and react to the client in a hostile manner. Rather, it is more therapeutic to discuss the feelings and any outbursts to determine the cause of the client's anger. Brief explanations of treatment plans and offering clients choices can be helpful. The nurse should note the kinds of events that tend to bring on inappropriate angry outbursts and assist the client in reacting in a more socially acceptable manner.

Nurses should avoid placing themselves in dangerous situations. If it is possible that the client may get out of control, the nurse should take precautions such as having other personnel present.

A care plan for an older schizophrenic is shown on p. 213. This client had a history of withdrawal and isolation and had to be encouraged to make contact with

Nursing Care Plan for an Older Adult with a Diagnosis of Schizophrenia

Assessment data	Nursing diagnosis and goals	Nursing interventions	Evaluation
Subjective "I don't need anything. People try to take my things. I can't leave my house—they'll come in. I don't have a car. I can't go anywhere. My daughter lives far away. She never comes to visit me."	Social isolation related to lack of trust as evidenced by staying home alone. **Short-term goals** 1. Client will invite nurse into home when nurse visits. 2. Client will talk with nurse for 15 minutes.	1. Send card to client informing him when visit will occur. 2. Visit client every other week. 3. Ask client if nurse can visit with him in his home for 15 minutes.	1. Card sent. 2. Visit made. 3. Client allowed nurse in home somewhat reluctantly. Nurse stayed 15 minutes. Client seemed tense.
Objective 80-year-old man lives alone in home. Wife died 15 years ago. He rarely leaves home. Keeps shades pulled over windows and doors locked. Goes to corner grocery once or twice a week. Little food in kitchen.	**Long-term goals** 1. Client will use public transportation to increase radius of excursions from home. 2. Client will accompany neighbor to senior citizen's center for meals and activities. 3. Client will make contact with daughter. 4. Client will form meaningful relationship with nurse.	4. Encourage client to talk. Ask open-ended questions. 5. Tell client about public transportation including special services for older people. 6. Provide a schedule for public transportation. 7. Describe senior citizen's center and schedule of activities. 8. In a few weeks encourage client to discuss daughter. 9. In a few weeks encourage client to make contact with daughter. 10. Listen to client. 11. Be on time for appointments with client.	4. Client answered questions. Did not volunteer information. 5. Client informed about public transportation but made no verbal comment. 6. Left bus schedule with him. Will talk about this again. 7. Informed client of senior citizen's center schedule. 8. Will implement later. 9. Will implement later. 10. Listened to client, although he said little. 11. Was on time for appointment.

others in order to meet his needs. The nurse worked with the client in his urban home.

❖ *Paranoid Personality Disorders*

The incidence of paranoid beliefs increases with age (Butler et al., 1991). The paranoid person has often gone through life developing few human relationships; as these few people die or move away, the aging person becomes more alone. Social isolation, illness, and the aging process tend to increase suspiciousness and paranoid thoughts (Burnside, 1988).

Characteristics

A person may have paranoid symptoms and not be diagnosed as having paranoid schizophrenia. The person with a paranoid disorder has a persecutory or grandiose delusion that influences mood, behavior, and thinking. The delusions of the schizophrenic are more bizarre and less systematized than are the delusions of the person with paranoid disorder. Wilson & Kneisl (1992) reported that elders are more prone than other age groups to have persecutory delusions. Even though paranoid persons may be resentful, belligerent, and generally unable to relate well to people, many live isolated in homes or apartments and are not hospitalized. Neighbors and relatives are mistrusted and may become a part of their delusions.

One 85-year-old woman living in a retirement center was referred by the manager to a psychiatrist because of repeated evidence of hallucinations and delusions. The older woman said several "foreign men and women" were after her. She said she heard them talking about her and constantly walking in the apartment above her and in the hall outside her apartment. She especially heard the women because they wore high heels. These comments might not sound particularly unusual in an apartment in a retirement center where the noises of others can be heard above and in the hall. The woman was well-groomed, friendly, and seemed alert. However, on further questioning she said that sometimes she had red spots on her arms because those people sprayed chemicals under her apartment door and through the keyhole. One morning she was found on a bed in an empty apartment. She said that those people had drugged her, picked her up during the night, and taken her into the other apartment. She had some skin problems and probably some beginning organic brain changes that could possibly have accounted for her concern about her skin and nighttime wandering. This situation demonstrates the complexity of mental problems imposed on physical problems in very old clients. This client threatened to shoot the people who were bothering her, and she did have a handgun in her apartment. Unfortunately, she refused further evaluation and treatment. Her family also refused to seek treatment for her, saying, "Mother has had these same beliefs for years." Fortunately, she moved out of the retirement center, because she was a potential threat to other residents.

In the person who suffers from chronic paranoid disorder or paranoid schizophrenia, the deeply rooted inability to trust others is based on long-standing insecurities that can often be traced to early childhood. However, it is believed that severe stress can produce paranoid disorders in later life (Butler et al., 1991). When the senses are unable to perceive accurately, details are filled in by the mind, and others may be accused of laughing at or talking negatively about the older person (Butler et al., 1991). It has also been observed that some medications seem to cause paranoid symptoms. An example is the male hormones taken in conjunction with antidepressants (Wilson & Kneisl, 1992). Many feelings of suspiciousness and paranoia are responses to relationships and situations in which the older person is made to feel powerless and unimportant (Ebersole & Hess, 1994). According to Wilson and Kneisl (1992), "Persecutory delusions may be a response of the elderly to a diminishing sense of self-mastery" (p. 882). When older people begin to lose independence and control, they may begin to believe that people are taking advantage of them. They then begin to reject their caregivers (e.g., family) in an effort to regain control over their own lives. Reality is the basis for suspicion and paranoia in many older people (Eisdorfer, 1980). The news media often relate instances in which others have plotted against older people to obtain their money or other belongings.

Paranoid reactions may be associated with dementia. Delusions are not systematized and often change. As dementia and other conditions improve, paranoid ideation also diminishes (Burnside, 1988).

Nursing Care

Paranoid persons are generally brought to the caregiver or health care facility by others rather than seeking help themselves. They believe that others have a problem or are causing problems; therefore paranoid persons usually have no incentive to seek or accept help. They are frequently angry about what is happening to them. One older patient diagnosed with paranoid schizophrenia was angry and verbally and physically abusive to those around her. She had long-term delusions, blaming her multiple problems on state and national elected officials who had been in office many years ago. She talked constantly but was difficult to understand because of severe tongue movements, most likely tardive dyskinesia caused by long-term psychiatric drug therapy. She was hospitalized for a short time for evaluation and revision of her medication regimen, but her ultimate prognosis was poor.

Since the paranoid person may not be motivated to cooperate, it may be necessary to obtain a history from significant others. As the person becomes less angry and anxious, additional details may be added by the paranoid older person.

When caring for a paranoid person, the nurse's long-term goal is to build trust. This is done by being scrupulously honest, by keeping appointments, by being kind but not too friendly or too nice, and by not being too reassuring. Clear communication and empathic listening are essential.

The aim of treatment for the paranoid person is to reduce anxiety. The nurse should try to understand the underlying anxiety and avoid threatening the person.

Trying to prove that delusions are irrational can be threatening. These belief systems have been developed in response to anxiety, and attempts to challenge them may increase anxiety. Instead the caregiver can listen without encouraging or reinforcing the delusional ideas. It is often best to make no comment.

Anxiety may be reduced by allowing the paranoid person to set limits on the closeness of relationships with the nurse and others. Whenever possible, the client should be allowed to determine the length and frequency of human interactions. Long contacts are not tolerated well. Personal space should be invaded with care and based on clues the caregiver receives from the paranoid person. The distance maintained by the person may decrease as trust increases.

Allowing the paranoid person to make as many decisions as possible without interfering with the rights and the care of others prevents unnecessary anxiety. Trying to force participation in group activities can cause unpleasant experiences for all involved. Offering the individual the opportunity to participate is a better approach.

Accurate perception of the environment through the senses is helpful in preventing suspiciousness. Glasses, hearing aids, color-coded walls, and large lettering can assist those with impaired sensory perception. Increasing lighting and decreasing sensory overload caused by unnecessary noise and activity allows impaired older adults to decrease confusion and tension.

The paranoid person may be generally angry, and the nurse should accept the angry attitude as a reaction to the person's perception of a threatening environment. It is best to acknowledge the anger without reacting with anger in turn and to accept criticism without becoming defensive. The nurse should be accepting of persons even though they are angry (Ebersole & Hess, 1994).

Families of paranoid persons need support and help to understand what is happening to the older family member. They should be involved in planning for the care of the paranoid person. It may be necessary for a family member to supervise the older person's taking of medication and follow-up care.

❖ *Anxiety Disorders*

Types

Anxiety disorders most commonly found in older adults are obsessive-compulsive disorder, generalized anxiety disorder, and phobic disorders. "*Obsessions* are persistent ideas, thoughts, impulses, or images that are experienced as intrusive and inappropriate and that cause marked anxiety or distress" (American Psychiatric Association, 1994, p. 418). "*Compulsions* are repetitive behaviors . . . or mental acts . . . the goal of which is to prevent or reduce anxiety or distress, not to provide pleasure or gratification" (American Psychiatric Association, 1994, p. 418). As the obsessive-compulsive person strives to control anxiety through ritualistic behavior, restrictions and demands may be placed on others in the environment. For example, an older woman was hospitalized in a psychiatric facility because of her disruptive rituals. In the hospital she would sit in only one chair in the group room. If she came into the room and someone was in her selected chair, she would leave and refuse to participate in activities. Her lengthy morning rituals related to bathing and dressing usually meant that she was late to scheduled appointments. Attempts to rush her increased her anxiety to the point where she was obviously frustrated and would begin to tremble. Others had to wait and make special adjustments in their own schedules to accommodate her. Obsessive-compulsive disorder in older adults may be associated with or predispose to depression. Also, it is sometimes seen in the person with dementia (Verwoerdt, 1980).

Generalized anxiety disorder is characterized by symptoms such as restlessness, fatigue, difficulty concentrating, irritability, muscle tension, and sleep disturbance (American Psychiatric Association, 1994).

Causes

Causes of anxiety in older adults are as varied as for any other age group. Sometimes the cause is obvious and a precipitating event can be identified. At other times a professional person such as a psychiatric or gerontological nurse may be needed to help the older person explore causes for the anxious feelings. Areas that often produce anxiety in older adults are declining health, the aging process, financial problems, changing housing arrangements, loss of loved ones, and lack of transportation.

Nursing Care

When providing care for anxious older patients, the caregiver must understand the unique and anxiety-producing life hazards that older people face. Limitations such as less reserve physical and emotional capacity or organic brain disease must be recognized.

Intervention may be as simple as listening to the older person describe the anxiety-causing event. Sometimes simply talking about an anxiety-producing event will put it into perspective and reduce the anxiety.

The degree of anxiety should be assessed. Mild anxiety can motivate a person to concentrate and learn (Wang, 1986). Moderate to severe anxiety causes discomfort, and efforts should be made to alleviate the uncomfortable feelings. Physical and emotional signs include increased pulse, elevated blood pressure, nausea and vomiting, gastrointestinal upset, headache, and excessive perspiration. In older people some symptoms, such as tremor, may be due to physical illness (Wang, 1986). Emotional indicators of anxiety are statements such as "I feel like something awful is going to happen to me," "I can't concentrate," and "I am really uptight." As the anxiety increases, feelings of helplessness increase, and the person becomes more dependent on significant others, including caregivers.

The calm presence of a trusted person is usually appreciated. The client who has ability to learn should be helped to identify anxiety as a feeling, and the nurse should note any relief behavior. Next the events preceding increased anxiety are discussed to discover the causes. These problem-solving techniques may identify the source of the anxious feelings; however, the person may not be able to determine exact causes. Nevertheless, measures should be taken to make the person more comfortable. Actions effective in dealing with or preventing discomfort should be identified and implemented. Wang (1986) notes that some older adults with anxiety disorders have limited ability to learn because of dementia or other organic problems, so this approach is not appropriate for them. Instead, calm reassurance from a caregiver is more helpful. Physical activity such as walking, jogging, and some sports can help alleviate anxiety. It should be purposeful and absorb the client's energy (Verwoerdt, 1980).

Symptoms of severe or panic anxiety include loss of reality, experiences such as delusions or hallucinations, extreme fright, inability to sleep or relax, and diaphoresis. This level of anxiety is physically dangerous and must be alleviated as soon as possible. Persons in automobile accidents or with delirium tremens have panic anxiety.

It is important to provide a safe, well-lighted, quiet environment with little stimulus to be misinterpreted, which increases anxiety. Verbal communication should be short and clearly stated. The short attention span precludes involved directions.

Persons experiencing moderate to panic level anxiety should be referred to a physician for evaluation for somatic and other types of therapies. Chronic high levels of anxiety reduce the quality of and zest for life. Efforts should be made to alleviate anxiety whenever possible.

A stable, familiar environment surrounded by those who care is important in anxiety prevention. Allowing the older person to set the pace for activities helps to avoid anxiety. Anticipating needs of older clients and helping them use community resources such as transportation and sources of balanced meals can also prevent anxiety.

It may be desirable to involve family members in anxiety prevention in older people. Family members may be resourceful in problem solution. Prompt anxiety reduction is necessary in some families because chronic or intense anxiety tends to drive others away from the older person at a time when they are most needed.

For the obsessive-compulsive older person, attempts to interrupt or hurry the behavior is seldom helpful. It is generally better to help the person feel loved and appreciated. Planning ahead to allow time for rituals and searching for their underlying causes may be productive.

Nursing intervention for phobic disorders includes anxiety-reduction techniques. The calm, reassuring attitude of the caregiver can help the phobic person feel some measure of control in most difficult or frightening situations. Also, brief discussions of phobic thoughts and the accompanying feelings of fear help the person to put uncomfortable situations in better perspective. Relaxation techniques are effective in reducing fear and anxiety. Behavior modification using desensitization therapy by a trained therapist is advocated for the person experiencing a phobic disorder.

❖ *Somatoform Disorders*

Hypochondriasis

Somatoform disorders such as hypochondriasis are frequently found in older clients. This group of disorders is characterized by complaints of physical symptoms with no medical condition that accounts for the symptoms (American Psychiatric Association, 1994). The symptoms "appear to be psychologically rather than physically caused" (Butler et al., 1991, p. 140). For example, a significant loss may have occurred leaving the person lonely. Somatic delusions composed of morbid content are not uncommon in older persons (Wilson and Kneisl, 1992).

Hypochondriasis occurs frequently among older clients, especially women. The person is preoccupied with the body or body parts and concerned that disease has invaded or that the body is not functioning properly. Symptoms are usually vague and relate to many different systems or parts of the body. Discussion by the client frequently focuses on somatic complaints; however, there appears to be little real concern or worry expressed. Instead, the older person discusses symptoms matter-of-factly and rarely develops insight into the hypochondriacal behavior. Some research suggests that hypochondriasis is a symptom of depression (Matteson & McConnell, 1988; Wilson & Kneisl, 1992). Hypochondriasis is often preceded by a significant life event such as retirement, change of residence, or change in a family relationship.

Complaints of aches and pains may be an attempt by the older person to deal with or to communicate a more basic anxiety or depression. It may be an unconscious attempt to identify with a deceased loved one by taking on similar physical symptoms (Butler et al., 1991).

Nursing Care

When the nurse is planning and providing care, a positive, trusting relationship must be established. Time limits for interactions should be set and generally maintained. If limits are ignored, the client may bring up new symptoms at the close of the designated time period to have the nurse stay longer (Busse, 1986).

At the first meeting it is important to complete a thorough history and health assessment. Initial physical complaints should not be ignored, and appropriate referrals should be made (Bruce & McNamara, 1992). Clients who were thought to be hypochondriaical have had symptoms ignored until they became seriously ill; some have actually died.

The impact of continual physical complaints on the family should be assessed. Noting reactions to determine if the older person is being rewarded by the family with undue attention or hostility can help in planning care (Matteson & McConnell, 1988).

It is important to be a good listener; however, continual complaining should not be rewarded. When possible the person should be encouraged to reminisce or discuss other topics of interest. A trusting relationship makes this easier.

The nurse should be alert for the possibility of overmedication when obtaining the history. It is not unusual that a hypochondriac has seen several physicians and received different medication prescriptions from each.

The nurse should avoid trying to convince the person that the illness is not real. Such action only makes the person more determined to persuade others of the real nature of the illness (Busse, 1986). The nurse should acknowledge that a problem exists but not offer a diagnosis or prognosis. Positive client behaviors and attitudes should be reinforced (Matteson & McConnell, 1988).

❖ *Summary*

All types of functional psychiatric problems are found in older adults. The nurse will provide care for these clients in both health care facilities and homes. It is important to be aware of the special circumstances, life events, and hazards of this developmental age group when planning and providing care.

Self-awareness is a major focus of nursing care; the interpersonal relationship is a key factor in helping the older person adjust and improve. It is important for the suspicious or paranoid person to develop a trusting relationship. When the schizophrenic uses illogical or symbolic communication, the nurse should attempt to understand and clarify meanings in a nonthreatening manner. Severely withdrawn clients may need help to meet basic needs for food and fluids. Mute patients should be encouraged to verbalize when ready.

Delusions and hallucinations should be assessed but not rewarded so that healthful coping skills are encouraged rather than sick behavior. Touch should be used with caution when caring for a schizophrenic patient because physical contact can be threatening. Physical activity and a planned daily schedule relieve anxiety, aid sleep, and improve self-esteem.

When dealing with an angry client, it is best not to personalize the anger. Encouraging socially appropriate expression of feelings is helpful. The nurse should avoid dangerous situations in which clients may lose control. Assistance should be sought from others as necessary.

The paranoid person should be allowed to make decisions whenever possible. This person should also set limits on the length and frequency of interactions with the caregiver. Personal space should be treated with respect. Aids for accurate sensory perception can help alleviate anxiety and suspicion. Many suspicious older people have hearing problems.

Anxiety is an uncomfortable feeling that is a common component in functional psychiatric diagnoses. Effective intervention reduces symptoms and increases quality of life. Interventions may be as simple as listening, companionship, and reassurance.

The degree of anxiety should be assessed. The person who experiences disruptive anxiety can be helped to identify problems that cause anxiety and to find more satisfactory ways of preventing and dealing with anxiety-producing situations. Persons with high levels of anxiety should stay in well-lighted rooms with little stimulation present. The environment should be safe. Communication should be short and simple.

Rituals of the obsessive-compulsive older person should not be interrupted. Planning to allow time for rituals and searching for the root causes of the anxiety producing the rituals may be helpful.

The hypochondriac should have an initial thorough health assessment and additional evaluation as new complaints develop. Complaints should not be rewarded. Attempts to convince the person that the illness is not real should be avoided. Positive client behaviors and attitudes should be reinforced.

With the care and concern of family and professionals, the older person with a functional psychiatric problem can be helped to achieve a more rewarding and satisfying life. Nurses can make a difference in meeting this goal.

❖ *References*

American Psychiatric Association. (1994). *Diagnostic and statistical manual of mental disorders* (4th ed.). Washington, DC: Author.

Bruce, M., & McNamara, R. (1992). Psychiatric status among the homebound elderly: An epidemiologic perspective. *Journal of the American Geriatrics Society, 40*(6), 561-566.

Buckwalter, K. (1992). Phantom of the nursing home. *Journal of Gerontological Nursing, 18*(9), 46-47.

Burnside, I. M. (1988). *Nursing and the aged* (3rd ed.). New York: McGraw-Hill.

Busse, E. (1986). Treating hypochondriasis in the elderly. *Generations, 10*(3), 30-33.

Butler, R., Lewis, M., & Sunderland, T. (1991). *Aging and mental health* (4th ed.). New York: Macmillan.

Ebersole, P., & Hess, P. (1994). *Toward healthy aging: Human needs and nursing response* (4th ed.). St. Louis: Mosby.

Eisdorfer, C. (1980). Paranoia and schizophrenic disorders in later life. In E. W. Busse & D. G. Blazer (Eds.). *Handbook of geriatric psychiatry* (pp. 329-337). New York: Van Nostrand Reinhold.

Hall, G. R., & Buckwalter, K. C. (1989). Diagnostic clues in the past. *Geriatric Nursing, 10*(4), 202-204.

Matteson, M. A., & McConnell, E. (1988). *Gerontological nursing: Concepts and practice.* Philadelphia: Saunders.

Naguib, M., McCuffin, P., Levy, R., Festenstein, H., & Alonso, A. (1987). Genetics markers in late paraphrenia: A study of HLA antigens. *British Journal of Psychiatry, 150*(1), 124-127.

Roth, M. (1987). Late paraphrenia: Phenomenology and etiological factors and their bearing upon problems of the schizophrenic family of disorders. In N. Miller & G. Cohen (Eds.). *Schizophrenia and aging* (pp. 217-234). New York: Guilford Press.

Strauss, J. (1987). Schizophrenia and aging: Meeting point of diagnostic and conceptual questions. In N. Miller & G. Cohen (Eds.). *Schizophrenia and aging* (pp. 3-8). New York: Guilford Press.

Stuart, G., & Sundeen, S. (1995). *Principles and practice of psychiatric nursing* (5th ed.). St. Louis: Mosby.

Verwoerdt, A. (1980). Anxiety, dissociative and personality disorders in the elderly. In E. W. Busse & D. G. Blazer (Eds.). *Handbook of geriatric psychiatry* (pp. 368-380). New York: Van Nostrand Reinhold.

Wang, H. S. (1986). Anxiety disorders. *Generations, 10*(3), 27-29.

Whanger, A., & Meyers, A. (1984). *Mental health assessment and therapeutic intervention with older adults.* Rockville, MD: Aspen.

Wilson, H. S., & Kneisl, C. (1992). *Psychiatric nursing* (4th ed.). Menlo Park, CA: Addison-Wesley.

Winokur, G., Pfohl, B. & Tsuang, M. (1987). A 40 year follow-up of hebephrenic-catatonic schizophrenia. In N. Miller & G. Cohen (Eds.). *Schizophrenia and aging* (pp. 52-60). New York: Guilford Press.

Chapter *9*

❖ *Substance-Related Disorders*

Maisie Schmidt Kashka
Sandra Helene Tweed

Substance abuse is a broad term that covers several patterns of drug taking. *Drug use* is the ingestion of medication for a legitimate purpose in the manner in which it is intended. *Drug misuse* is the ingestion of medication for a reason other than that for which the medication is designed, or ingestion of the drug in a manner other than that for which it is intended. *Drug abuse* is the most serious form of substance abuse. It refers to inappropriate drug ingestion in such a way that the individual's functioning, relationships, or both are disrupted to some degree. DSM-IV (1994) describes substance dependence as "a cluster of cognitive, behavioral, and physiological symptoms indicating that the individual continues use of the substance despite significant substance-related problems" (p. 176). In the past, physical addiction received heavy emphasis as the major criterion for a diagnosis of substance abuse. However, current thought among clinicians is that psychological dependence on a particular drug or drugs is a sufficient criterion for a diagnosis of substance abuse. With the newer approach, drug abuse is considered to be present when an individual's lifestyle or relationships are disrupted. Therefore the amount of a substance ingested is not as important as the effect that ingestion has on the person's life and functioning.

❖ *Prevalence*

Substance misuse and abuse is a complicated issue in older adults for the following reasons: (1) they receive a greater proportion of prescribed drugs, (2) they have more reasons for needing medications, and (3) they have a diminished tolerance for most drugs. Although persons over 65 are only 11% of the population, they consume 25%

to 33% of all prescribed drugs (Closser & Blow, 1993). About 75% of persons over the age of 65 use some kind of medication, one third of which are over-the-counter medications. Inappropriate use of prescription and over-the-counter drugs most commonly is drug misuse rather than drug abuse. An increasing number of medications prescribed for older adults are psychoactive agents. Older adults take more antidepressants and antianxiety (minor tranquilizer) drugs than other age groups. This is particularly dangerous among older adults who also drink because of the synergistic effect of these drugs with alcohol. These synergistic effects can lead to accidents and oversedation; oversedation in turn can lead to aspiration pneumonia (Closser & Blow, 1993).

Maddox (1988) summarized data collected by the National Institute of Mental Health and made the following seven assertions concerning alcohol use among older people in the United States:

1. Older individuals, particularly women, are more likely than younger individuals to abstain from alcohol, and many of those who abstain in later life have been abstinent all of their lives.
2. Alcohol use declines in the later years, particularly after age 60.
3. Although approximately 5% of the adult population exhibit patterns of alcohol abuse, the rates are greatest among men of all ages, but far less for older men. In fact, alcohol-related problems are lower in old age than at any other time in the adult life cycle.
4. Socioeconomic class appears to play a role in alcohol abuse patterns, at least among adults in general, with more abuse seemingly exhibited by individuals of lower socioeconomic status. However, whether this observation is valid in the older adult population is questionable.
5. The rates of alcoholism in the older adult population exhibit great variability, so much so that great caution must be used in interpreting any assertions regarding the rate of alcoholism in this age group.
6. The onset of alcohol abuse after age 65 is rare because most problem drinkers in the later years established their problematic drinking behavior before age 65.
7. The best evidence available suggests that alcohol abuse among older adults is low.

This last assertion is challenged by other authorities. Closser and Blow (1993) believe the rate of alcohol abuse among older adults is probably higher because of (1) the use of screening measures developed for young, not older, adults, (2) lack of identification of alcohol abuse symptoms by health care professionals and patients, and (3) greater stigma attached to reporting alcohol abuse among this group (p. 205). Especially with older adults, professionals often confuse the symptoms of alcohol abuse with manifestations of other mental or physical disorders (Kela, Kosberg, & Joyce, 1984).

While Maddox (1988) maintains that there will be no evidence that the rate of alcoholism will increase as the present middle-aged population ages, Alexander & Duff (1988), Closser and Blow (1993), and Glantz and Backenheimer (1988) disagree. These authors believe alcohol use in the present older cohort has always been light, at least partially because they grew up with a strong temperance tradition. They further assert that as the heavier-drinking current middle-aged and young adult cohorts (who were brought up in a more permissive atmosphere) age, the rates of abuse of alcohol and other substances will most likely increase.

Although the rate of substance abuse among older adults is relatively low compared with that of the overall adult population, the substance *most* abused is alcohol. The older alcohol abuser tends to be a man who comes for treatment with many chronic, debilitating illnesses that are a direct result of long years of alcoholism (Garland, 1983). Estimates of alcoholism in older adults range from 2% to 10% (Mendelson & Mello, 1985; Pascarella, 1981). Whittington (1988) challenges both the 2% and the 10% estimates and asserts that there are no reliable estimates of the rate of alcoholism among the older population. Closser and Blow (1993) report that the National Institute of Mental Health's Epidemiological Catchment Area (ECA) statistics suggest that among community-dwelling individuals 65 and over 14% of the men and 1.5% of the women abuse alcohol. They assert that in clinical settings (hospitals, clinics, and nursing homes) the rate is much higher and state that reported rates of current alcoholism among older adults varies from 15% to 58%. They conclude that alcoholism among older adults is hidden, underidentified, and underreported. Closser and Blow (1993) state that "there is emerging evidence that alcoholism among the elderly is a significant and growing health problem in this country" (p. 205).

There are also conflicting opinions regarding the rate of alcoholism among older women. Liptzin (1987) suggests that older men have alcohol or drug dependence rates of 3% to 4% and older women have a negligible rate. There may be fewer older women alcoholics, but they exhibit a gender vulnerability to alcohol because "alcoholic women die 15 years earlier than nonalcoholic women and have death rates 50% to 100% higher than alcoholic men" (Chatham, 1987, p. 17). In addition, older women alcoholics are stigmatized more than men alcoholics, which compounds the isolation and difficulty in getting women to obtain treatment.

One of the difficulties in obtaining a firm estimate of the rate of alcoholism in older adults is the isolation of the older alcoholic person because of decreasing social contact. Older adults usually are no longer employed at full-time jobs and because of widowhood may live alone. Therefore they have contact with far fewer people than at any other period in their lives. Typically alcohol use declines with age, so that some individuals who have a history of heavy drinking during earlier years may drink far less in later years because of their impaired ability to metabolize alcohol and the physical sequelae of a lifetime of alcohol abuse. Alcoholism is a life-threatening illness, and many alcoholics who survive to old age are in a severely impaired physical condition. Although alcohol abuse is not restricted to any one category of older individuals, "those elderly persons associated with the highest rate of problem drinking or alcoholism show a typical social profile of being widowed, divorced, or single men who have experienced difficulty with the police and who live in impoverished areas" (Mendelson & Mello, 1985, p. 128). However, Alexander and Duff (1988) report that the heaviest drinkers in the retirement communities are also the heaviest social drinkers, those who drink both socially and alone. This suggests that their pattern of alcohol use may be apparent to others in their social setting.

Opiate abuse is even less visible because it tends to occur among a hidden group of urban older adults and is sometimes found in older Asian-Americans. Since most opiate addicts use less as they age, and since the opiates do not cause some of the serious complications of alcoholism, this population does not as often come to the attention of health care providers. Older opiate abusers are sometimes encountered in methadone maintenance programs. In a New York City methadone maintenance clinic the average age of black clients was 30.4 years and the average age of Chinese clients was 64.9 years (Reed, 1981, p. 759).

❖ *Causes*

It is tempting to assume that causes of substance abuse fit into neat categories, particularly within an age group. However, certain causative factors are more prevalent in some age groups than others. For example, losses, loneliness, and physical illness are more likely to be causes of alcohol abuse for older people than for younger individuals.

Losses

Losses increase dramatically as people age. Many older persons have lost their lifetime significant relationships, prized personal possessions, financial security, rewarding employment, and physical health. Depending on the number and rate of losses individuals encounter, their internal emotional resources, and their interpersonal support system, these losses may be overwhelming. Thus loss of significant emotional attachments leads some older persons to seek the chemical numbing provided by alcohol. For individuals who develop this pattern of coping, the pain of their later years may become unbearable without the chemical relief of alcohol or another tranquilizing drug. Essentially, such individuals use self-medication to relieve psychological pain. For some of these older persons, alcohol will become the friend they no longer have.

Loneliness

Loneliness usually results from the losses discussed in the preceding section. The loneliness of old age may both cause substance abuse and prevent its detection. The very isolation that precipitates the abuse also hides it. However, Alexander & Duff (1988) emphasize that although there are some older individuals who use alcohol in a solitary fashion, their study, which examined the relationship between alcohol use and social isolation in older people, found that "the more isolated individuals are the least likely to drink heavily. . . . Socially gregarious individuals make up the bulk of the heavy drinkers" (p. 60). On the other hand, Caroselli-Karinja (1985) believes that life changes in older adults increase their vulnerability to using drug and alcohol as a means of coping.

Physical Illness

Concerns about declining physical health lead some older individuals to use over-the-counter medications. This can be further complicated by limited resources that prevent them from seeking medical help for physical problems. For some older individuals, it may be financially less expensive in the short term to self-medicate.

❖ Types of Substance Abuse

Alcohol

Any discussion of alcohol use in the older adult is complicated by the controversy regarding the potential benefits of moderate alcohol use throughout the life span, particularly in old age (Kastenbaum, 1988). Zimberg (1978) challenges the suggested physiological benefits of alcohol use. He believes that any benefits of alcohol use are a result of the socialization that accompanies alcohol use and not the chemical itself. He suggests that other means should be found to increase socialization in the older population. Kastenbaum (1988) reviewed and conducted studies on the moderate use of alcohol in older people and reported that the results of alcohol use were positive and that alcohol seemed to serve both a facilitating socialization function and a physiological function. Kastenbaum also found that some individuals who used wine in moderation had improved sleep quality, positive mood changes, improved concentration, improved coordination of thought, improved free recall memory, and greater self-confidence. Naturally, such results should be approached with caution. Alcohol intake should not be encouraged in older adults with any history of alcohol abuse or any health problems or current medications that could be complicated by alcohol ingestion. It should be further emphasized that the subjects in Kastenbaum's studies were very carefully chosen individuals who would not have been harmed by the alcohol intake. Clearly, encouragement of alcohol use in older adults remains controversial because alcohol has a prolonged and more intense effect in this age group. In fact, spontaneous remission sometimes occurs in older alcohol abusers, since the body's response to alcohol intake is often unpleasant as a result of aging (Zimberg, 1978).

The physiological changes that occur with aging are particularly important for older people who use alcohol or other drugs. According to Lamy (1988), these changes include (1) a reduction in the intracellular and extracellular fluids, which makes less volume available for the distribution of water-soluble drugs such as alcohol; (2) decreased kidney function affecting the body's need both to excrete and to preserve fluids; (3) alteration in the liver's ability to metabolize drugs; (4) probable increased permeability of the blood-brain barrier, leading to increased sensitivity of the brains of older people to drugs and alcohol; (5) increased potential for drug-induced orthostatic hypotension as a result of cardiovascular changes; and (6) reduced ability of the stomach to secrete the mucus that protects the stomach lining from the toxic effects of drugs.

All of these changes mean that older adults are particularly sensitive to alcohol and have decreasing tolerance (Closser & Blow, 1993). Lifelong drinkers who have used but not abused alcohol may find as they age that they drink less and experience more of alcohol's effects. The changes brought on by aging also cause the alcohol withdrawal syndrome to be much more severe. Closser and Blow suggest that the central nervous system seems to lose ability to respond in a flexible manner to toxins such as alcohol. Thus an older person who has used alcohol all his or her life may in old age for the first time experience a severe withdrawal. Closser and Blow caution that alcohol detoxification is also more dangerous, as oversedation with benzodiazepines used to treat alcohol withdrawal may also cause falls and/or aspiration pneumonia. Most older alcoholics should be detoxified in an inpatient setting. Cutezo and Dellasega (1992) suggest that "Medicare coverage reimburses patients for alcohol rehabilitation because providing physical and psychological support for the elderly person during this period is critical" (p. 22). It is unknown whether changes in national health care policy will affect this reimbursement. If a person must be detoxified at home, the family must be educated about the withdrawal syndrome, and nursing support is essential (Cutezo & Dellasega, 1992).

As stated previously, one difficulty involved with identifying and intervening with the older alcoholic is that some individuals are isolated from the social groups that might draw attention to compulsive alcohol use. Some older abusers of alcohol tend to drink alone or in family groups. Middle-aged alcoholics often enter treatment programs because their drinking interferes with their job performance and thus comes to the attention of employers, who can propel the alcoholic into treatment. Since many older persons do not have full-time employment, this means of identification and motivation for treatment is missing. However, potential loss of visitation of grandchildren can be a powerful motivator to propel older alcoholics into treatment (Lindblom, Kostyk, Tabisz, Jackyk, & Fuchs, 1992). Many older alcoholics are protected by relatives who fear the stigma of having their parent or other relative labeled as an alcoholic. In addition, when older alcoholics do come to the attention of the health care system, they are often misdiagnosed or treated ineffectively. They also may lack information about treatment programs or lack the financial resources to pay for treatment if it is available (Mendelson & Mello, 1985).

Thibault and Maly (1993) suggest three primary reasons that alcoholism is often not diagnosed in older adults: (1) Most older persons still feel the effects of alcohol even when they drink less, and physicians usually use quantity consumed as an abuse indicator. (2) Older persons' physical symptoms overlap with their alcohol abuse symptoms. (3) The age-related stereotype interferes with health care professionals perceiving the symptoms of alcohol abuse, or if they do perceive the symptoms, the professionals tend to believe the problem is not great enough to require treatment.

Some older persons who abuse alcohol do not fit the social profile of the older poor, less educated, lower socioeconomic man (Maddox, 1988). Mendelson and Mello (1985) identify three types of older adult problem drinkers and alcoholics: early-onset, late-onset, and intermittent alcoholics. Pascarella (1981) estimates that two thirds of older alcoholics belong to the first group, and the remaining third are alcoholics who developed problems with drinking in later life. Both men and women are susceptible to alcohol abuse at all life stages. Although there are more male than female alcoholics at all ages, Pascarella (1981) asserts that there is a greater proportion of women who are alcoholics in later life. Very little research data documents actual rates of alcohol abuse among older women. Glantz and Backen-heimer (1988) believe the ratio of men to women alcoholics among older people is 4:1. However, they expect that ratio to change, since younger women drink more heavily than did the women presently over 65.

Types of Alcoholics

EARLY-ONSET ALCOHOLICS.   Some older individuals have abused alcohol for most of their adult lives and may be termed survivors, since many of their alcoholic cohorts have long since died. Although at this stage of their lives they may be abstinent or nearly so, they exhibit symptoms of prolonged alcohol abuse, especially cirrhosis of the liver and brain damage. Because of their medical problems, such individuals are often encountered in inpatient medical care settings, where myriad presenting symptoms may mask past or present alcohol abuse. Intellectual deterioration and dementia are often symptoms of long-term alcohol abuse. Lamy (1988) pointed out that alcoholic patients of any age show more signs of mental deterioration than their nonalcoholic cohorts. In general, alcoholic patients are also more likely to exhibit gastrointestinal disturbances, cardiovascular problems, coagulation disorders, and increased susceptibility to infections (Lamy, 1988). However, Schuckit and Miller (1976) found a lower rate of cardiac disease in older alcoholic patients than in older psychiatric and medical patients. They suggested that the lower rate may be a result of the fact that "so many alcoholics die at younger ages from accidents and suicide in addition to cancer and lung disorders, that fewer of them remain at risk for cardiac disorders" (p. 751). A more recent study (Hermos, LoCastro, Bouchard, & Glynn, 1986) found that cardiovascular disease, (especially ischemic heart disease), was apparently influential in causing a decrease in problem drinking in the later years. Whether the change in drinking habits altered mortality rates among the subjects in the study was not clear. What seems apparent is that although alcoholism or problem drinking may no longer be manifested in the older person's life, it may be one of the antecedent risk factors for physical illness in old age. Therefore, individuals with a lifelong pattern of alcohol abuse more likely will be physically ill. In addition, they often will display various personality disturbances and lack the ability to successfully relate interpersonally with other people. This group of older alcohol abusers may not have any interpersonal support system, since their drinking may have long ago separated them from those who once had been significant others. For early-onset alcoholics, the underlying cause of their alcoholism remains hidden in their personal history and is usually not especially helpful in the treatment. Their alcoholism is a long-established behavior pattern that has affected significant portions of their lives and relationships. If they are abstinent at this period of their lives, withdrawal is not an issue. If they are still drinking, severe life-threatening withdrawal must be of real concern to the nurse.

LATE-ONSET ALCOHOLICS. Late-onset alcoholics generally began drinking problematically after the age of 40, usually in response to loss. Unlike the early-onset group, who may or may not be presently drinking, late-onset alcoholics usually continue to drink. However, because they have been drinking for fewer years, the physical complications of alcohol abuse tend to be less severe. This group of alcoholics also will tend to exhibit fewer personality and behavioral disturbances, since they probably have positive personality and behavioral strengths that predate the onset of alcohol abuse. The cause of the initial pattern of alcohol abuse is recent enough that it may be an issue that can be handled in a therapeutic setting, particularly if unresolved losses are a precipitating factor. Some previously social drinkers may fall into addictive drinking as a result of loneliness, depression, or simply too much unstructured time. As they drink to relieve boredom, the addiction occurs. Depending on their rate of current alcohol use, physical dependence may be present. If there is physical dependence, these individuals are subject to alcohol withdrawal syndrome.

INTERMITTENT ALCOHOLICS. The third group of older alcoholics, (or problem drinkers), use alcohol for its central nervous system depressant effects. They use alcohol as an antianxiety agent, to relieve stress. The pattern of alcohol abuse exhibited by this group is one of binges during periods of high stress followed by periods of abstinence or moderate drinking. Usually the precipitating cause of alcohol abuse is fairly obvious and can be dealt with in therapeutic settings. Intermittent alcoholics need to learn better methods of handling stress. For those who are abstinent between binge periods, physical addiction may not be an important factor.

Treatment

Unfortunately, the older alcoholic has been considered a poor risk for treatment. However, according to Pascarella (1981), older alcoholics, in contrast to younger alcoholics, appear to respond rapidly to treatment once they are sober and medically stable. Not only do older alcoholics respond as well as younger alcoholics in traditional programs, their treatment has even greater potential for success when they are treated in a peer age group (Closser & Blow, 1993). Treatment with disulfiram (Antabuse) is not recommended for older persons because many are not physiologically capable of handling the adverse reactions that occur with accidental or intentional alcohol ingestion (Lamy, 1988). Except for the caution about the use of disulfiram, the medical treatment of the older alcoholic does not differ appreciably from that of the younger abuser; it includes treatment with thiamine, folic acid, vitamins, magnesium sulfate, electrolytes, and an antianxiety agent to reduce the chance of withdrawal seizures (Lamy, 1988). However, because older alcoholics are more medically complex, their stay in a treatment program is usually longer. The older alcoholic often needs other kinds of health services during treatment because of the combined physical effects of the chemical disease and the aging process (Closser & Blow, 1993).

One of the most popular and successful modes of treatment is Alcoholics Anonymous. An AA group that includes other older individuals who are dealing with alcohol-related problems may be a particularly good choice for individuals with late-onset alcoholism related to loss and stress. Mendelson and Mello (1985) believe that the older alcohol abuser is often best treated in a community hospital or nursing home instead of a traditional alcoholism treatment center. AA is an effective alternative treatment for some older alcoholics (Closser & Blow, 1993; Thibault & Maly, 1993). Self-help groups such as AA tend to combat boredom and social isolation and promote social support. Zimberg (1978) emphasizes that time for informal socializing is an important part of any substance abuse treatment for older clients. Moos and Finney (1984) emphasize the need to perceive the older individual with alcohol abuse problems differently from the younger alcoholic person, and they remind health caregivers that the older population is a heterogeneous group. Therefore, treatment should be both age-specific and individual-specific. Older patients should be carefully matched to the treatment method that will best meet their needs, which may or may not be a traditional chemical dependency treatment.

A nurse may be reluctant to confront a person who may be alcoholic or a family member because of concern that the client or family may become defensive and angry. However, this confrontation may be made easier when the nurse recalls that this is an issue of physical and emotional health, not a moral issue. Lindblom et al. (1992) point out that the health care professional who does not act becomes an enabler of drinking. It is unrealistic to wait for the alcoholic to ask for help or exhibit motivation for treatment. The substance-abusing person is usually either in denial regarding the abuse or honestly ignorant of the disease. Nurses unfamiliar with chemical dependency treatment can seek assistance from colleagues in the chemical dependency field until they are comfortable confronting patients with substance abuse issues.

Treatment of alcoholism in older adults is based on the same principles as for other age groups. Alcohol intake must be restricted or stopped, depending on the seriousness of the condition, the absence or presence of physical dependence, or both. In the presence of the latter, complete abstinence may be the realistic goal for rehabilitation.

Older persons whose alcoholism is recent generally respond well to therapeutic interventions. They are likely to remain in treatment, and they particularly benefit from social and interpersonal interventions. Furthermore, the natural decline in the desire for alcohol that usually accompanies advancing age favors positive outcomes. Although persons who began drinking early in life and continue to drink excessively into old age tend to have a less favorable prognosis, even they will show improvement when abstinence is achieved and other life problems are addressed (Estes, Smith-DiJulio, & Heinemann, 1980).

The medical hospital is the most common type of treatment facility for the older alcoholic. Older persons most commonly seek treatment for medical problems, not only because these tend to increase with advancing age, but also because family and job pressures are no longer motivations for encouraging the older alcoholic to seek treatment (Mishara & Kastenbaum, 1980).

Although this picture of the addicted older person may be unattractive, one might continue to ask what realistic alternatives are available in a society that so often places care and concern for older adults near the bottom of its social priority list. This rationale is not intended as a defense for alcohol abuse in old age, but it does suggest that some caution be exercised before automatically concluding that the use of alcohol in old age is itself a fundamental problem. Instead, it can be seen as a simplistic and less than optimal response to other problems that are much more fundamental. From the practical standpoint, the latter view may lead to more attention focused on the causes of alcoholism than on the problem drinker per se (Mishara & Kastenbaum, 1980).

An alternative approach derives from a sociocultural framework. Emphasis is given to the life events that may lead to problem drinking. Intervention frequently emphasizes bolstering social support networks or helping the individual to cope better with losses and stresses (Mishara & Kastenbaum, 1980). With older alcoholics, specific group treatment focusing on grief and/or aging is often helpful (Closser & Blow, 1993). The importance of peers as counselors to the older person cannot be overemphasized. Older adults need to share life experiences and are much more open to the need for reminiscence and life review than are younger persons, who are more present or future oriented. Unfortunately, no comparative research focuses directly on the differential benefits or liabilities of various treatment methods for younger and older alcoholic adults. Furthermore, there has not been adequate attention directed to individual differences among older problem drinkers.

Reports from Canada (Holmstrom, 1990; Lindblom et al., 1992) describe specific community outreach projects aimed at providing services to older adults who are abusing alcohol or drugs. The focus of these programs is on alcohol, opiate, and benzodiazepine abuse. Lindblom et al. describe the Elders Health Program as a community demonstration program providing identification, intervention, and treatment for such individuals. Older adults over 65 seeking emergency department treatment were screened for substance abuse. In a 2-year period, 68 persons were identified and treated through this program. Holmstrom reports on two similar programs in Canada, one of which is available to persons 55 and older. These programs suggest that the older adult can benefit from treatment based in the community, which differs from that used with middle-aged and young substance abusers. Holmstrom suggests that the older person may not meet the admission criteria for an inpatient program because of concurrent medical problems and difficulty with activities of daily living. Further, older adults have a slowed pace that may not respond to the usual schedule of traditional inpatient treatment programs.

Older adults are also often reluctant to reveal personal problems in a public forum, an expectation of patients in traditional treatment. The Canadian programs often treat the alcoholism as a secondary problem and focus first on other needs such as housing. This is in direct contrast to the approach with younger alcoholics, which considers abuse the primary problem (Holmstrom, 1990). These community-based programs may well serve as models for future substance abuse programs aimed at older persons.

Opiates

Although opiate abuse is not usually perceived as a problem in older adults, it is found in certain cohort groups. Tamayo and Haglund (1981) investigated drug use and treatment programs among Asian-Americans and found that opiates were the drug of choice for 89% of their small sample (57 subjects, average age 56.5 years). Methadone maintenance was the preferred treatment for the subjects in this study. Opiate abuse entails some different medical and treatment issues from those of alcohol abuse. First, alcohol is a legal drug, whereas the opiates can be obtained only by prescription. This means that opiate abusers are legally considered criminals. Second, lifelong opiate addiction (if the supply is pure and the route of use is uncontaminated) does not present the life-threatening physical problems encountered with alcohol abuse. Therefore the Asian-Americans who abuse the opiates may not exhibit physical symptoms that might alert the health care provider to the addiction. Opiate addiction in this cohort is an example of the role of culture in the choice of the abused substance. However, drug of choice is more often the result of the interaction between social class and availability than a function of ethnicity.

Another population of opiate abusers is urban opiate addicts, or typical street addicts. Although surveys of methadone maintenance programs include only a small number of persons over age 60, projections indicate that these numbers will increase dramatically in the future because of the growing number of urban addicts in our present population. As these middle-aged addicts reach old age, they may cause a dramatic increase in the numbers seeking admission to such programs; some authorities suggest a doubling or tripling effect (Petersen, 1988). There are few reports in the literature about treatment for older opiate abusers other than methadone maintenance programs. Apparently, opiate abuse among older adults is a small and largely ignored issue.

Crack Cocaine

The first report of crack addiction in an older person appeared in the literature in 1991 (Nambudiri & Young, 1991). This is the case of a 64-year-old Hispanic man who began using crack 6 months before he was admitted to the hospital with chest pain, auditory hallucinations, and persecutory delusions. This history did not reveal past chemical dependency, although he was an occasional user of alcohol and marijuana. Initial treatment produced relief of symptoms, but 3 months after discharge the family reported he was again using crack and exhibiting psychotic symptoms. With the increasing use of crack and its highly addictive potential, health professionals will most likely continue to see increasing numbers of cocaine users, some of whom will be older adults.

Prescription and Over-the-Counter Medications

Many drugs are prescribed to help older persons cope with some of the effects of aging. For example, as the need for sleep decreases and/or the quality of sleep declines, older adults may take sedatives such as the benzodiazepines. Older persons who have chronic pain due to age-related changes in the musculoskeletal system may use analgesics such as propoxyphene (Darvon). These psychoactive drugs have the potential to addict. Older persons may misuse prescribed drugs simply because they do not understand the need to take the medications as prescribed. Further, they may misunderstand or have difficulty reading the directions. Misunderstanding the effects and use of a drug with addictive properties can cause the older person to become an inadvertent substance abuser.

Older women are at particular risk for misuse of psychoactive prescription drugs. Data suggest that physicians are more likely to prescribe these medications for women than for men (Glantz & Backenheimer, 1988). Such practices by physicians place older women at risk for dangerous drug interactions. Glantz and Backenheimer (1988) state that "elderly women appear to be at greater risk for physician-perpetuated drug abuse involving prescription psychoactive drugs than any other age by gender group" (p. 21).

It is estimated by Wetter (1981) that one fifth of all patients entering geriatric services have problems caused by prescription drugs. These older patients have often taken legally prescribed medications in a nonrecommended manner or without proper medical supervision and may have supplemented prescribed medications with over-the-counter drugs. Another estimate is that 10% of all geriatric hospital admissions are actually the result of adverse drug reactions (Gordon & Preiksaitis, 1988). The incidence of these adverse reactions increases with age; patients over age 80 have twice the incidence as those under age 60. Such adverse reactions may initially be seen as mental confusion or mental decline, and if they are not properly recognized, further psychotropic medication may be prescribed and exacerbate the problem. Pascarella (1981) believes that substance misuse in older adults tends to occur in the direction of overuse; the overused substances tend to be central nervous system depressants, with 80% to 90% of acute drug reactions in older individuals stemming from misuse of psychotropic drugs. Whittington (1988) disagrees: "When older people do decide to use drugs in ways that doctors have not recommended, it is usually to take fewer pills rather than more" (p. 6). It is certainly true that medication use in the older population, both prescription and over-the-counter, is complicated by the fact that older people often have complex medication regimens, multiple illnesses and symptoms, multiple prescribers (more than one physician), and sensory and cognitive impairments (Shimp & Ascione, 1988). Chenitz, Salisbury, and Stone (1990) assert that in most cases of abuse of prescription drugs the person does not see himself or herself as a drug abuser. The addiction, usually inadvertent, begins with legitimate use. Thus the individual may have difficulty perceiving use of the drug as misuse or abuse. Because some older adults who abuse prescription drugs do so for pain relief, it is important to note that the drug use itself can prolong the chronic pain. According to Morse (1988), "the majority of patients treated for the disorder of prescription drug abuse and chronic pain seem to have an improvement in their painful condition when the drug use is discontinued" (p. 265). Another concern is that over-the-counter or prescribed medications that contain alcohol, narcotics, or minor tranquilizers (antianxiety agents) can jeopardize the sobriety of a previously addicted client.

Nicotine

Cessation or avoidance of smoking has been identified as the single most important behavior that American women could practice to improve their health (Alexander, 1987). In 1985, lung cancer replaced breast cancer as the leading cause of death among women. With that increase, cessation of cigarette smoking became a leading public health goal. The incidence of emphysema has more than doubled in older women (Johnson, 1987). Between 1966 and 1976, smoking tended to decrease overall for men of all ages but only for women over 45 (Garland, 1983). Women may be particularly vulnerable to nicotine addiction because men metabolize nicotine faster than women; this leads to the phenomenon of women becoming addicted more easily than men even if they smoke less, finding cessation more difficult and reporting more severe withdrawal (Johnson, 1987). Therefore, smoking cessation may be particularly difficult for older women addicted to nicotine.

As with alcohol and opiate use, smoking tends to decrease with age. However, there remain older smokers who are at high risk for medical disorders related to their use of nicotine. As with chronic alcohol abusers, many lifelong addicts to nicotine will not have survived to old age, since over 350,000 premature deaths a year are associated with cigarette use (Ray & Ksir, 1993). Those who have survived will most likely come to the attention of health care professionals because of serious chronic health problems stemming from smoking. Sadly, although some older adults can benefit from smoking cessation programs, many are never able to quit, even when they are in the latter stages of smoking-related illnesses. These discouraging facts should not lead health care professionals to give up trying to assist the older nicotine addict in cessation efforts. Rather, these individuals should be encouraged to try different programs and regimens until they find the treatment strategy best suited to their needs.

Caffeine

In our culture, caffeine is found primarily in coffee, tea, soft drinks, and chocolate. Caffeine has a stimulant and mood-elevating effect at any age. It produces some opposing physiological effects; therefore, it is difficult to predict the effect of caffeine at lower intake levels. There have been differing reports as to whether it produces more negative or positive effects (Ray & Ksir, 1993). There are various patterns of caffeine use; one such pattern points to men, smokers, and whites as being more likely to use coffee (Garland, 1983). A recommended course for the nurse to follow with regard to caffeine use in older adults is to assess the amount of caffeine consumed over the course of a day and to assess whether any of the older patient's symptoms might be a result of excessive caffeine intake.

❖ *Nursing Process*

Because addictions nursing is a subspecialty within psychiatric nursing, the American Nurses' Association's Council on Psychiatric/Mental Health Nursing and Council on Medical-Surgical Nursing Practice and the National Nurses Society on Addictions have formulated standards to guide the practice of nurses working with clients who have substance abuse problems. These standards, shown in Box 9-1, are a guide for all phases of the nursing process (American Nurses' Association and National Nurses Society on Addictions, 1988).

Assessment

Nurses are in prime positions for identifying the older person who has an alcohol problem. Because family and job problems tend to become less relevant as reasons to motivate the older alcoholic to seek treatment, medical problems and health issues tend to be the primary ways an older person who has an alcohol or other drug problem may be identified (Mishara & Kastenbaum, 1980). Thus nurses in either outpatient or inpatient settings are positioned to identify the older alcoholic (Hoffman & Heinemann, 1986). However, although the alcoholic is in a health care setting, the substance abuse is often not diagnosed. In older adults, alcoholism, if diagnosed at all, is usually not the primary disease (Closser & Blow, 1993). If an older person exhibits withdrawal symptoms while being treated for a medical condition, the symptoms may be attributed to the medical condition or aging rather than alcohol or drug withdrawal. Nurses alert to the possibility of substance abuse in older persons may thus be the first health professional to look beyond the obvious medical condition and see the hidden substance abuse problem. Cutezo and Dellasega (1992) state that nurses are crucial to the identification of alcoholism in patients: "No other health professionals have the same opportunity for direct assessment and timely intervention" (p. 19). Nurses who are aware of the potential for substance abuse in older persons can incorporate substance abuse screening into their assessment. For example, the nurse on an orthopedic unit should consider alcohol abuse as a possible precipitating factor for an older patient with a broken hip resulting from a fall. The medical-surgical nurse working with a recently admitted confused older person should consider alcohol withdrawal as a possible cause of the client's confusion. The psychiatric nurse working with a depressed older client should thoroughly assess the possibility of alcoholism in this client. The community health nurse who consistently finds the older individual unkempt and noncompliant with medication and diet might consider alcohol abuse as a possible factor.

Box 9-1 **Addictions Nursing**

   I. The nurse uses appropriate knowledge from nursing theory and related disciplines in the practice of addictions nursing.

  II. Data collection is continual and systematic and is communicated effectively to the treatment team throughout each phase of the nursing process.

 III. The nurse uses nursing diagnoses congruent with accepted nursing and interprofessional classification systems of addictions and associated physiological and psychological disorders to express conclusions supported by data obtained through the nursing process.

  IV. The nurse establishes a plan of care for the client that is based upon nursing diagnoses, addresses specific goals, defines expected outcomes, and delineates nursing actions unique to each client's needs.

   V. The nurse implements actions independently and/or in collaboration with peers, members of other disciplines, and clients in prevention, intervention, and rehabilitation phases of the care of clients with health problems related to patterns of abuse and addiction.
   A. The nurse uses the "therapeutic self" to establish a relationship with clients and to structure nursing interventions to help clients develop the awareness, coping skills, and behavior changes that promote health.
   B. The nurse educates clients and communities to help them prevent and/or correct actual or potential health problems related to patterns of abuse and addiction.
   C. The nurse uses the knowledge and philosophy of self-help groups to assist clients in learning new ways to address stress, maintain self-control or sobriety, and integrate healthy coping behaviors into their life-style.
   D. The nurse applies knowledge of pharmacological principles in the nursing process.
   E. The nurse provides, structures, and maintains a therapeutic environment in collaboration with the individual, family, and other professionals.
   F. The nurse uses therapeutic communication in interactions with the client to address issues related to patterns of abuse and addiction.

  VI. The nurse evaluates the responses of the client and revises nursing diagnoses, interventions, and the treatment plan accordingly.

Continued.

Box 9-1 **Addictions Nursing—cont'd**

VII. The nurse's decisions and activities on behalf of the clients are in keeping with personal and professional codes of ethics and in accord with legal statutes.

VIII. The nurse participates in peer review and other staff evaluation and quality assurance processes to ensure that clients with abuse and addiction problems receive quality care.

IX. The nurse assumes responsibility for his or her continuing education and professional development and contributes to the professional growth of others who work with or are learning about persons with abuse and addiction problems.

X. The nurse collaborates with the interdisciplinary treatment team and consults with other health care providers in assessing, planning, implementing, and evaluating programs and other activities related to addictions nursing.

XI. The nurse participates with other members of the community in assessing, planning, implementing, and evaluating community health services that attend to primary, secondary, and tertiary prevention of addictions.

XII. The nurse contributes to the nursing care of clients with addictions and to the addictions area of practice through innovations in theory and practice and participation in research, and communicates these contributions.

From American Nurses' Association (1988). *Standards of Addictions Nursing Practice with Selected Diagnoses and Criteria* (pp. 5-23) Kansas City: Author; with permission.

Even in the retirement home, according to Holmstrom (1990), nurses should be aware that symptoms of substance abuse can be incorrectly attributed to aging; such symptoms include "unsteadiness, missing meals, over-sleeping, accidents and falls" (Holmstrom, p. 8). These examples are not meant to imply that alcoholism is the *only* explanation for these situations, but alcoholism is a *possible* explanation that nurses and other health professionals too often fail to consider. Failure to consider alcoholism as a precipitating factor of many health problems for the older person is particularly distressing when one realizes that alcoholism is a treatable illness, especially when identified in its early stages. Thus it is an illness for which hope and recovery can be offered to the older person, unlike many other chronic illnesses with which older persons must cope.

As a first step, the alcoholic must be identified. As previously stated, nurses and other health professionals often miss the opportunity to identify the older alcoholic. There are a number of reasons for blinders. One is low awareness regarding the possibility of alcoholism in older adults. Another is feeling uncertain and helpless about what to do if an older person is identified as alcoholic (Tweed, 1989). A third reason is negative attitudes toward alcoholic persons in general or a combined negative attitude toward older persons and alcoholism. Another reason for blinders may be the attitude that an older person should be allowed to do whatever he or she wants to do with the remainder of his or her life, even if it is self-destructive. Nurses and other health care professionals often have misperceptions about alcoholism and substance abuse. These misperceptions include (1) not realizing that treatment of substance abuse can be successful, particularly in the older individual, (2) believing that confrontation is only effective with the younger substance abuser, and (3) believing that the older alcoholic must reach bottom before he or she can benefit from treatment.

It is important to remember that approximately one third of older alcoholics are in the early phase of alcoholism, even though they are in the later phase of their life. Therefore, positive outcomes from early intervention are just as possible for the older alcoholic person as for one who is younger. Nurses should be aware that a crisis involving physical health is a major precipitating factor that may force an older alcoholic to face honestly the negative consequences of drinking for the first time. Awareness of this fact can assist the nurse to perceive the responsibility of the health care professional in identifying and confronting the older substance abuser.

Assessing the Older Alcoholic

Cahalan, Cisin, and Crossley's classic 1969 work identified the following nine constellations of symptoms indicative of alcoholism for the general population:

- Symptoms developed as a result of drinking, such as debilitating hangovers, blackouts, memory loss, and shakes
- Psychological dependence on alcohol, defined as the inability to conduct normal everyday tasks without drinking or planning one's life around drinking
- Health problems related to alcohol use, including accidents resulting from drinking and existing health problems compounded by drinking
- Financial problems related to alcohol use
- Problems with spouse or relatives as a result of alcohol use
- Problems with friends or neighbors as a result of alcohol use
- Problems on the job as a result of drinking
- Belligerence associated with drinking
- Problems with police or the law as a result of drinking

These symptom constellations are not mutually exclusive. Williams, Carruth and Hyman (1973) defined problem drinkers as persons with difficulties in three or more of these nine-symptom constellations.

However, identifying alcoholism in older persons is more difficult than it is in younger persons (Estes et al., 1980). For example, older people may have some of these symptom constellations without anyone knowing they are problem drinkers. As stated earlier, some survey results suggest that older persons tend to drink either alone or in family groups (Cahalan et al., 1969). Thus these symptoms in older persons are less likely to be noticed than with younger people who drink in public places. Family members and close friends may shield the older person's drinking and deny a problem. Thinking of grandmother or grandfather as an alcoholic may seem unfair and unacceptable. For this reason, when family members express concern about an older adult's drinking, the health care professional should take their concern very seriously and assess for substance abuse. Some older alcoholic persons live alone, and no one is aware of their drinking practices. Cutezo and Dellasega (1992) point out the similarities between age- and alcohol-related changes in body systems (p. 20). Further, age-related changes can be exaggerated by alcohol use. Short-term memory loss can arise from either aging or alcohol use and is compounded when both are present. Another example is the increased incidence of arthritis and gout as one ages and the increase in uric acid blood levels related to alcohol use. The similarities between the symptoms of aging and the symptoms of alcohol use make it imperative that nurses include history of substance use and abuse when conducting assessments.

Thibault and Maly (1993) suggest that when an older person has the following symptoms, he or she should be assessed for alcohol abuse (p. 160):

1. Difficulty in performing activities of daily living
2. A history of injuries due to falls
3. Lack of self-care resulting in a neglect of appearance
4. Impairment of short term memory and attention span
5. Symptoms of depression, including thoughts of suicide
6. Anxiety
7. Incontinence and/or diarrhea
8. Insomnia

All of these symptoms may be due to numerous other causes; even so, assessment of such symptoms should include a thorough and careful history of alcohol use.

In contrast to the middle-aged alcohol abuser, job and family problems often are not motivating factors for an older person who seeks treatment. As suggested earlier, potential loss of grandchild visitation can be a powerful motivator with older adults (Lindblom et al., 1992). Older women in particular are likely to have lost their spouse, so current marital problems are not likely to be a precipating factor in this group. Williams, Carruth and Hyman (1973) suggest that many older individuals are not diagnosed or treated as problem drinkers because they have avoided contact with agencies that could provide care, stopped contact with agencies before their drinking problem was detected, or managed to receive treatment for other symptoms while their alcohol-related problems remained undetected and untreated. This last reason for nondetection is especially disturbing because it reflects an assessment failure by the nurse or other health professionals.

Still another factor making identification of the older alcoholic problematic is the fact that the quantity consumed may not be a useful indicator. In the older person, even *moderate* amounts of alcohol may have serious effects on behavioral and physiological functioning (Estes et al., 1980; Closser & Blow, 1993). It is known that quantity and frequency of drinking change with age, and even minimal drinking may have implications for health in older adults (Cahalan et al., 1969). However, Willenbring and Spring (1988) identified what they consider maximum amounts of alcohol that are reasonable and safe for older persons. They consider two drinks per day or three drinks per occasion as reasonable for a 55- to 75-year-old man. For men over 75 years of age, one drink per day and two per occasion are considered safe amounts. However, they caution that "it is not clear that a safe dose exists for women at any age" (Willenbring & Spring, 1988, p. 31).

A further impediment to identifying alcoholism in older adults is the fact that diagnostic criteria have been established for use with middle-aged populations and therefore may not be appropriate for older people (Mishara & Kastenbaum, 1980). For example, tremors and disorientation, signs of physical addiction that occur during withdrawal, may be ongoing conditions in older adults and unrelated to alcohol use.

Health problems in older adults may compound the difficulty of recognizing alcohol problems. Various diseases and psychological conditions can mimic symptoms of alcoholism. General physical deterioration, malnutrition, mental deterioration, and social isolation may be attributed to the effects of age instead of the consequences of heavy drinking. Alcohol may also cause problems for the older person without progressing to physical addiction. For example, confusion, staggering gait, and drowsiness should prompt assessment for alcohol problems. Careful assessment by the nurse is necessary to clarify whether alcohol use or abuse or some other disease process is the cause of such symptoms (Estes et al., 1980).

Because the signs of alcoholism in older adults are more subtle than in younger persons, more in-depth assessments are necessary to identify alcohol problems in this age group (Zimberg, 1978). This is partially a result of the lack of awareness regarding how functioning is compromised in older adults by their drinking (Blose, 1978). In addition, intentional distortions and blackouts may make self-report information unreliable, necessitating careful questioning and when possible obtaining data from more reliable sources such as family members. Although lack of awareness, distortion, and blackouts are also typical of younger alcoholic persons, these symptoms seem particularly pronounced in the older alcoholic person (Estes et al., 1980).

Health Problems

When accidents or falls occur more frequently in older persons than might be expected, alcohol abuse should be considered as a possible factor (Glatt, 1978). Bruises on legs or arms caused by bumping into furniture when intoxicated also indicate the possibility of alcohol abuse by an older person. Bruises are observed more frequently in older than in younger persons because of the effects of intoxication coupled with declining motor skills (Estes et al., 1980). Burns on the hands or chest that result from falling asleep while smoking are another important observation for nurses to make because they may indicate alcohol abuse. Other physical signs of alcohol abuse in the general population that also apply to the older person include puffy eyes or face (unaccounted for by uremia or allergy), flushed face, enlarged nose with prominent veins, reddened conjunctivae, noctural diaphoresis, insomnia, and impotence (Criteria Committee, 1972; Estes et al., 1980). Although any single sign or symptom does not conclusively indicate alcoholism in the older person, astute observation of such characteristics should alert the nurse to the possibility of an alcohol problem and to the appropriateness of exploring the client's drinking history (Tweed, 1989).

Tremulousness should arouse suspicion of alcohol abuse. The older person who requires assistance with bathing or brushing teeth may experience shakes caused by alcohol overuse and withdrawal. Although confusion may be a function of brain disease or a symptom of Wernicke's encephalopathy, it may also be a sign of alcohol intoxication or withdrawal. Rosin and Glatt (1971) cited an 80-year-old woman who became confused after surgery. The patient had brought liquor with her to the hospital without telling hospital staff, but she was unable to reach the bottle because of her physical incapacity, and so she developed acute alcohol withdrawal. Severe symptoms that occur during alcohol withdrawal such as tremulousness, hallucinations, seizure activity, or delirium tremens should alert the nurse to assess for alcohol abuse.

Older alcoholics have an increase in various health problems. In a study of older hospitalized alcoholics compared with a nonalcoholic cohort, hematemesis and hematuria were significantly higher in the alcoholic group of patients (Funkhouser, 1977-1978). In another study, chronic obstructive lung disease occurred with greater frequency in older alcoholics than in a younger group (Schuckit & Miller, 1976). Malnutrition is another possible indication of alcohol overuse in older adults. Older persons who show changes in weight, notably loss of weight, changes in appetite, abdominal distress, vomiting, or altered bowel habits may be satisfying their appetite with alcohol instead of food, resulting in vitamin deficiencies, blood dyscrasias, and behavioral disturbances (Estes et al., 1980). These alcohol-related illnesses should alert the nurse to assess for alcohol abuse.

Persons with chronic alcoholism often have experienced numerous hospitalizations and major illnesses (Eckhardt et al., 1981). Although almost every organ of the body is finally affected by alcoholism after years of uncontrolled drinking, certain body systems are more susceptible to damage than others. The major illness usually associated with alcoholism is cirrhosis of the liver; over 90% of the cases of cirrhosis in the United States are related to alcohol abuse (Lewis, 1980). However, there may not be a particularly high rate of cirrhosis among older people because chronic alcoholics with cirrhosis may have died relatively young. Another effect of chronic alcoholism that may be conclusive of addiction is organic brain syndrome; therefore the nurse should perform a mental status examination to explore possible organic mental impairment (Chafetz, 1983; Gaitz & Baer, 1971).

Illnesses that should alert the nurse are alcoholic hepatitis, pancreatitis in the absence of cholelithiasis, and gastrointestinal problems such as gastritis, esophagitis, and chronic diarrhea (Abbott, Goldberg, & Becker, 1974; Shropshire, 1975). Hematological disorders such as anemia and clotting disorders are possible signs of alcoholism (Criteria Committee, 1972). Cardiovascular disease is also associated with heavy drinking (Brody & Mills, 1978), and a problem with alcohol abuse is a possibility in clients with such problems. Infections such as pneumonia and other medical conditions such as hypertension and diabetes that do not respond to treatment should also alert the nurse to the possibility of alcohol abuse (Eckhardt et al., 1981). A high percentage of trauma clients have a history of problem drinking (Parkinson, Stephensen, & Phillips, 1985); thus nurses should consider alcohol abuse with these clients, especially when they are older.

Physical findings that indicate possible alcoholism are peripheral neuropathy, enlarged liver, gynecomastia, cardiomyopathy, and arrhythmia not associated with arteriosclerotic heart disease (Eckhardt et al., 1981). Tachycardia and elevated blood pressure should also alert the nurse to the possibility of heavy alcohol use.

Tolerance to the effects of alcohol is another physiological manifestation that the nurse must assess, although in the older alcoholic person, reverse tolerance is more likely to be a problem. Tolerance is the gradual increase in the amount of alcohol necessary to produce the same effect as did the first drink. Increasing the tolerance allows individuals to consume larger quantities of alcohol without appearing intoxicated. A sign of alcoholism in its advanced stages and in older adults is a decrease in previously high tolerance levels; this occurs in the more chronic phase of alcoholism and in the older person because of the inability of the liver to detoxify alcohol.

Unexpected or untoward effects of drugs may result from the concomitant intake of alcohol and other drugs. Alcohol interacts with many other drugs, affecting their absorption, metabolism, storage, and utilization. In older adults, alcohol combined with prescription drugs such as tranquilizers, antihypertensive agents, anticoagulants, digitalis, diuretics, insulin, or iron preparations is of particular concern. When alcohol is used in addition to prescription drugs, the potential for psychological and physiological disturbances is intensified. Meticulous assessment of the kinds and amounts of drugs the person is using in combination with alcohol is essential to the prevention of serious consequences.

Psychosocial Problems

Schuckit and Pastor (1978) identified three common problems that are important for the nurse to assess in the older alcoholic. First, they observed that depression is almost invariably present in older alcoholics as a result of the pharmacological effects of alcohol and the social isolation caused by a drinking lifestyle. Since depression is a transitory effect that may disappear after abstinence, it does not necessarily indicate that the older alcoholic suffers from an affective disorder. Second, they observed that the clinical picture of alcoholics can mimic schizophrenia. Symptoms such as auditory hallucinations or delusions may appear but will most likely resolve after a period of abstinence. Third, they depicted alcoholics as being in a state of confusion and disorientation. Therefore, it is important to realize that a seemingly confused older person who has alcohol-related problems may actually be suffering from a transitory acute organic brain syndrome that will disappear when the alcohol problem is treated. Furthermore, this picture of organic brain syndrome may relate to other common problems among alcoholics, such as vitamin deficiencies (especially thiamine), general ill health, and inadequate nutrition.

Social isolation may be a distinct indicator of alcohol overuse for the older person. Older people who watch television all day and drink as they watch, in preference to interacting with other people, are suspect for alcohol abuse. Older alcoholic persons report minimal social participation compared with older nonalcoholic persons. This is most pronounced with respect to sharing of personal life experiences with others, including close friends and relatives (Rathbone-McCuan, 1988). Those who have lost family and friends feel loneliness even more acutely. Bereavement, an important cause of depression in middle and later life, also may precipitate excessive drinking (Rosin & Glatt, 1971).

Assessment Approaches

Identifying alcohol abuse in the older person would be easier if the older person or a family member would mention to the nurse their concern about alcohol abuse. However, this is rarely the case because of denial, which is part of the disease process of alcoholism, and possibly because of lack of awareness that drinking may be causing adverse health and behavioral consequences. Therefore, if the nurse can assess specific health and psychosocial problems associated with alcohol misuse, taking the identification of alcohol abuse out of the realm of judgment and accusation and into the realm of objective fact, assessment and intervention will be more effective (Seixas, 1982).

Probably most important in the assessment process (in addition to alertness to the possibility of alcohol problems in the older person and knowledge of how to evaluate presenting problems) are nurses' attitudes and acceptance when they explore the drinking history with clients (Tweed, 1989). It is very important that the nurse communicate to older persons a sensitivity to their special needs and concerns. The quality of the relationship that develops and the assessment process itself may hinge on the nurse's ability to communicate this sensitivity (Estes et al., 1980).

The nurse should seek detailed information about the client's pattern of alcohol use in the process of assessing any older client. The assessment should be oriented toward examining the reasons for the effects of alcohol use instead of making a judgment (Chafetz, 1983). If there is a significant other person in the client's life, this person should be included in the assessment if possible (Tweed, 1989). Because many liquid medications contain alcohol in high concentrations, assessment of alcohol use must include these over-the-counter drugs as well. A history of use of liquid antihistamines and cold remedies should be part of the assessment (Morse, 1988). Also, because use of these medications can impair the sobriety of a client who is in recovery, the nurse must carefully assess previous addiction in clients. This assessment can serve a teaching function if older clients who are in recovery do not know the danger of using medications that contain alcohol and other addicting drugs.

Reed (1976) suggests that an assessment of the client's use of alcohol can be easily incorporated into every nursing history if the interviewer asks the following three questions regarding drinking: "How often?" "How?" "How much?" She states that the responses to these three questions allow the nurse to make an informed judgment about whether future assessment of the client's use of alcohol is necessary. During assessment for an alcohol problem in an older person, a fourth question should be asked in a nonthreatening, nonjudgmental way: "What are your reasons for drinking?" If the reasons include loneliness, lack of anything else to do, grief, depression, nerves, or dull pains, then the nurse should further explore the possibility of an alcohol problem. Conversely, if the older person's reason is socialization (depending on his or her circumstances and health conditions), this may be an indication of more healthy use of alcohol for some older people (Estes et al., 1980).

Pacing the interview so that the older person has ample time to respond is particularly important when talking with an older alcoholic individual, since it may be difficult for him or her to recall recent events. Being responsive to nonverbal cues such as facial expressions, gestures, and postures will probably aid the information-gathering process. The nurse should speak clearly and slowly and use appropriate language to convey a sense of interest and importance and of wanting to be understood. The use of touch is a highly appropriate means of conveying warmth and making contact; older people generally are less inhibited by touch than younger persons and respond to it positively (Blazer, 1978). Because of older persons' possible hearing and visual losses, nurses should position themselves so that it is possible for clients to hear and see them as clearly as possible. All these approaches tend to contribute to a more effective assessment of the older person. It is also important to remember that approaches must be individualized—not every older person has sensory deficits (Estes et al., 1980).

Nursing assessment of the person's total situation, including psychosocial and physiological states with subsequent identification of major problems, must be addressed. The findings of the assessment interview should be shared with the patient, and with his or her participation, management strategies should be identified and implemented (Estes et al., 1980).

Nursing diagnoses, Expected outcomes, Interventions, and Evaluation

Interventions with the older alcoholic person should be based on thorough nursing assessments resulting in appropriate nursing diagnoses and specific expected outcomes. Interventions should be tailored to the individual client as much as possible, considering the person's age, substance use and abuse history, family situation, and social circumstances. Interventions with older alcoholic persons can occur at several levels. Lindblom et al. (1992) believe intervention should begin at level 1, which is the least intrusive. At level 1 the nurse voices concern to the individual about substance use and encourages the client to seek help. The individual's social system can be encouraged to voice concerns as well. At level 2 the natural social system confronts the individual and states the consequences of the behavior and encourages the client to seek help. The most invasive intervention, level 3, occurs when a professional coordinates the intervention, bringing all the interested parties and the alcoholic together in a meeting with the goal of breaking through the denial and getting the person into treatment. With older persons this last intervention is often not needed. Lindblom et al. (1992) reported that out of 68 patients identified as needing some form of treatment, only 4 needed a level 3 intervention. Examples of application of the nursing process to the care of older alcoholic persons are presented in the following case histories and care plans.

Case Study **Ms. Vickers**

Ms. Vickers is a 66-year-old retired high school English teacher who lives alone. For years she lived with her dearest friend and fellow school teacher, Lucille Merck, in the apartment in which she now resides. Her friend died 19 years ago. Although Ms. Vickers maintained friendships with other friends, in the past few years all of her close friends have either moved out of the state after retirement, entered retirement housing, or died. Although she corresponds with those who have moved, she does not have enough money to travel for visits or make long-distance telephone calls. She states that she does not write them very often any more because "there is less and less to write about." Playing golf used to be a hobby that she enjoyed, but since Ms. Merck died and other friends moved away, she no longer plays golf.

Ms. Vickers has one living relative, a nephew who lives in another state. Their primary contact is at holiday times. She has not seen her nephew for several years; their contact now is limited to occasional correspondence and telephone calls on birthdays and holidays.

Ms. Vickers' major pastime is reading, but she goes to the library less frequently and now subscribes only to the weekend newspaper and one magazine. Several years ago she volunteered as a leader in a book discussion group at the senior citizen center, but she had a brief illness when the group started and someone else was asked to lead the group.

After Ms. Merck's death, Ms. Vickers would drink a glass of wine every night to help her feel better and to help her sleep. She now has wine in her orange juice every morning and sometimes has wine and a cracker for lunch instead of bothering to fix anything. She has her groceries and liquor delivered.

There are four other tenants in her building; all are younger and employed full time. Although they are pleasant and exchange brief conversations when they pass in the hall, they do not socialize with each other. The young man next door does stop by her apartment every Saturday to see if she needs anything. Sometimes he will drop by with a new mystery he has read because he knows that she enjoys such books.

Ms. Vickers is 5 feet 4 inches tall and weighs 125 pounds. She appears somewhat older than her 66 years. She smiles infrequently, her facial expression is somewhat sad, and she speaks slowly and softly.

One morning several weeks ago she fell and broke her leg. She was found lying on her kitchen floor by her neighbor, who saw that her apartment was darkened when he returned from work and heard her moans when he knocked on the door to check on her. She was hospitalized for several days and was sent home after a referral to the visiting nurse association, who visited daily for the first week and are now coming once a week. Nancy Johnson is the nurse assigned to Ms. Vickers. They have formed a close relationship that is in the working phase, and Ms. Vickers has begun to talk with Ms. Johnson regarding her feelings of loneliness and unresolved grief about Ms. Merck's death. Ms. Vickers points out objects around the apartment that belonged to Ms. Merck and states that she was never able to put them away even though they serve as constant, painful reminders of the absence of her friend.

After being assigned to Ms. Vickers, Ms. Johnson did a careful assessment with particular attention to the potential for alcohol or drug abuse, since the staff nurses in the hospital had noted other bruises on her extremities. It was also noted that on the second hospital day, Ms. Vickers began to have symptoms of tremulousness and had difficulty sleeping. The hospital staff attributed this to anxiety, but Ms. Johnson believes these symptoms might be signs of a mild alcohol withdrawal; this further confirms the need to assess for alcohol or drug use.

Ms. Vickers at first denied any problems with alcohol, stating that she only drank "a little wine now and then." On closer questioning and after being given information about the effect that even small amounts of alcohol can have on older individuals, she began to admit how much wine she had regularly consumed. She also began to talk about her loneliness and expressed the belief that her "life was over" and it was "too bad that people have to keep on living after there is nothing left to live for." Ms. Johnson assessed Ms. Vickers for suicidal ideation; although she said that she no longer finds any enjoyment from life, Ms. Vickers denied any plan to commit suicide.

After Ms. Johnson completed her assessment of Ms. Vickers, she developed a comprehensive nursing care plan on page 248.

Nursing Care Plan for Ms. Vickers

Assessment data	Diagnoses, goals, expected outcomes	Nursing interventions	Evaluation
Subjective "After Lucille died, I found that it helped me sleep if I had some wine every evening; I guess I just started drinking it more and more regularly. I never connected drinking wine with alcoholism. I would never have drunk hard liquor." "I haven't had any wine since we talked about this but I am finding that I miss it a lot. Probably if I didn't know you were coming to check up on me every week and would be asking about my drinking, I would go ahead and at least have a drink in the evening."	**Primary diagnosis** Substance abuse (alcohol) **Long-term goal** Patient will not use alcohol as a coping device. **Nursing diagnoses** 1. Knowledge deficit related to concept of alcoholism as a disease and effect of alcohol upon older individuals.	1a. Use part of visit each week to discuss alcoholism with patient, particularly stressing the effect of alcohol in older individuals. 1b. Leave printed information with patient and review following week. 1c. Discuss the role of AA in assisting individuals with alcohol problems.	Ms. Vickers was receptive to Ms. Johnson's care plan and did agree to attend an AA meeting, since Ms. Johnson went with her and the meeting was an open informational meeting in which Ms. Vickers was not expected to share her own problems with alcohol.
Objective 66-year-old white woman who appears older than stated age. 5'4", 130 pounds. Weight 1 year ago was 150 pounds. Left lower leg in walking cast, toes pink, warm to touch, nail beds indicate adequate perfusion. Fading bruises on right leg and left forearm. Small 1 cm scar from recent abrasion on right hand.	**Expected outcomes** 1a. Patient will verbalize the signs and symptoms of alcoholism. 1b. Patient will characterize alcoholism as a disease. 1c. Patient will discuss the effects of alcohol on older individuals. 1d. Patient will state that she has a problem with alcohol.	1d. If patient consents, accompany patient to an open AA meeting whose membership is composed primarily of older adults. 1e. Talk with patient about having an AA visitor come to her home to discuss the organization.	Ms. Vickers agreed to have Ms. Johnson contact AA and ask a representative to visit with her in her home. Following the visit, Ms. Vickers began to attend this group and did get a sponsor.

Subjective

"My life is over; the person I was closest to is dead and all my other friends have moved."

"It's too bad that people have to keep on living after there is nothing left to live for."

Nursing diagnoses

2. Grieving, dysfunctional related to death of close friend and companion.

Expected outcomes

2a. Patient will verbalize her feeling of loss regarding her friend.

2b. Patient will share some of the memories of her friend with the nurse.

2c. Patient will begin to make decisions about some of her friend's former possessions regarding which should be given away or kept as special reminders.

2a. Encourage patient to discuss her feelings about the loss of her friend.

2b. Discuss with patient some of the steps of the grieving process, ask her to assess her current status in grieving process.

Ms. Vickers' grief over Ms. Merck continued, and Ms. Johnson did not feel that Ms. Vickers had successfully resolved it, but because of the resolution of the other problems, the grief issue was not actively pursued.

Ms. Vickers stated "I guess I will always miss Lucille very much, but I don't think about it as much since I am so busy these days."

Objective

Ms. Vickers is avoiding relationships with other people.

Nursing diagnoses

3. Social isolation related to moving of friends and lack of any other social group.

Long-term goal

Patient will be socially involved with others.

Expected outcomes

3a. Patient will attend an AA group comprised of other older alcoholics.

3a. If patient is receptive to AA, accompany her to an open AA meeting.

3b. Support and encourage patient to become involved with AA.

3c. If patient does not choose to become involved with AA, encourage her to find another social group in which she can become involved.

Ms. Vickers attended an AA meeting with Ms. Johnson. She did meet some other older adults from her neighborhood and expressed surprise at the friendly, supportive atmosphere that existed at the meeting.

Continued.

Nursing Care Plan for Ms. Vickers—cont'd

Assessment data	Diagnoses, goals, expected outcomes	Nursing interventions	Evaluation
	3b. Patient will ask for an AA sponsor.	3d. Obtain a list of other social groups available for retired individuals in her neighborhood; particularly search for a group for retired single professional women.	Ms. Vickers did decide to visit the group and join it. Later she became a sponsor herself and was very active in AA.
	3c. Patient will attend AA meetings of this group at least once a week.	3e. Discuss with patient the role that social isolation plays in alcoholism and other substance abuse problems.	
	3d. Patient will call sponsor when she feels particularly lonely or wants to have a drink.		
	3e. Patient will begin to work the 12 steps.		
	3f. Patient will attend another social function of her choice (perhaps with a fellow AA member).		
	3g. Patient will verbalize that she has found someone with whom she can play golf after her leg heals.		
	3h. Patient will investigate the possibility of volunteering some of her teaching and English skills.		
	3i. Patient will state that she feels less lonely.		

Subjective

"I don't really care about doing anything."

Nursing diagnoses

4. Hopelessness related to pessimistic view of future.

Expected outcomes

4a. Patient will verbalize plans for the future.

4b. Patient will no longer verbalize hopelessness about growing older.

4c. Patient will discuss meaningful activities in which she has become involved.

4a. Continue to assess patient for suicidal ideation.

4b. Continue weekly visits, make more frequent contact if hopelessness seems to intensify.

4c. Discuss with patient the role that hopelessness plays in alcoholism and other substance abuse problems.

4d. Reinforce to the patient her strengths, but allow her to express her negative feelings.

4e. Explore with patient how she would like to change her life, encourage her to identify ways that she could make those changes, and assist her in setting realistic goals.

Ms. Vickers increased her involvement with other people and made realistic future plans.

Continued.

Nursing Care Plan for Ms. Vickers—cont'd

Assessment data	Diagnoses, goals, expected outcomes	Nursing interventions	Evaluation
Subjective "I don't feel like I have anything to offer."	**Nursing diagnoses** 5. Self-esteem, situational low. **Expected outcomes** 5a. Patient will indicate involvement in an activity that uses her special skills and talents.	5a. Assist patient in a realistic assessment of her strengths and talents. 5b. Assist patient to identify some meaningful ways that she can continue to share her knowledge and expertise from her teaching profession. 5c. Obtain a list of agencies needing retired professional volunteers, perhaps a program like an adult literacy program.	Ms. Vickers became involved in the adult literacy program and felt positive about her contributions to other people's learning. She began to feel better about herself and what she had to offer other people.

Case Study **Mr. and Mrs. Anderson**

Mr. Anderson is a 70-year-old retired executive; his wife is 68 years of age. He held a very responsible position with a large firm for 35 years before retirement. He lived his life with much intensity and was known by his family and associates as a workaholic. Alcohol was always part of the Andersons' social life. They used to exhibit a pattern of moderate to heavy drinking in social situations, often entertaining business associates. Sporadically Mr. Anderson would drink too much, but his behavior was never socially unacceptable. Mr. Anderson had never encountered any negative consequences of drinking.

Mrs. Anderson has been a housewife all her life. She married her husband when she was 24, after her graduation from a small Catholic college for women. The Andersons had five children, all of whom are grown with families of their own. The children remain close to their parents and each other. The entire family sees each other on holidays and birthdays.

Four years ago the Andersons moved to a retirement community in a southern state. They quickly became a part of the social setting of this community and they frequently entertain, both in their home and at the country club in the subdivision.

Although Mr. Anderson's drinking has not increased substantially at parties from his preretirement days, he routinely becomes so inebriated that his wife must drive him home. At the last family celebration, Mr. Anderson fell asleep on the couch after several drinks. A daughter-in-law commented to Mrs. Anderson that he certainly couldn't hold his liquor very well anymore. In addition, Mr. Anderson has a drink every morning and wants Mrs. Anderson to have a morning drink with him. She refuses and works instead on her quilting or one of her other hobbies. Mrs. Anderson has almost stopped drinking entirely because she has become very concerned about her husband's behavior and use of alcohol. They have recently had some unpleasant arguments regarding his alcohol use. Mr. Anderson insists that he doesn't drink any more now than he ever did and says that he enjoys alcohol and it has never been a problem for him.

Before retirement, Mr. and Mrs. Anderson had a satisfying sexual relationship; however, sexual activity has almost stopped. Mrs. Anderson sometimes feels very alone and wishes they had never moved to the retirement community because she believes that these problems would never have developed if they had "stayed home."

Mr. Anderson's sole leisure activity in the past was tennis. Although there are tennis courts available at the club and active play takes place between residents of the retirement community most of the time, Mr. Anderson has stopped playing entirely. Mrs. Anderson thinks he seems unhappy and has encouraged him to play tennis again, but when she mentions it, he accuses her of trying to get him out of the house.

One of the services offered at the senior citizen center is a blood pressure check every month. Mrs. Anderson's blood pressure was very high one month and she returned to have it retaken. The nurse noticed that Mrs. Anderson

Continued.

Case Study   **Mr. and Mrs. Anderson—cont'd**

---

seemed sad, and after noting that her blood pressure was 160/100, she told her that she was exhibiting some hypertension and referred her to a physician for follow-up. When the nurse informed Mrs. Anderson about her hypertension, Mrs. Anderson burst into tears and said to the nurse, "I just don't know what to do. I wish we had never moved here; my husband is worrying me to death."

The nurse spent the next hour with Mrs. Anderson to give her an opportunity to discuss her feelings and to gain information about the situation. After the interview the nurse informed Mrs. Anderson that she would be making a referral to the physician regarding both Mrs. Anderson's hypertension and Mr. Anderson's apparent problems with alcohol. In addition, the nurse told Mrs. Anderson that she will arrange a meeting with the physician, the alcohol counselor, the nurse, and Mrs. Anderson to discuss ways to deal with Mr. Anderson's drinking behavior.

After the meeting, the nurse formulated a comprehensive care plan to guide her interventions with the Anderson family (see p. 255).

Nursing Care Plan for Mr. and Mrs. Anderson

Assessment data	Diagnoses, goals, expected outcomes	Nursing interventions	Evaluation
Subjective Mrs. Anderson: "My husband seems to have a drink in his hand all the time." "We argue more and more about everything, especially his drinking. He said he doesn't have a problem—that he doesn't drink any more than he ever did." Mr. Anderson: (to nurse during home visit) "I don't know what you are talking about. I don't have a problem with alcohol. That's just my wife's idea." **Objective** Mrs. Anderson: Blood pressure 160/100. Tearful when discussing husband. Affect sad, anxious, depressed. Mr. Anderson: Hostile when questioned about alcohol intake. Florid complexion. Tremors noted in hands. (Patient seen in early AM; had not had any alcohol yet.)	**Primary diagnosis** Substance abuse (alcohol) **Long-term goal** Patient will participate in alcoholism treatment and will remain abstinent. **Nursing diagnoses** 1. Knowledge deficit related to disease of alcoholism and effect of alcohol on older adults. **Expected outcomes** 1. Patient will verbalize signs and symptoms of alcoholism. 1b. Patient will characterize alcoholism as a disease. 1c. Patient will discuss effects of alcohol on older individuals. 1d. Patient will state that he has a problem with alcohol abuse. 1e. Patient will agree to undergo treatment for his alcohol problem. 1f. Patient will agree to enter a hospital to undergo detoxification.	Coordinate a confrontation in which Mr. Anderson will be confronted (in a loving manner) with the facts and potential consequences of his drinking and its effects on his family, especially Mrs. Anderson. The aim of the intervention will be to persuade Mr. Anderson to enter hospital for detoxification and subsequent treatment and AA participation. Those present at the confrontation should include Mr. and Mrs. Anderson, their children, substance abuse counselor, physician, and nurse. Whether or not Mr. Anderson chooses to enter treatment, Mrs. Anderson should be encouraged to attend Al-Anon meetings on a regular basis.	Following the intervention, Mr. Anderson did agree to enter the local community hospital for detoxification. He detoxified safely, without incident, and was discharged 1 week later. While in the hospital he was referred to AA and the initial contact was made and the first meeting attended. He continued to attend AA meetings after discharge and saw a substance abuse counselor on an outpatient basis. Six months later, Mr. Anderson was still abstinent. Mrs. Anderson began attending Al-Anon when Mr. Anderson entered the hospital and she continued to attend weekly.

Continued.

Nursing Care Plan for Mr. and Mrs. Anderson—cont'd

Assessment data	Diagnoses, goals, expected outcomes	Nursing interventions	Evaluation
Subjective Mrs. Anderson: "We argue more and more about everything, especially his drinking: he said he doesn't have a problem—that he doesn't drink any more than he ever did." "I never used to have to drive him home from parties because he had too much to drink." "I just don't know what to do." Mr. Anderson: (to nurse during home visit) "I don't have a problem with alcohol. It's just my wife: she isn't willing to let me just enjoy my retirement. I worked hard to earn all this and I ought to be able to enjoy it any way I want to."	**Nursing diagnoses** 2. Family processes, altered related to alcohol abuse. **Long-term goal** Patient and wife will report improved marital relationship. **Expected outcomes** 2a. Mrs. Anderson will attend Al-Anon. 2b. Mr. and Mrs. Anderson will report improved communication. 2c. Mrs. Anderson will verbalize her own patterns of enabling behavior. 2d. All family members will verbalize acceptance of Mr. Anderson's alcohol problem. **Nursing diagnoses** 3. Powerlessness related to reluctance to admit alcohol abuse. **Expected outcomes** 3a. Mr. Anderson will admit that he is an alcoholic. 3b. Mr. Anderson will verbalize that his feeling that he is powerless over his drinking is part of the disease process of addiction. 3c. Mr. Anderson will verbalize knowledge of the 12 steps.	2a. Encourage Mrs. Anderson's participation in Al-Anon. 2b. Refer Mr. and Mrs. Anderson for marital counseling if marital problems continue. 3a. Encourage Mr. Anderson's participation in AA after hospital discharge.	Mrs. Anderson did attend Al-Anon and reported that she benefited from this experience and understood the ways in which spouses sometimes enable the alcoholic's drinking. Mrs. Anderson reported that their marital situation was much improved and felt they did not need further counseling about the marriage. Mr. Anderson continued to attend AA meetings after hospital discharge.

Subjective

Mrs. Anderson:
"We used to have a close physical relationship, but that's gone now."

Mr. Anderson:
"Retirement isn't as relaxing as I thought it would be for me."

Nursing diagnoses

4. Sexual dysfunction related to unknown cause (probable cause: alcohol abuse).

Expected outcomes

4a. Mr. and Mrs. Anderson will verbalize the effect of alcohol on sexual functioning.
4b. Mr. and Mrs. Anderson will report improvement in their physical relationship.

Nursing diagnoses

5. Adjustment, impaired related to retirement.

Long-term goal

Patient will engage in leisure activities that he enjoys.

Expected outcomes

5a. Mr. Anderson will begin to participate in his recreational sport, tennis.
5b. Mr. Anderson will verbalize his feelings regarding retirement.

4a. Discuss with Mr. and Mrs. Anderson the effects of alcohol on sexual functioning (e.g., inhibition of erection).
4b. Discuss with Mr. and Mrs. Anderson the importance of touching and holding each other without specific sexual expectations.

5a. Discuss with Mr. Anderson recreational activities in which he might be interested in participating. Explore with him friends and acquaintances with whom he could participate in these activities.
5b. Encourage Mr. Anderson to discuss his thoughts and feelings about retirement. Help him identify any difficulties he is having accepting retirement as well as the possible factors that go along with it.

Mr. and Mrs. Anderson expressed understanding of the effects of alcohol on sexual functioning.
Mr. and Mrs. Anderson reported that they were slowly reestablishing their physical relationship with each other and that they were closer than they had been in recent years.

Mr. Anderson did begin to participate in tennis and other leisure and recreational activities at the club.
Mr. Anderson began to discuss his feelings about his retirement.

Continued.

Nursing Care Plan for Mr. and Mrs. Anderson—cont'd

Assessment data	Diagnoses, goals, expected outcomes	Nursing interventions	Evaluation
Subjective Mr. Anderson: "I've been a successful businessman all my life. I don't have a problem with alcoholism. That's just my wife's idea."	**Nursing diagnoses** 6. Noncompliance related to denial of alcoholism. **Expected outcomes** 6a. Mr. Anderson will admit his alcohol problem. 6b. Mr. Anderson will agree to inpatient detoxification followed by outpatient counseling and participation in AA.	Coordinate a confrontation (described in preceding section). If Mr. Anderson does not enter treatment, continue to meet with him and Mrs. Anderson on home visits and help Mr. Anderson identify his drinking behaviors and their effect on Mrs. Anderson. Also, discuss the effects of alcohol intake on older persons.	Mr. Anderson did enter treatment.
Subjective Mr. Anderson: "I feel a little shaky but I'm OK." **Objective** Mr. Anderson Pulse on admission = 90 BP on admission = 150/90	**Nursing diagnoses** 7. Sensory-perceptual alteration related to alcohol withdrawal syndrome. **Expected outcomes** 7a. Mr. A. will agree to enter hospital for detoxification. 7b. Mr. A. will not experience delirium tremens during withdrawal period. **Nursing diagnoses** 8. Injury, high risk for related to alcohol withdrawal syndrome. **Expected outcomes** 8a. Mr. Anderson will detoxify in hospital setting. 8b. Mr. Anderson will detoxify safely.	7 and 8. On inpatient unit, carefully assess Mr. Anderson's drinking history, including amount of alcohol consumed per day and time of last drink. Closely monitor Mr. Anderson's vital signs and signs of agitation or restlessness. Administer sedative medication appropriately. Provide quiet and calm environment.	Mr. Anderson did detoxify safely in the hospital and did not experience delirium tremens.

❖ Summary

The prevalence of substance abuse is not extremely high in older adults because drinking usually decreases after age 60 and because chronic alcoholics usually do not survive into old age. Nevertheless, the consequences of substance abuse are devastating for the older person and his or her family. The older addicted person may be isolated and lonely. Often it is the nurse who has the first opportunity and responsibility for identifying the problem, because the health care system is the first point at which the older person is most likely to appear with symptoms that can be attributed to alcoholism or substance abuse if the nurse is perceptive and assesses for this possibility. Treatment is usually successful with older substance abusers, particularly those who began abusing substances later in life. Therefore the prognosis is hopeful, and health care professionals should approach this problem with a positive attitude.

❖ References

Abbott, J. A., Goldberg, A. A., & Becker, C. E. (1974). The role of a medical audit in assessing management of alcoholics with acute pancreatitis. *Quarterly Journal of Studies on Alcoholism, 35,* 272.

Alexander, D. F. (1987, July/August). Women's physical health and well-being. Proceedings of the National Conference on Women's Health. *Public Health Reports Supplement,* pp. 9-11.

Alexander, F., & Duff, R. W. (1988). Drinking in retirement communities. *Generations, 12*(4), 58-62.

American Nurses' Association and National Nurses Society on Addictions. (1988). *Standards of addictions nursing practice with selected diagnoses and criteria.* Washington, DC: Author. Nurses' Association.

American Psychiatric Association. (1994). *Diagnostic and statistical manual of mental disorders: DSM-IV* (4th ed.). Washington, DC: Author.

Blazer, D. (1978). Techniques for communicating with your elderly patient. *Geriatrics, 33*(11), 79-84.

Blose, I. L. (1978). The relationship of alcohol and aging and the elderly. *Alcoholism: Clinical and Experimental Research, 2,* 17.

Brody, J. A., & Mills, G. S. (1978). On considering alcohol as a risk factor in specific diseases. *American Journal of Epidemiology, 107,* 462-466.

Cahalan, D., Cisin, I. H., & Crossley, H. M. (1969). *American drinking practices.* New Brunswick, NJ: Rutgers Center for Alcohol Studies.

Caroselli-Karinja, M. (1985). Drug abuse and the elderly. *Journal of Psychosocial Nursing, 23*(6), 25-30.

Chafetz, M. E. (1983). *The alcoholic patient: Diagnosis and management.* Oradell, NJ: Medical Economics Books.

Chatham, L. R. (1987, July/August). Issues related to alcohol, drug use and abuse, and mental health of women. Proceedings of the National Conference on Women's Health. *Public Health Reports Supplement,* pp. 17-18.

Chenitz, W. C., Salisbury, S., & Stone, J. (1990). Drug use and abuse in the elderly. *Issues in Mental Health Nursing, 11,* 1-16.

Closser, M., & Blow, F. (1993). Recent advances in addictive disorders: Special populations: Women, ethnic minorities, and the elderly. *Psychiatric Clinics of North America, 16*(1), 199-209.

Criteria Committee, National Council on Alcoholism: Criteria for the diagnosis of alcoholism. (1972). *Annals of Internal Medicine, 77,* 249-258; *American Journal of Psychiatry, 129,* 127-135.

Cutezo, E., & Dellasega, C. (1992). Substance abuse in the homebound elderly. *Home Healthcare Nurse, 10*(1), 19-23.

Eckhardt, M. J., Harford, T. C., Kaelber, C. T., Parker, E. S., Rosenthal, L. S., Ryback, R. S., Salmoiraghi, G. C., Vonderveen, E. & Warren, K. R. (1981). Health hazards associated with alcohol consumption. *Journal of the American Medical Association, 246,* 648-666.

Estes, N. J., Smith-DiJulio, K., & Heinemann, M. E. (1980). *Nursing diagnosis of the alcoholic person.* St. Louis: Mosby.

Funkhouser, M. (1977/1978). Identifying alcohol problems among elderly hospital patients. *Alcohol Health and Research World, 2,* 27.

Gaitz, C. M., & Baer, P. E. (1971). Characteristics of elderly patients with alcoholism. *Archives of General Psychiatry, 24,* 372-378.

Garland, L. M. (1983). Gerontologic nursing. In G. Bennett, C. Vourakis, & D. Woolf, (Eds.). *Substance abuse: Pharmacologic, developmental, and clinical perspectives.* New York: Wiley.

Glatt, M. M. (1978). Experiences with elderly alcoholics in England. *Alcoholism: Clinical and Experimental Research, 2,* 23.

Glantz, M., & Backenheimer, M. (1988). Substance abuse among elderly women. *Clinical Gerontologist, 8*(1), 3-26.

Gordon, M., & Preiksaitis, H. G. (1988). Drugs and the aging brain. *Geriatrics, 43(5),* 69-78.

Hermos, J. A., LoCastro, J. S., Bouchard, G. R., & Glynn, R. J. (1986). Influence of cardiovascular disease on alcohol consumption among men in the normative aging study. In G. Maddox, L. N. Robins, & N. Rosenberg (Eds.). *Nature and extent of alcohol problems among the elderly* (pp. 117-133). New York: Springer.

Hoffman, A., & Heinemann, E. (1986). Alcohol problems in elderly persons. In N. J. Estes & M. E. Heinemann (Eds.). *Alcoholism: Development, consequences, and interventions.* (2nd ed.) St. Louis: Mosby.

Holmstrom, C. (1990). Substance abuse in the elderly. *Psychiatric Nursing, 31*(1), 6-8.

Johnson, E. M. (1987, July/August). Substance abuse and women's health. Proceedings of the National Conference on Women's Health. *Public Health Reports Supplement* (pp. 42-48).

Kastenbaum, R. (1988). In moderation: How some older people find pleasure and meaning in alcoholic beverages. *Generations, 12(4),* 68-73.

Kela, L. A., Kosberg, J. I., & Joyce, K. (1984). The alcoholic elderly client: Assessment of policies and practices of service providers. *The Gerontologist, 24*(5), 517-521.

Lamy, P. P. (1988). Actions of alcohol and drugs in older people. *Generations, 12(4),* 9-13.

Lewis, D. C. (1980). Diagnosis and management of the alcoholic patient. *Rhode Island Medical Journal, 63,* 1-5.

Lindblom, L., Kostyk, D., Tabisz, E., Jackyk, W., & Fuchs, D. (1992). Chemical abuse: An intervention program for the elderly. *Journal of Gerontological Nursing, 18*(4), 6-14.

Liptzin, B. (1987). Women's health: Issues in mental health, alcoholism, and drug abuse: Mental health and older women. *Public Health Reports Supplement* (pp. 34-38).

Maddox, G. L. (1988). Aging, drinking, and alcohol abuse. *Generations, 12(4),* 14-16.

Maddox, B., Robins, L. N., & Rosenberg, N. (1984). *Nature and extent of alcohol problems among the elderly.* New York: Springer.

Mendelson, J., & Mello, N. (1985). *The diagnosis and treatment of alcoholism.* New York: McGraw-Hill.

Mishara, B. L., & Kastenbaum, R. (1980). *Alcohol and old age.* New York: Grune & Stratton.

Moos, R. H. & Finney, J. W. (1984). A systems perspective on problem drinking among older adults. In G. Maddow, L. Robines, & N. Rosenberg, (Eds.). *Nature and extent of alcohol problems among the elderly* (pp. 151-167). New York: Springer.

Morse, R. (1988). Substance abuse among the elderly. *Bulletin of the Menninger Clinic, 52*(3), 259-268.

Nambudiri, D. & Young, R. (1991). A case of late-onset crack dependence and subsequent psychosis in the elderly. *Journal of Substance Abuse Treatment, 8,* 253-255.

Parkinson, D., Stephensen, S., & Phillips, S. (1985). Head injuries: A prospective, computerized study. *Canadian Journal of Surgery, 28,* 79-83.

Pascarella, E. F. (1981). Drug abuse and the elderly. In J. Lowinson & P. Ruiz (Eds.). *Substance abuse: Clinical problems and perspectives* (pp. 752-757). Baltimore: Williams & Wilkins.

Petersen, D. M. (1988). Substance abuse, criminal behavior, and older people. *Generations, 12*(4), 63-67.

Rathbone-McCuan, E. (1988). Promoting help-seeking behaviors among elders with chemical dependencies. *Generations, 12(4),* 37-40.

Ray, O., & Ksir, C. (1993). *Drugs, society, and human behavior* (6th ed.) St. Louis: Mosby.

Reed, J. A. (1981). A socio-cultural comparison of lifestyles and survival differences between Chinese and black addicts on methadone in New York City. In A. J. Schecter (Ed.). *Drug dependence and alcoholism: Social and behavioral issues* (pp. 757-768). (vol. 2). New York: Plenum.

Reed, S. W. (1976). Assessing the patient with an alcohol problem. *Nursing Clinics of North America, 11*(13), 483-492.

Rosin, A., & Glatt, M. M. (1971). Alcohol excess in the elderly. *Quarterly Journal of Studies on Alcohol, 32,* 53-59.

Schuckit, M. A. & Miller, P. L. (1976). Alcoholism in elderly men: A survey of a general medical ward. *Annals of the New York Academy of Sciences, 273,* 558-571.

Schuckit, M. A. & Pastor, P. A. (1978). The elderly as a unique population: Alcoholism. *Alcoholism: Clinical and Experimental Research, 1,* 31-38.

Seixas, F. A. (1982). Criteria for the diagnosis of alcoholism. In N. J. Estes & M. E. Heinemann (Eds.). *Alcoholism: Development, consequences, and interventions.* (2nd ed.) St. Louis: Mosby.

Shimp, L. A., & Ascione, F. J. (1988). Causes of medication misuse and error. *Generations, 12(4),* 17-21.

Shropshire, R. W. (1975). The hidden faces of alcoholism. *Geriatrics, 30*(3), 99-102.

Tamayo, J. V. & Haglund, R. M. (1981). Drug treatment for the elderly abuse. In A. J. Schecter (Ed.). *Drug dependence and alcoholism.* New York: Plenum.

Thibault, J., & Maly, R. (1993). Recognition and treatment of substance abuse in the elderly. *Primary Care, 20*(1), 155-165.

Tweed, S. H. (1989). Identifying the alcoholic client. *Nursing Clinics of North America, 24*(1), 13-32.

Wetter, R. E. (1981). A drug education program for the elderly. In A. J. Schecter (Ed.). *Drug dependence and alcoholism.* New York: Plenum.

Whittington, F. J. (1988). Making it better: Drinking and drugging in old age. *Generations, 12*(4), 5-7.

Willenbring, M. & Spring, W. D. (1988). Evaluating alcohol use in elders. *Generations, 12*(4), 27-31.

Williams, E. P., Carruth, B., & Hyman, M. M. (Eds.). (1973). *Alcohol and problem drinking among older persons.* Springfield, VA: National Technical Information Service.

Zimberg, S. (1978). Diagnosis and treatment of the elderly alcoholic. *Alcoholism: Clinical and Experimental Research, 2,* 27.

Chapter 10

❖ *Inpatient Geropsychiatric Nursing in a General Hospital*

Joan M. Wagner

Treatment on an inpatient geropsychiatric unit can help the older person with an acute mental health problem to achieve important health and quality of life goals. The goals of geropsychiatric care include optimizing the patient's general functioning and physical health status, preventing institutional care, enhancing self-esteem, decreasing the suffering caused by the patient's mental illness or behavioral problem, and enhancing the family caregiver role (Abraham et al., 1990). The treatment of an acute mental health problem in the geriatric patient mandates a holistic perspective in which the patient's mental, physical, social, functional, and spiritual well-being are addressed; the use of a traditional model of disease- or symptom-focused care is inadequate and may be useless for the multifaceted, interacting problems of the geriatric patient.

Mental health problems that can be treated on a geropsychiatric unit include severe depression, neurobehavioral problems of a dementing illness, sudden onset of confusion, dependence on pain medication, functional disorders, anxiety, and obsessive-compulsive disorders. A geropsychiatric inpatient program requires a staff that has the appropriate knowledge and skills to care for these patients, is highly motivated to work with these patients, and can work collaboratively.

Geropsychiatric inpatient units have existed in state psychiatric hospitals and in veterans' hospitals for many years, although treatment efforts were limited. Lazarus (1976) described a psychiatric program for older patients, established at the Psychiatric Institute of Michael Reese Hospital in 1968, that provided intensive psychiatric treatment, including group therapy. He reported that problem behaviors in these patients, some of whom had organic brain disorder, showed improvement in response to group pressure. The program was established because of the difficulty of the older patients with the regular therapeutic program, which appears to have been geared to young adults.

Interest in the establishment of geropsychiatric units in acute-care general hospitals has been accelerating since the early 1980s. Geropsychiatric units can be viewed as one type of *medical-psychiatric unit,* which integrates psychiatric and medical care for a specific population (Stoudemire & Fogel, 1986). A defining characteristic of such a unit is the concurrent management of the patient's medical condition with the psychiatric problem. Inpatient geropsychiatric units serve the older person who has an acute psychiatric condition that requires inpatient care. Because the older person may have a chronic illness or a physical health problem in addition to the psychiatric condition, a geropsychiatric unit must provide for these needs. This chapter describes such units.

❖ *Strategic Planning and Marketing*

The inpatient geropsychiatric unit requires the support of the hospital, the medical staff, and the community as well as the cooperation of an interdisciplinary team. Some factors that at first glance may appear to have little bearing on care can have a strong influence on the unit's success. The reasons for this derive from the nature of geriatric clinical care.

Health care professionals, especially but not exclusively physicians, who have not studied gerontology may not understand how psychiatric care can help older persons (Greene, 1985). Because physicians admit patients to the hospital, this lack of knowledge is a barrier to the admission of persons who could benefit from such care. Without the cooperation of the hospital's staff physicians, patients may not be admitted to a geropsychiatric unit even though they have mental health problems that can be treated there. This does not mean that physicians are opposed to geropsychiatric care, only that they may not understand the kinds of problems that can be treated, how to identify appropriate patients, and what the physician role on a geropsychiatric unit is. One purpose of a marketing plan is to address these issues.

Other barriers to mental health care are ageist attitudes, for example, that the older person is inappropriate for mental health care, that mental health resources are wasted on the older adult, and that nothing can be done to improve the mental health of the older adult (Moak, 1990). These attitudes exist both within the general population and among some health care professionals. The marketing plan of a geropsychiatric unit must include a means of providing appropriate information to counter such beliefs and attitudes.

Such problems must be addressed, because patients in need of geropsychiatric services are not likely to seek these services on their own; usually a family or institutional caregiver recognizes the need for specialized mental health care. Mental health services and care tend not to be in demand the way high-tech health care is, so families as well as physicians must be aware of the kinds of problems appropriate for a geropsychiatric unit and the kind of help available there. Without attention to these issues, the geropsychiatric unit may not serve the population in need of its services and may be shut down for lack of patients. The assumption is that family caregivers, physicians, and others who understand the help available will use the facility appropriately and provide a population of patients adequate to maintain the unit's existence.

A comprehensive plan for developing an inpatient geropsychiatric unit is developed from answers to the following questions:

◆ Is the region large enough and does it have enough individuals 60 and over to support a geropsychiatric unit?
◆ Do family practice physicians and internists on the hospital's medical staff have older patients in their practices? Do these physicians recognize a need for mental health services for their older patients? Will they admit geriatric patients from their practice who are in need of intensive psychiatric care?
◆ Is there a geropsychiatrist or a psychiatrist with an interest in practicing with older patients on the hospital's medical staff who is willing to serve as the unit's medical director or support the establishment of a geropsychiatric unit?
◆ Does the hospital already have an inpatient psychiatric service? What is the status of the medical, nursing, and hospital staff's acceptance of a specialized psychiatric unit in addition to any already in existence?
◆ Is there an inpatient geropsychiatric unit in the immediate area? If there is, will the area support another such unit? How will the new unit differ from the existing one?
◆ Will the unit function under the Prospective Payment System (PPS) or under PPS-exempt status? Are there state licensing, certificate-of-need or other requirements? If the unit is to be PPS exempt, do hospital and nursing management know how to apply for exempt status, know Medicare requirements, and understand the effect of the unit on the hospital's financial status?
◆ Is there a nursing leader available with credentials and experience in geropsychiatric, geriatric, or gerontological nursing?

♦ Are qualified, experienced nursing, social services, and recreational therapy staff available?
♦ Is there a designated area within the hospital with appropriate care and support areas? Is the time frame for establishing the unit known?

Answers to these questions will form the basis of a marketing plan. Marketing in this discussion is defined as activities that promote education, outreach, and consumer satisfaction in groups having an interest in a geropsychiatric unit. These groups or constituencies are as follows:

♦ Present, former, and prospective patients
♦ Family caregivers of older people
♦ Psychiatrists and other physicians on a hospital's medical staff
♦ Nursing homes
♦ Home health agencies
♦ Other hospital departments

Other small but important constituencies are hospitals without psychiatric units, rural hospitals, community mental health centers, residential service providers to older people (boarding homes, retirement homes), members of the aging network such as the local Office on Aging and senior centers, private practitioners with older clients (psychologists, social workers, nurses), law enforcement agencies, judges, mental health officials, and attorneys. The nurse researching the community for groups or individuals who have an interest in service to older clients will find many such examples. The marketing plan should provide for outreach to these constituencies.

Family caregivers of older people, including spouses, siblings, and middle-aged children, have a vital interest in identifying appropriate resources for the assessment and treatment of their care recipients; reaching these family caregivers is an important objective of the marketing plan.

An example of a marketing plan for a geropsychiatric unit is shown in Box 10-1. A marketing plan provides for the unit's and hospital's objectives. In a time of unprecedented change in the health care delivery system this means not only providing the highest quality of patient care but also being concerned with the needs of unit constituencies such as physicians, agencies, and the community in general. The concerns of these groups are a basis for making organizational changes that can lead to more satisfied consumers (Strasen, 1987).

Responsibility for implementing the unit's marketing plan should be assigned to a specific staff member, with a designated amount of time allocated for marketing efforts. Portions of the plan that call for liaison and meetings with individual physicians are best implemented by the unit's nursing leader, because a strong clinical background is necessary for discussing admission criteria and screening procedures. The implementation of the marketing plan, including provisions for suggestions of physicians, creates an opportunity to develop collaborative, collegial relationships

Box 10-1   **Marketing Plan**

 I. Medical staff: psychiatrists, other physicians
     A. Individual meetings to review and explain
         1. Admission criteria
         2. Types of problems treated and examples of appropriate clients
         3. Treatment program and modalities
         4. Patient identification and preadmission screening
         5. Concurrent medical management
     B. Medical staff meetings for physician orientation

 II. Hospital marketing
     A. Orientation of clinical nursing departments to topics above
     B. Orientation of all other hospital departments
     C. Ongoing orientation for new hospital employees

III. Community outreach and visibility
     A. Individual calls with administrative, clinical staffs
         1. Nursing homes
         2. Home health agencies
     B. Calls on other constituency representatives
         1. Rural hospitals
         2. Hospitals without psychiatric units
         3. Retirement homes, boarding homes
         4. Attorneys, law enforcement officials, judges, mental health officials
     C. Community visibility
         1. Institutional membership in groups and organizations serving older people: Council on Aging, Alzheimer's Association
         2. Representation at health fairs and similar events
         3. Hospital-based special education and service efforts: caregiver classes, support groups

 IV. Other marketing activities
     A. Marketing budget
     B. Design, drafting of appropriate materials and literature
     C. Marketing meetings
     D. Media efforts and materials

between the unit's interdisciplinary staff and hospital physicians who admit or follow patients on the unit (Turner, 1990). While initial contact with a physician may be made by the nurse responsible for marketing the unit, all unit staff must be committed to this kind of staff-physician relationship; otherwise marketing efforts will have a very limited effect.

❖ *Admission*

Admission Criteria

While an upper age limit is not usually necessary, some thought should be given to a minimum age. This can range from 50 through 70 years of age, depending on treatment goals. Without an age criterion, questions will continually arise about the appropriateness of particular persons for admission.

Patients must have a psychiatric diagnosis and problems of such severity that inpatient care is indicated. Behaviors and conditions that meet these criteria are those that make the patient a danger to self or others. Some examples are suicidal threat, psychotic symptoms, and physically aggressive or assaultive behavior.

The patient's physical and medical condition must allow active participation in therapy. Stable chronic illness does not preclude such participation, nor does dependency in activities of daily living.

Preadmission assessment to determine appropriateness for admission in regard to medical condition requires direct patient assessment and history taking. While assessment information obtained from health care practitioners and agencies may be helpful, it is not a good substitute for direct assessment. Reliance on the assessments of others can create acute problems when a patient arrives at the geropsychiatric unit and admission to a medical unit is determined to be necessary instead. The following information will help to identify patients whose medical needs should be addressed prior to their admission to the geropsychiatric unit.

- Is the patient under a physician's care, and when was the patient last seen by the physician? Are there any health problems? What medications is the patient taking?
- What kinds of care is the caregiver providing? Insulin injection? Dressing? Other medications? What else?
- How has the patient been feeling physically? Do physical symptoms indicate a need for medical attention?
- What is the baseline of physical health as described by the patient or caregiver? Is the patient at or near this baseline, or does available information indicate a possible physical health problem in addition to the mental health problem?

Patients on a hospital medical unit may be assessed for their potential to participate in the geropsychiatric treatment program on the basis of answers to the following questions:

- If the patient has been on a medical unit, is the intensive or aggressive part of the medical treatment completed? Vital signs should have been stable for several days and the patient out of bed for some of the day. The patient should not need intravenous therapy for hydration or nutrition.

- ◆ Have treatment goals for the medical problem been reached?
- ◆ If the patient is recovering from surgery, is there evidence of increasing ambulation?
- ◆ What are the patient's mobility and functional levels at the time of the assessment, and what is the potential for the immediate future? If the patient has been acutely ill for several weeks and is very weak or debilitated, his or her strength may have to improve before an intensive psychiatric regimen can be initiated.

Examples of patients who are appropriate for admission to a geropsychiatric unit are described below.

- ◆ Mr. Vang, age 83, has been on the medical unit for several days. His multiple somatic symptoms have been medically evaluated and no physical basis for them found. Evaluation by the consulting psychiatrist reveals that Mr. Vang is clinically depressed, and Mr. Vang agrees to enter the geropsychiatric unit for treatment of the depression.
- ◆ Mrs. Means, age 69, was admitted to a nursing home 9 months ago after she was found to have Alzheimer's disease. Although still ambulatory, she has rapidly deteriorated mentally and no longer can communicate verbally. In the nursing home she has struck clients who come near her and has become combative with nursing staff when they attempt to provide care. After obtaining the family's consent the nursing home social worker called the geropsychiatric unit to request a preadmission screening.
- ◆ Mrs. Penn, age 75, has been living with her daughter, who is her caregiver. When Mrs. Penn sees babies and other persons she becomes extremely agitated; this agitation creates severe management problems for her caregiver daughter. Mrs. Penn's daughter contacts the family physician to describe the behavior, and after an evaluation of Mrs. Penn at an office visit, the physician recommends admission to the geropsychiatric unit.
- ◆ Mrs. Grant, age 80, lives next door to her daughter. She is subject to severe anxiety, palpitations, and nocturnal sleeplessness. She has begun calling her daughter on the telephone up to 20 times a day in an attempt to obtain relief from her anxiety. Her daughter calls the hospital's client information line and is referred to the geropsychiatric unit.
- ◆ Miss Binn, age 77, is in a rural hospital recovering from a self-inflicted gunshot wound. Although her wound is healing well, Miss Binn is clearly depressed, and the hospital's social worker is arranging for discharge care. The social worker contacts the geropsychiatric unit to request a preadmission screening for the patient.
- ◆ Mr. Brown, age 83, is arrested by the police in his home town after brandishing a gun at them. At his court hearing he is offered either jail or a psychiatric evaluation and chooses the latter. He is referred to the geropsychiatric unit by a mental health official in the community.

Persons not appropriate for admission include those with dementia who need acute care for a medical condition such as pneumonia or a fractured hip, comatose or bedridden patients, those in isolation, those whose only need is nursing home placement, and those who have no behavioral problem but whose family caregiver is in need of respite.

During their hospital stay, medically stable geropsychiatric patients may be diagnosed with clinical problems requiring strenuous tests (e.g., intravenous pyelogram, barium enema) or treatment such as intravenous or enteral therapy. Clinical nursing judgment and consultation with the primary physician may be required in these situations to set priorities for treatment.

Admission Routes

The most frequent route of admission to a geropsychiatric unit is direct admission by a psychiatrist or other physician on the hospital's medical staff. The patient admitted by the internist or family practitioner is likely to be a private patient and may come to the hospital directly from the physician's office. The patient admitted by a geropsychiatrist is likely to be a referral from a physician or some other source. In either case, the patient has been assessed for admission.

Some patients come from other units in the hospital: medical, surgical, cardiac, rehabilitation, or emergency department. Older individuals may be taken to a hospital's emergency department after being found wandering in the community, for behavior problems that families are unable to manage, or by caregivers who can no longer tolerate difficult behaviors. Such patients may be referred to the geropsychiatric unit if their medical condition permits. In some instances the patient has had a psychiatric evaluation that identified a problem appropriate for treatment on the geropsychiatric unit; in others the nurse, recognizing the nature of the problem, suggested to the physician that either a psychiatric consultation or a preadmission screening by the staff of the geropsychiatric unit be done. Identification of geriatric patients by hospital nursing and clinical staff members is an important link to mental health care, including inpatient geropsychiatric care. In these situations follow-up by geropsychiatric unit staff consists of preadmission screening to determine whether the patient meets admission criteria. Admission may be arranged after consultation with the patient's physician.

These typical referral patterns to a geropsychiatric unit show that physicians, health care providers, and the community at large must be aware of the unit as a resource to be able to make referrals. All staff members of the geropsychiatric unit must listen carefully to the call from the community, obtain relevant information from the caller, do at least a preliminary telephone screening, and refer the caller to the most appropriate source of help, whether or not that help is in the geropsychiatric unit. A cooperative working relationship among the unit's interdisciplinary staff, physicians, and hospital staff is essential.

❖ *Assessment of the Patient*

Psychiatric and Medical Evaluation

The psychiatric evaluation includes a description of the problem for which the patient is being admitted. Information is usually obtained both from the patient and from family members. All problem behaviors and symptoms and their effect on the patient's ability to function and on the family are specified. Additional information is the patient's psychiatric history; medical history; mental status and neurological examinations; drug and alcohol history; medications, including psychotherapeutic medications previously used by the patient; and their effectiveness or failure. The evaluation also includes a diagnostic formulation and suggested treatment plan for the hospital stay (Silver & Herrmann, 1991).

Diagnostic information includes psychiatric and medical diagnoses, and personality disorders, psychosocial stressors, and an assessment of the patient's functioning stated as a numerical score (GAF, or Global Assessment of Functioning). These data are organized as axes, with each axis providing a different but necessary perspective on the patient. Box 10-2 depicts the organization of this information. The patient's strengths and disabilities are also included in the psychiatric evaluation.

A medical history and physical examination by an internist or family practitioner form the basis for an overall evaluation of the patient's physical health status. Screening tests may be done to determine whether psychiatric symptoms are due to a physical illness (Alessi & Cassel, 1991; Patterson & LeClair, 1989). Identification of health problems or illnesses of the geriatric patient is necessary for the patient to achieve optimal health. An abrupt behavior change or decompensation in a patient who has been diagnosed with Alzheimer's disease may be a sign of a physical illness or problem (Barry & Moskowitz, 1988). For all these reasons, evaluation of the patient's physical health is essential. Appropriate tests are shown in Box 10-3.

Box 10-2   **DSM-IV Multiaxial System**

Axis   I   Clinical disorders
Axis II   Personality disorders, mental retardation
Axis III   General medical conditions
Axis IV   Psychosocial and environmental problems
Axis   V   Global assessment of functioning

Adapted from American Psychiatric Association (1994). Diagnostic and statistical manual of mental disorders (4th ed.). Washington, D.C.: Author, p. 25; with permission.

Box 10-3 **Screening Tests to Rule out Reversible or Treatable Cause of Dementia**

Blood count	Thyroid function
Chemistry panel	Electrocardiogram
Urinalysis	Chest x-ray film
Syphilis serology	Drug levels
Vitamin B_{12} and folate	

Admission Geropsychiatric Nursing Assessment

The geropsychiatric nursing assessment presents a holistic and pragmatic view of the patient at the time of admission. In addition to the behavior or problem for which the patient requires treatment, it is essential to assess the patient's physical health, functional abilities, family concerns, legal status, and risk status. An outline of assessment areas is shown in Box 10-4.

Physical health history and assessment are essential to establish a baseline for the patient. Other important information includes allergies, height, weight, temperature, and blood pressure. Detailed medication information and behavior should include prescription and over-the-counter medications. Since an overall review of medications is done during hospitalization, it is important that these be recorded.

Mental status assessment may be completed from a structured questionnaire, direct questioning, or from responses to other questions. The questions about reason for hospitalization, however, should be asked directly of the patient. This response will provide insight into the patient's perception of the hospital experience.

The functional assessment should include all personal and instrumental activities of daily living. Personal activities of daily living include bathing, dressing, toileting, walking, continence, and feeding; instrumental activities of daily living are those considered necessary for independent living, such as shopping, food preparation and cleanup, use of the telephone, transportation, and managing finances. The use of a scale or instrument is helpful.

Information about the patient's legal status is necessary to protect his or her rights, including obtaining appropriate consent for admission to the hospital. Patients' and families' wishes about confidentiality in regard to the hospitalization must be noted and implemented.

A discussion of the use of restraints may or may not be indicated. The purpose of initiating a discussion of this topic is to learn the patient's and family's feelings about safety measures in general when prevention of injury is an issue.

Caregiver information is obtained for several reasons. First, the patient and caregiver may have different perspectives on what the patient can and cannot do.

Box 10-4 **Areas of Nursing Assessment at Time of Admission**

I. Health history and physical assessment
   A. Major illnesses and hospitalizations in recent years
   B. Review of body systems and physical assessment
   C. Temperature, pulse, respirations, blood pressure, height, weight
   D. Allergies
   E. Prescription and over-the-counter medications
      1. Medication name, dosage, schedule
      2. Prescribing physician
      3. Duration of time medication has been taken
      4. Problem for which the medication was prescribed
      5. Date of last appointment with prescribing physician

II. Mental status assessment
   A. Orientation to place, time, persons
   B. Appearance
   C. Comprehension
   D. Speech
   E. Memory
   F. Insight
   G. Affect
   H. Indications of hallucinations, delusions, suicidal threat or ideation, potential for injury to self or others
   I. Reason patient is coming to the hospital in own words

III. Functional assessment
   A. Ability to perform activities of daily living
   B. Assistive devices or equipment used at home
   C. Glasses, hearing aids
   D. Daily routine as provided by the client

IV. Patient's rights and legal status
   A. Power of attorney, conservatorship, guardianship status
   B. Advance directive status
   C. Confidentiality regarding calls from family members and others
   D. Visitor restrictions
   E. Admission and treatment consent signatures
   F. Discussion of restraints

V. Caregiver and discharge planning information
   A. Name of person accompanying patient to the hospital; identifying information, including relationship to patient, telephone number

Continued.

> *Box 10-4*   **Areas of Nursing Assessment at Time of Admission—cont'd**
>
>   B. Description of care provided for patient
>   C. Names of relatives who are in regular contact with patient, whether or
>   not they are aware of the admission
>   D. Family conflict regarding care or hospitalization of patient
>   E. Patient's and family's tentative discharge plan
>   F. Name of family physician and date of last appointment
>
> VI. Risk assessment
>   A. Falling
>   B. Wandering
>   C. Smoking
>   D. Memory deficit

Cognitively impaired patients often do not perceive themselves as having disabilities even though they need a great deal of assistance. Second, caregiver information is necessary for discharge planning. Assessment of caregiver stress or burden may indicate an appropriate discharge plan. Third, caregiver participation is essential if the discharge plan is to be implemented.

Family information such as the patient's children and their knowledge of the hospitalization helps to determine the potential for problems during the hospital stay. Whether or not there is family conflict, the patient's children may have different ideas about what constitutes appropriate treatment; to the extent that relationships between the patient, family members, the patient's physician, and the hospital staff can be clearly understood in advance, problems may be avoided.

The family physician is noted because the patient will probably be returning to the care of that physician after discharge from the hospital.

The final assessment areas are those in which the degree of risk in several areas is assessed, so that appropriate nursing measures may be instituted. These areas include the risk of falling and wandering away from the unit, safety problems due to smoking, and agitation or other problems because the patient is forgetful. Some patients forget that the family has brought the patient to the hospital and insist on going home.

Social Service Assessment

The patient and family are interviewed by a social worker to assess the family's reaction to the illness and the patient's perception of his or her condition. Information is also obtained about the patient's living situation, family and other social support systems, financial resources, use of community resources, and any legal, ethical, or other problems that may affect the patient and his or her functioning. A tentative discharge plan is formulated and discussed with the patient and family.

Nutritional Assessment

Elements of a nutritional assessment include a review of the patient's medical history and physical examination; laboratory test values; dietary history, including usual eating patterns and food preferences; height, weight, and skinfold measurements; type of assistance needed with eating; and identification of nutritional problems. When the nutritional assessment is completed, by a registered dietitian, recommendations can be made for the treatment plan.

Recreational Therapy Assessment

The recreational assessment provides information about hobbies, interests, use of leisure time, and abilities to pursue them. The recreational therapist uses this information to plan activities appropriate in terms of functioning and interest and geared to the reason for hospitalization.

Other Assessments

The assessments described above form the core of the interdisciplinary assessment of the patient; many patients also require other evaluations to address specific problems.

Additional medical specialists may be required to evaluate a patient. These may include a neurologist, cardiologist, dermatologist, gastroenterologist, and podiatrist, for example. The purpose of the evaluation may be diagnosis (e.g., possible normal pressure hydrocephalus, possible basal cell carcinoma), selection of appropriate treatment for a heart condition, or treatment of a condition affecting the patient's functioning (e.g., ingrown toenail or painful bunion).

When a patient has mobility problems, a physical therapy assessment can help determine the nature of the problem and identify the appropriate intervention. Indications for a physical therapy assessment include unsteady gait not clearly attributable to a specific cause, inability to walk for more than a short distance in a patient who seems to have the potential for greater mobility, and painful mobility of joints due to chronic osteoarthritis.

Patients who have problems with speech, verbal comprehension, or swallowing may benefit from an evaluation by a speech pathologist. This evaluation can help determine the most appropriate approaches and interventions for communicating with the patient and for the most effective feeding techniques in those with swallowing difficulties.

Questions may arise about the patient's ability to perform activities of daily living when the unit's functional assessment protocols do not provide adequate answers. In these instances an evaluation by an occupational therapist can identify specific functional abilities and suggest the most appropriate level of care following discharge from the hospital.

❖ *Treatment Modalities*

Therapeutic Environment

An inpatient geropsychiatric unit is a therapeutic environment for older persons with mental health or psychiatric problems of such severity that hospitalization is indicated. Such a unit, a physically separate area in an acute-care hospital, encompasses sleeping areas; patient lounges; visiting, dining, and therapeutic activity areas; support areas (e.g., nurses' station, medication and utility rooms); and offices for the staff. The conceptual model is a *therapeutic community* in which all aspects of the environment—physical, interpersonal, and cultural—are designed to promote the patients' recovery or well-being (Leach, 1982).

The physical environment accommodates the needs arising from the aging process and promotes safety and functioning in cognitively impaired patients. Adequate light without glare, color contrast between walls and floor, and no inappropriate patterns on walls, draperies, and furniture are examples of important features.

A therapeutic environment is safe for patients (Kreigh & Perko, 1983; Schultz & Dark, 1982). Safety should include planned measures for the prevention of falling, injuries due to wandering and accidents, and smoking safety. Other safety concerns include suicide prevention, drug withdrawal precautions, and seizure precautions.

The nursing staff of a therapeutic environment must know about the needs of older patients, be skilled in the application of techniques and interventions appropriate for geriatric patients, and function as members of an interdisciplinary team.

A policy of street clothes for patients instead of hospital garb or pajamas creates an atmosphere of wellness and normality; such an atmosphere helps to foster appropriate behavior and is good for morale. When patients take their meals in a community dining room, mealtime becomes a time of socialization and enjoyment. The implicit cues in this type of setting can help even a severely impaired patient behave more appropriately.

Psychopharmacology

Psychotherapeutic medications include major tranquilizers, antidepressants, minor tranquilizers or antianxiety agents, and lithium. Age alone is not a contraindication to the use of these classes of medication, nor is age alone an indication for their use when behavior is perceived as troublesome by others (e.g., wandering or repetitive behavior). The treatment goals for use of psychotherapeutic medication are alleviation of symptoms, maintenance of the improvement, and prevention of relapse (Young & Meyers, 1991).

Group and Individual Psychotherapy

Group psychotherapy offers significant benefits to older persons (Baker, 1985). Group therapy can provide peer support and encouragement, feedback from others, confrontation about negative or disruptive behaviors, and a shared appreciation of the problems associated with aging, including the need for a change in the level of care required. The type of group psychotherapy appropriate for a particular patient will depend on his or her cognitive and functional status, individual needs, and motivation. Patients who have been functioning independently and who are not cognitively impaired may benefit from group therapies that use verbal and intellectual skills and interpersonal processes. For those whose memory or verbal communication skills are impaired, therapies such as music and reminiscence can engage the patient's attention and abilities to meet specific treatment goals. In a group setting patients can listen and talk to others and enjoy the social situation (Greene, Ingram, & Johnson, 1993).

Individual psychotherapy may be indicated for patients in especially difficult situations or who have unresolved grief, family conflict, or unaddressed issues from childhood such as physical or sexual abuse.

Other Therapies

Other activities to which patients respond positively include reminiscence groups, music therapy (Charatan, 1989), exercise or movement therapy (Paillard & Nowak 1985), pet therapy (Wilson & Netting, 1983), and pleasurable individual activities (Teri & Logsdon, 1991).

Patient and Family Education

At some point during the hospital stay, the patient (if appropriate), the family caregiver, and other family members should attend a scheduled individual conference to receive information about the patient's care and to discuss any necessary action. At this conference discussion focuses not only on the diagnosis but also on the meaning of that diagnosis for the patient's behavior and the problem that required the admission to the hospital. For example, when the patient has a diagnosis of dementia, the family needs to understand that what they may have interpreted as stubbornness or irascibility may actually be inability to understand or respond appropriately. During this discussion the therapist may offer suggestions for minimizing the problems of home care. Depending on the diagnosis, the family can also be invited to discuss care in the future, for example, the possibility of nursing home care. Finally, this conference allows families to ask questions that may have arisen during the hospitalization.

Discharge Planning

Discharge planning is routine for every patient; the effectiveness of brief hospitalization depends on a successful discharge planning strategy. Elements of this strategy include patient and family understanding that hospitalization will be brief, the initiation of discharge planning on admission, and focused goal-oriented treatment planning and implementation with target dates for each goal. Interdisciplinary treatment team members work together to structure the hospital stay and treatment to meet treatment goals on schedule.

❖ Treatment Planning

Because the presentation of illness in older patients may be nonspecific or vague (e.g., loss of appetite, fatigue, frequent falls), a well-defined strategy to identify and address problems and improve the patient's condition during a brief hospital stay is required. Such a strategy begins with clear admission criteria and a screening procedure in which problems appropriate for inpatient treatment are identified. Treatment planning begins when the patient is admitted. The assessments completed by the treatment team form a database that is used to identify problems, set goals, and measure progress.

Nurcombe (1988) described stabilization and brief hospitalization as useful concepts for treatment planning. Stabilization, the improvement of a clinical problem sufficiently for the patient to be treated less intensively or restrictively, is a major goal of brief hospitalization.

Brief hospitalization is necessitated by reimbursement policy; that is, payment for the hospital stay is limited, and treatment must be accomplished within this time. This period may be as brief as 2 weeks. Treatment planning of necessity must be highly focused to achieve goals in this amount of time.

The problem for which the patient is admitted is defined not only as the psychiatric symptom but as behavior that results in harm to the patient or to others and makes inpatient care necessary. Nurcombe (1988) defined this as a "pivotal problem" of the hospitalization. It is this problem that must be stabilized before discharge. Stated differently, a pivotal problem is a symptom and its effect on the patient's functioning and on the caregiver.

Pivotal problems are reframed as goals. Appropriate interventions and goals are determined by the interdisciplinary treatment team, assigned to specific team members for implementation, and evaluated regularly.

A hospitalization of approximately 2 weeks can be divided into three stages: admission and orientation, working or middle stage, and discharge (Box 10-5).

These stages reflect an uncomplicated stay in which the initial and continuing treatment responses are positive and there are no complicating medical conditions or legal, ethical, family, or discharge problems. In some situations the stay is even briefer. This may be the case if the patient responds very quickly to treatment, is highly motivated, is independent in activities of daily living, and has an adequate social support system.

Box 10-5 **Stages of Brief Hospitalization**

I. Admission and orientation (approximately 2 to 3 days)
   A. Patient and family oriented to unit
   B. Admission assessments performed
   C. Tentative discharge plan formulated
   D. Therapy begins

II. Working or middle (approximately 8 to 10 days)
   A. Therapeutic activities
   B. Initial treatment team meeting; pivotal problems identified and addressed
   C. Treatment plan reviewed with patient and family
   D. Coordination of psychiatric and medical goals
   E. Therapies and interventions implemented by team members
   F. Discharge plan discussed with patient and family; implementation pursued as necessary
   G. Regular treatment team meetings continue, with response to treatment and potential for further improvement evaluated

III. Discharge (approximately 1 to 2 days)
   A. Discharge date set; discharge plans settled
   B. Discharge instructions to patient and caregiver prepared and implemented
   C. Patient-staff and patient-patient relationships concluded

---

These problems can affect length of hospital stay:

◆ Lack of response to first psychotherapeutic medication (antidepressant, major tranquilizer); second or third attempt required.
◆ Medical problems requiring extensive evaluation or management, for example, occult gastrointestinal bleeding, pneumonia.
◆ Puzzling or complicated symptoms requiring additional medical consultants.
◆ Dysfunctional family: family members have widely differing perceptions of the situation, disagree on appropriate treatment and discharge plan; the hospital stay provides a stage for acting out this conflict.
◆ Nursing home placement is indicated but timely arrangements cannot be completed (bed not available, application for Medicaid or other program takes time).

During treatment team meeting, assessment data are reviewed with all team members present and suggestions from all members are considered. Team meetings are held at regular intervals, and all team members involved in the patient's care should attend. A successful treatment team meeting requires that patient assessment data be reviewed before the meeting (Box 10-6). This preparatory review indicates the need for follow-up (e.g., to obtain a urine culture and sensitivity when the admission urinalysis was abnormal) and encourages a holistic look at the patient. Examination of behavior patterns over several days can reveal problems that are not evident on any one day: the patient may be losing weight, constipated, or consistently isolating himself or herself from others. Without a review of such data, opportunities for maximizing therapeutic benefit may be overlooked.

❖ *Nursing Interventions*

Structural

Surveillance
Confused ambulatory patients should be allowed to move about the unit freely. Their safety necessitates ongoing surveillance by staff. Surveillance includes observation and extends to the collection of data about the patient from primary and secondary sources (Dougherty & Molen, 1985). These data may be used as a basis for clinical decision making.

Ongoing surveillance will provide clues to patients' needs in many daily activities. Patients may need assistance at mealtimes, at intervals during the day such as for going to the bathroom, and when they appear uncomfortable. Surveillance by all nursing staff will also help to identify usual behavior and communications patterns, facilitating problem identification. Data obtained by nursing staff in ongoing patient surveillance form the basis for planned and impromptu nursing interventions.

Reality Orientation
A prominently featured reality orientation board in community areas helps to keep patients aware of date and other orienting information. Verbal reality orientation by the nurse may also be helpful: "This is City Hospital, Mrs. Smith." Printed signs identifying the hospital by name in each bedroom and in community areas provides ongoing orientation to place. Clocks and calendars strategically placed throughout the unit also aid in orientation to time.

The use of reality orientation techniques and interventions does not imply that recall of this information is necessarily a goal. A cognitively impaired patient may be distressed at being unable to recall this information. Orienting information should be provided if a situation warrants it or if a patient requests it; it is not something the patient needs to learn and remember.

The use of signs, labels, and pictures to identify areas and their use is also reality orientation. "Bathroom," "clothes closet," and "dining room" are signs that help patients find their way about the unit.

Box 10-6 **Interdisciplinary Treatment Team Meeting**

  I. Evaluation of assessment data
    A. Patient's response to hospitalization reviewed
    B. Medical problems and effect on treatment goals assessed
    C. Laboratory values and other diagnostic test results reviewed, with any necessary follow-up noted
    D. All assessments by treatment team reviewed and problems brought to their attention
    E. Patient's status evaluated for treatment goals and to optimize functioning
       1. Ability to perform personal activities of daily living
       2. Appetite, daily nutritional intake
       3. Weight pattern since admission
       4. Waking and sleeping patterns
       5. Appearance and informal socialization
       6. Continence
       7. Mobility
       8. Skin condition
       9. Use of restraints
    F. Participation in therapeutic activities
    G. Family's involvement in treatment
    H. Discharge plan and status

 II. Individualized treatment planning
    A. Pivotal problems listed on treatment plan
    B. Therapies, interventions, and goals for all clinical problems specified
    C. Responsibility for specific interventions assigned
    D. Evaluation dates for each treatment goal noted on treatment plan

III. Subsequent team meetings
    A. Progress toward goals reviewed
    B. Status of medical problems noted, especially their effect on patient's functioning and on discharge plan
    C. Status of all problems on treatment plan and estimated potential for improvement reviewed
    D. Aftercare plan and discharge plan
    E. Evaluation of patient's status, including any changes since previous meeting and their significance for discharge plan
       1. Nutritional status
       2. Weight compared to admission weight
       3. Appearance, informal socialization
       4. Continence
       5. Mobility
       6. Skin condition
       7. Use of restraints

Consistency

While treatment is based on an individualized plan, the patient's daily schedule should have a certain amount of predictability. Consistent mealtimes are one basis of stability; scheduled activities such as group and movement therapy are another. Daily dressing and grooming, regular vital signs, taking medications, and visiting hours also create a sense of structure in the day. All of these activities, occurring at approximately the same time each day, help to promote a sense of order and predictability.

Systematic, Ongoing Nursing Assessment

While a patient's physical condition is usually stable on admission to a geropsychiatric unit, it may change. Careful, regular physical and mental assessment of the patient is necessary to detect small changes that may indicate clinical problems. Changes in skin color, cardiac irregularities, pain, dizziness, or changes from the previous assessment should be monitored carefully and reported to the patient's physician as indicated. Careful assessment is also necessary to determine whether changes signify altered physical condition, a physiological response to psychotherapeutic medication, or anxiety, to name a few possibilities. Regular assessment is also necessary to determine iatrogenic nursing problems such as constipation, impaction, marginal dehydration, skin breakdown, and functional incontinence. If the patient requires diagnostic tests for which strenuous preparation is necessary (e.g., barium enema), nursing assessment will also be necessary to determine the need for additional rest, rehydration, and nutrition.

Unplanned Nursing Interventions

Any group of patients will be engaged in varying activities at any time. They will be at different stages of hospitalization and have different problems and perceptions of their situations. For their individual needs to be met and reconciled with interdisciplinary treatment goals, unplanned interventions may be necessary as surveillance reveals that a problem is in the making. A one-time intervention may be necessary to avert or solve such problems. These are examples of unplanned interventions:

- ◆ Elicit cooperation for a test or procedure
- ◆ Assist with a phone call to a relative
- ◆ Assess a patient who has fallen
- ◆ Comfort or stay with a patient who is upset or crying
- ◆ Intervene in a conflict between patients
- ◆ Answer the family members' questions
- ◆ Help a patient to put clothes on correctly

Individualized Nursing Interventions

Managing Aggressive Behavior

Severe agitation and verbal or physical aggression in a cognitively impaired patient are managed with a combination of techniques. Reducing external stimuli by placing the patient in a quiet environment, avoidance of comment and requests, and addressing the patient's stated or implied need are initial responses to the behavior. Sclafani (1986) described five levels to manage behavior, beginning with environment planning, then verbal intervention, a team approach, pharmacological intervention, and mechanical restraint.

Reminders and Behavior Shapers

Over time, gentle reminders and requests for responses such as "please" and "thank you" can bring about surprising changes in the patient's behavior. Statements of rules and expectations, given calmly by the nurse, are another way of eliciting appropriate behavior.

Special Protocol

Special interventions such as suicide precautions, neuromuscular malignant syndrome management, and seizure and withdrawal precautions are implemented as needed. Protocols for preventing falls, injuries, and wandering should also be used.

❖ *Other Clinical Issues*

Even though a patient's physical condition was medically stable at the time of admission, a sudden change in condition may require a transfer to a medical unit. This is one reason that careful, ongoing nursing assessment is necessary; subtle physical changes are often detected in nursing assessments. Changes in the patient's condition should be reported to the attending physician and psychiatrist. After transfer to a medical unit the patient may be readmitted to the geropsychiatric unit following medical stabilization if psychiatric treatment goals have not been achieved.

A patient's need for medical or physical treatment need not preclude admission to a geropsychiatric unit. A person requiring oxygen therapy may still participate in therapy if oxygen can be provided; similarly, enteral tube feeding can be continued during treatment for depression. Decisions about admission for patients with such needs are a matter of policy and of nursing assessment of the patient's physical condition. Psychiatric nurses who are accustomed to a general adult clientele sometimes have difficulty in accepting the relatively frail health of the geropsychiatric patient. However, therapy often improves the patient's physical as well as mental health.

The effectiveness of nursing interventions should be assessed on the basis of the patient's response. An intervention that increases agitation or is generally upsetting is clearly not appropriate. Reality orientation is sometimes a problem in this regard. While attempts to orient a patient are generally desirable, these attempts should not be allowed to develop into repetitive correction. It may be more desirable to allow patients to state their perception of reality without comment or with only noncommittal remarks if a response is needed.

Confrontation of the cognitively impaired patient should also be avoided because it is likely to have an adverse effect. Attempts to obtain explicit agreement to take a bath or to engage in other necessary activities should be avoided; instead, a matter-of-fact statement of specific direction may be used: "Come with me, Mr. Barnes."

Physician admission orders should include provision for the information listed in Box 10-7.

Geropsychiatric nurses as well as family members sometimes hear unfeeling and even cruel comments about patients whose appearance or behavior may be upsetting. Often such comments must be understood as an expression of the speaker's own fear of disability or death.

❖ *Evaluation of the Concept*

The Patient's Perspective

Treatment on an inpatient geropsychiatric unit makes mental health care available to persons who otherwise would encounter barriers to such care.

Most inpatient psychiatric units serve a general adult population that is physically healthy and independent in activities of daily living. But the geriatric patient may not be independent in activities of daily living or in robust health, and so may be denied admission even though the mental health problem is appropriate for inpatient care. This is especially likely to be the case if the person is incontinent or in the later stages of dementing illness. The geropsychiatric unit serves older persons who might not otherwise obtain appropriate mental health care.

Box 10-7 **Physician Admission Orders**

Name of admitting psychiatrist or physician and admitting diagnosis
Medical physician to follow patient and condition for which it is requested
Laboratory tests
Imaging and other examinations
Assessments to be performed (usually social services, nutrition, and activities or recreational therapy)
Diet and physical activity
Unit protocols regarding vital signs, weight, lying and standing blood pressure, community meals, and participation in therapeutic activities
Privilege or activity status
Bowel regularity protocol
Medications (listed individually)

If the geriatric patient is admitted to a unit that serves a general adult population, participation in therapeutic activities may be limited because activities are geared to adults whose cognitive, perceptual, and motor skills are stronger. The geriatric patient may have some degree of vision or hearing difficulty and may not have the energy or stamina of younger adults and therefore not participate fully in the program. He or she therefore may miss out on potentially beneficial activities and be reinforced in the belief that he or she cannot keep up with others.

In group psychotherapy the older person may lack the experience or verbal skills to express his or her life stage concerns to the group, may resist attending, or may not be encouraged or required to attend at all. This may be because the staff considers that the older person does not fit in with the others or believes that age makes change or improvement impossible.

In none of these situations is there a conscious intent on anyone's part to provide less than optimal care, but that can be the unintended consequence. Since a geropsychiatric unit is designed for the older patient, these problems are much less likely to occur.

The Physician's Perspective

The physician who follows the patient for concurrent medical management during the hospital stay may find medical management facilitated in several ways. First, treatment team members make informed suggestions to the physician about the patient's functioning; second, medical management may be facilitated by requests or suggestions from the psychiatrist or other team members; third, the family's needs for support are shared; and fourth, discharge planning is provided. Many physicians who follow patients on a geropsychiatric unit develop a strong appreciation for this collaborative approach to care.

The Family Caregiver's Perspective

Family members often realize that the patient's mental status may be related to the number of medications he or she is taking or to his or her multiple medical problems yet be unable to obtain a comprehensive assessment of the patient. In their search for mental health care, family members may encounter ageism, therapeutic nihilism, and ignorance. "He's just getting old" and "there's nothing to be done" are not infrequent responses heard by a concerned family member seeking help for unexplained confusion or forgetfulness. The family often appreciates the holistic and comprehensive approach that characterizes a geropsychiatric unit.

The Hospital's Perspective

A geropsychiatric unit expands the hospital's array of services and becomes a valuable community resource. If the unit operates under an exemption from PPS/DRG guidelines, the hospital's financial position may also be strengthened.

❖ *Quality Management*

The quality management plan should incorporate the varied clinical problems of a geriatric population, psychiatric treatment issues, standards of care, utilization review issues, legal and ethical issues, and the satisfaction of as many of the unit's constituencies as can be reasonably obtained. The quality management plan can provide essential information about care. It must also include action taken to solve identified problems.

Clinical issues include safety of patients, safe medication, and outcomes of care. Appropriateness of admissions as defined in policy, appropriate discharge planning, and length of stay are utilization review issues. A most important aspect of care is the prevention of iatrogenic problems (Gorbien et al., 1992; Steffl & Rowell, 1984). The quality management plan should address the patient's status at discharge in regard to these issues. Iatrogenic problems include mobility deficits, weight loss, dehydration, skin lesions, incontinence, constipation, and impaction.

Legal issues include protection of patients' rights. Consent for admission and informed consent for special procedures require meticulous care and documentation because many patients are confused.

Measures of satisfaction with care and functioning should be developed for as many of the unit's constituencies as possible. At a minimum, evaluations by patients and their family caregivers, by psychiatrists and physicians who admit or follow clients on the unit, and by agencies referring patients for admission should be obtained on a regular and systematic basis.

In addition to geropsychiatric nursing issues, the quality management plan should include indicators used by the hospital's medical-surgical nursing unit for intravenous therapy, enteral feeding, bladder catheter care, and other measures that reflect general quality of care.

Quality indicators are also necessary for interdisciplinary interventions such as social services and recreational or occupational therapy. Depending on the administrative structure, these indicators may be used by a particular department (e.g., social services) or by the unit's nursing manager.

❖ *Resources*

Networking

Because the family is the long-term care provider for so many older adults, family caregivers are the experts on care and therefore an important resource to health care professionals. Networking in the form of membership in advocacy groups such as the Alzheimer's Association can help keep the nurse in touch with family caregivers and their concerns in a situation separate from care.

Networking with others in geropsychiatry and in psychiatric care can provide a feeling for the state of the art as others are developing it. Networking creates helpful relationships and promotes the sharing of useful information. Some possibilities are meetings, telephone conferences, and newsletters. Membership in any part of the *aging network* in a community—persons, agencies, professionals, and institutions that provide services for older people or that have an interest in this age group—is useful.

Educational Resources

The wide array of educational resources includes workshops, books, and audiovisual materials on many aspects of the care of older adults, but resources in geropsychiatric nursing are limited.

❖ *Future Trends and Research Needs*

Projections of population figures indicate that the absolute and relative numbers of the older population will continue to increase until the year 2040 (Longino, Soldo & Manton, 1990). According to Conwall et al. (1989), given the incidence of coexisting medical and psychiatric illness in this population and the resources of acute care hospitals, geropsychiatric care will continue to have an important place there. Other factors that can be expected to influence the continuing growth of geropsychiatric units in acute care hospitals include the trend toward specialized units for the care of older patients, the need to maintain census levels, and reimbursement policies that make such units financially advantageous.

There is a pressing need for research in geropsychiatric nursing because strategies and interventions applicable to the general adult population are often not appropriate for geriatric patients. Additionally, the physical health problems of this population create needs that must be addressed concurrently. Clinical experience will soon demonstrate to the geropsychiatric nurse the inappropriateness of some traditional psychiatric nursing interventions with cognitively impaired patients (e.g., providing information, stating an observation or reality, restatement and reflection). However, verbal techniques deemed untherapeutic in general adult psychiatric nursing (Haber, 1992) sometimes have a very positive effect on these patients. Giving direction or advice, changing the subject, and making stereotypical comments are useful techniques. But the nurse seeking research reports on tested nursing interventions with these patients will have very little success.

Other areas of identified research need are nursing interventions for specific problems such as disruptive behavior and physical problems such as falls, incontinence, and nutrition maintenance. Models and strategies are needed for home care of patients, staff education, reduction of disability in patients, and identification of an appropriate knowledge base for practice (Duffy, Hepburn, Christensen & Brugge-Wiger, 1989).

The effectiveness of interdisciplinary geriatric assessment and consultation programs (Thomas, Brahan, & Haywood, 1993; Cole, Fenton, Engelsmann, & Mansouri, 1991; Carty & Day, 1993) has been reported more frequently than that of geropsychiatric inpatient units (Kujawinski et al., 1993).

Areas of research needed for inpatient units include appropriate kinds of nursing treatment goals, length of stay required to achieve treatment goals, patient and family needs during hospitalization, quality of life issues, and nursing management of combined physical and psychiatric problems.

Research demonstrating the effectiveness of inpatient geropsychiatric units could help to determine the most appropriate strategies for care during hospitalization and provide evidence of positive outcomes. Research data are needed to validate improved cognitive, affective, and functional status, lower morbidity and mortality rates following discharge, cost reduction, improved quality of life for the patient and caregiver, and improved physical health.

❖ *Summary*

Inpatient geropsychiatric units in acute care hospitals have been established in increasingly large numbers since the early 1980s. At first they were called combined medical-psychiatric units. Geriatric patients were admitted for simultaneous treatment of medical and psychiatric problems; coexistence of these problems is characteristic of a geriatric patient population.

The strategic and marketing plans for a geropsychiatric unit must provide for the education of constituencies with an interest in the unit, so that persons with problems appropriate for admission can be identified. These constituencies include medical staff physicians, agencies that serve an older population such as nursing homes and home health agencies, and family caregivers of older adults. A marketing plan contains the means and methods for reaching these constituencies.

A therapeutic environment for geropsychiatric patients is safe, has physical features that facilitate the functioning of sensorially and cognitively impaired patients, and is staffed with nurses and other professionals who understand the patients' needs and who function as members of an interdisciplinary treatment team. Other treatment modalities include psychopharmacology, concurrent medical management of physical health problems, group psychotherapy, recreational therapy, patient and family education, and discharge planning. Treatment planning is focused, intensive, and geared to a hospital stay of approximately 14 days. All therapeutic efforts are directed toward stabilization of symptoms, or pivotal problems. These are the problems that require inpatient treatment; their stabilization makes treatment at a less intensive level possible.

Treatment team members meet regularly to review each patient, to determine interventions for problems, and to assign responsibilities and goals for them. Preparation for team meetings includes review of assessment data and the use of these data to evaluate the patient's progress during the hospital stay.

The hospital stay begins with the orientation or admission stage, in which the patient and family get acquainted with the unit staff and with the program; the patient is assessed and begins therapy. In the middle, or working, stage of hospitalization, pivotal and other problems are identified, the treatment plan and goals are reviewed with the patient and family, the discharge plan is pursued, and the patient continues therapy. In the discharge stage, preparations are made for discharge from the hospital on the day the team determines that maximum progress toward treatment goals has been achieved.

Structural nursing interventions are implemented by the nurse as part of the unit's therapeutic milieu. Surveillance, reality orientation, consistency of routine, and ongoing systematic nursing assessment are structural interventions appropriate in a geropsychiatric unit. Unplanned nursing interventions are done as the need arises. Eliciting a patient's cooperation to complete a test, helping with a personal care need, or responding to an implicit emotional need are examples of unplanned interventions. Individualized nursing interventions are required by a patient to solve a particular clinical problem such as aggression.

The quality management plan reflects the problems of an older patient population, including iatrogenic nursing problems, mental health issues, clinical nursing standards, utilization review issues, patient and family satisfaction with care, and interdisciplinary issues.

Networking with other professionals and with family caregivers in the community is an important resource for the geropsychiatric nurse, as is membership in groups with a special interest in the older population.

Research in geropsychiatric nursing is needed to identify effective nursing interventions, because many of the interventions in psychiatric nursing are not appropriate for the cognitively impaired. Research is also needed in management of behavior problems, home care, staff education, strategies to reduce excess disability in patients, and an appropriate knowledge base for practice. Finally, research is needed to determine the most effective treatment strategies during a brief hospital stay and to validate treatment effectiveness with outcome measurements such as improved functioning, cost effectiveness, and improved quality of life.

❖ References

Abraham, I. L., Fox, J. M., Harrington, D. P., Snustad, D. D., Steiner, D. A., Abraham, L. H., & Brashear, H. R. (1990). A psychogeriatric nursing assessment protocol for use in multidisciplinary practice. *Archives of Psychiatric Nursing, 4*(4), 242-259.

Alessi, C. A., & Cassel, C. K. (1991). Medical evaluation and common medical problems. In J. D. Sadavoy, L. W. Lazarus, and L. F. Jarvik (Eds.). *Comprehensive review of geriatric psychiatry* (pp. 171-195). Washington, DC: American Psychiatric Press.

Baker, N. J. (1985). *Journal of Gerontological Nursing, 11*(7), 21-24.

Barry, P. P., & Moskowitz, M. A. (1988). The diagnosis of reversible dementia in the elderly: A critical review. *Archives of Internal Medicine, 148*(9), 1914-1918.

Carty, A. E. S., & Day, S. S. (1993). Interdisciplinary care: Effect in acute hospital setting. *Journal of Gerontological Nursing, 19*(3), 22-32.

Charatan, F. B. (1989). Practical benefits of music therapy. *Geriatric Consultant, 8*(2), 27-28.

Cole, M. G., Fenton, R. R., Engelsmann, F., & Mansouri, I. (1991). Effectiveness of geriatric psychiatry consultation in an acute care hospital: A randomized trial. *Journal of the American Geriatrics Society, 39*(12), 1183-1188.

Conwall, Y., Nelson, J. D., Kim, K., & Mazure, C. M. (1989). Elderly patients admitted to the psychiatric unit of a general hospital. *Journal of the American Geriatrics Society, 37*(1), 35-41.

Dougherty, C. M., & Molen, M. T. (1985). Surveillance. In G. M. Bulecheck & J. C. McCloskey (Eds.). *Nursing interventions: Treatments for nursing diagnoses* (pp. 301-315). Philadelphia: Saunders.

Duffy, L. M., Hepburn, K., Christensen, R., & Brugge-Wiger, P. (1989). A research agenda in care for patients with Alzheimer's disease. *Image, 21*(4), 254-257.

Gorbien, M. J., Bishop, J., Beers, M. H., Norman, D., Osterweil, D., & Rubenstein, L. Z. (1992). Iatrogenic illness in hospitalized elderly people. *Journal of the American Geriatrics Society, 40*(10), 1031-1042.

Greene, J. A. (1985). Health care for older citizens: Overcoming barriers. *Journal of the Tennessee Medical Association, 78*(5), 289-293.

Greene, J.A., Ingram, T. A., & Johnson, W. (1993). Group psychotherapy for patients with dementia. *Southern Medical Association Journal, 86*(9), 1033-1035.

Haber, J. (1992). Therapeutic communication. In J. Haber, A. Leach, P. Price-Hoskins, & B. F. Sileleau (Eds.). *Comprehensive psychiatric nursing* (4th ed.). St Louis: Mosby.

Kreigh, H. Z., & Perko, J. E. (1983). *Psychiatric and mental health nursing: A commitment to care and concern.* Reston, VA: Reston.

Kujawinski, J., Bigelow, P., Diedrich, D., Kikkebusch, P., Korpan, P., Walkzak, J., Maxson, E., Ropski, S., & Farran, C.J. (1993). Research considerations: Geropsychiatry unit evaluation. *Journal of Gerontological Nursing, 19*(1), 5-10.

Lazarus, L. W. (1976). A program for the elderly at a private psychiatric hospital. *The Gerontologist, 16*(2), 125-131.

Leach, A. M. (1982). Environmental and alternative therapies. In J. Haber, A. M. Leach, S. M. Schudy, & B. F. Sideleau (Eds.). *Comprehensive psychiatric nursing* (2nd ed.) (pp. 377-392). New York: McGraw-Hill.

Longino, C. F., Soldo, B. J., & Manton, K. (1990). Demography of aging in the United States. In K. F. Ferraro (Ed.). *Gerontology: Perspectives and issues* (pp. 19-41). New York: Springer.

Moak, G. S. (1990). Improving quality in psychogeriatric treatment. *Psychiatric Clinics of North America, 13*(1), 99-111.

Nurcombe, B. (1988). Goal-directed treatment planning and the principles of brief hospitalization. *Journal of the American Academy of Child and Adolescent Psychiatry, 28*(1), 26-30.

Paillard, M., & Nowak, K. B. (1985). Use exercise to help older adults. *Journal of Gerontological Nursing, 11*(7), 36-39.

Patterson, C., & LeClair, J. K. (1989). Acute decompensation in dementia: Recognition and management. *Geriatrics, 44*(8), 20-26.

Schultz, J. M., & Dark, S. L. (1982). *Manual of psychiatric nursing care plans.* Boston: Little Brown.

Sclafani, M. (1986). Violence and behavior control. *Journal of Psychosocial Nursing, 24*(11), 8-13.

Silver, I. L., & Herrmann, N. (1991). History and mental status examination. In J. Sadavoy, L. W. Lazarus, & L. F. Jarvik, (Eds.). *Comprehensive review of geriatric psychiatry* (pp. 149-169). Washington, DC: American Psychiatric Press.

Steffl, B. M., & Rowell, G. (1984). Unintentional injury and immobility: Hazards and risks in old age. In B. M. Steffl, *Handbook of gerontological nursing* (pp. 481-497). New York: Van Nostrand Reinhold.

Stoudemire, A., & Fogel, B. S. (1986). Organization and development of combined medical-psychiatric units: 1. *Psychosomatics, 27*(5), 341-345.

Strasen, L. (1987). *Key business skills for nurse managers.* Philadelphia: Lippincott.

Teri, L., & Logsdon, R. G. (1991). Identifying pleasant activities for Alzheimer's disease patients: The pleasant events schedule-ad. *The Gerontologist, 31*(1), 124-127.

Thomas, D. R., Brahan, R., & Haywood, B. P. (1993). Inpatient community-based geriatric assessment reduces subsequent mortality. *Journal of the American Geriatrics Society, 41*(2), 101-104.

Turner, S. O. (1990). Dealing with medical staff: It's time to do it differently! *Nursing Management, 21*(2), 52-53.

Wilson, C. C., & Netting, F. E. (1983). Companion animals and the elderly: A state-of-the-art summary. *Journal of the Veterinary Medical Association, 183*(12), 1425-1428.

Young, R. C., & Meyers, B. S. (1991). Psychopharmacology. In J. Sadavoy, L. W. Lazarus, & L. F. Jarvick (Eds.). *Comprehensive review of geriatric psychiatry* (pp. 435-467). Washington, DC: American Psychiatric Press.

Chapter *11*

❖ *Mental and Behavioral Problems in the Nursing Home*

Mildred O. Hogstel

The mental and behavioral problems of nursing home residents have received limited systematic assessment and nursing intervention. However, these problems cause major concerns for nursing home staff, other residents, and often residents' families. Sometimes the behaviors are so dangerous that they are a physical threat to the residents themselves, to other residents, and to nursing home staff.

There are many causes of behavioral problems in older adults in the nursing home setting. The cause may be physiological, such as a neurological disorder, or the problem may be a continuation of a lifelong mental or emotional problem. For example, some people diagnosed as having schizophrenia in young adulthood are now being cared for in nursing homes as they become older and are unable to cope with their physical and mental problems. Regardless of the medical diagnosis, however, many behavioral problems of residents in nursing homes may be caused by maladaptation to the aging process or maladaptation to the institutional (nursing home) environment. Severe depression, confusion, or anger often occurs when an older person has difficulty adapting to the increasing physical limitations of old age or adapting to the loss of home, personal freedom, and possessions when relocating to a nursing home. This anger, depression, or both can result in multiple behavioral problems. One blind 84-year-old woman who had been in a nursing home for about 1 month exhibited several behavioral problems. She was severely agitated, crying, and screaming. After the nurse talked with her for a while, she said that she "had a new home, a new doctor, no telephone, and no friends." It must be particularly difficult for a blind person, who was very accustomed to one environment, to be placed in such a situation.

Research on relocation of older adults during the 1950s found that moving an older person from one environment to another increased the emotional stress for that person. Research in the 1960s proposed that relocation could increase the incidence of death. Research in the 1970s showed that dissatisfaction was more prevalent than death and that the person's response was based on control of events (for example, if there was a better orientation to the new environment, there was less chance for a decrease in mental status). In a study of adjustment to the nursing home, Brooke (1989) identified the first phase (6-8 weeks) as the most difficult with residents expressing death wishes and fears of insanity.

Changes in the health care delivery system in the 1980s and 1990s have increased movement for older adults (from home to hospital for short stays to a nursing home and sometimes back home again), which causes increasing problems of adaptation. A stable, supportive environment is important to the well-being of most older adults, especially those who become increasingly dependent. When older people are moved several times in a few weeks, adapting to a new environment can be difficult and cause behavioral problems if specific interventions to help them adapt to the new environment are not implemented.

Because nursing staff care for residents 24 hours a day year after year and physicians only see the residents at intervals, nurses in nursing homes have a unique responsibility and challenge to assess the mental and behavioral problems of each resident and implement appropriate nursing interventions. Therefore the nursing home staff should carefully assess reasons for the behavioral problems of their residents and implement creative, effective, and safe nursing interventions.

However, nurse aides, who give most of the bedside nursing care, do not have the education to understand the complex psychological and disruptive behavior of the residents (Smith, Buckwalter, & Albunese, 1990). In some instances they have responded to a resident's anger, hostility, and aggressive behavior with their own aggressive behavior, resulting in physical or psychological abuse of the resident.

❖ Prevalence of Mental and Behavioral Problems

Research on the mental and behavioral problems of nursing home residents is very recent. Kane (1986) noted that "the prevalence of depressed affect, anxiety, rage and withdrawal is high among nursing home residents" (p. 237).

When discussing innovations in nursing home care, Levenson (1987) stated that nursing homes in the future will broaden their services to include increased availability of psychiatric services. He noted that "the proportion of surviving elderly with some degree of mental impairment is increasing markedly, and many of these people are winding up in nursing homes" (p. 77). He also reported that increasing numbers of nursing home residents are having "cognitive, emotional, or behavioral dysfunctions, such as agitation, aggression, wandering, depression, or withdrawal . . . causing some management or treatment problems" (p. 74).

Lucas, Steele, and Bognanni (1986) reported that abnormal behaviors "most often complained about by nursing home personnel . . . include wandering and pacing, abnormalities of eating and sleeping, incontinence and uncooperativeness, irritability, and violence" (p. 14). They also noted that the nurse must determine the exact behavior in order to decide on the right intervention, based on the underlying cause. For example, pacing may be a sign of agitation or depression, whereas wandering may simply be an attempt to go home (p. 14). They also noted that continuing in-service education for all nursing home staff on the care of the mentally ill is essential (p. 15).

Data from the 1987 National Medical Expenditure Survey conducted by the United States Department of Health and Human Services, Division of Medical Expenditures (Mental Health Status, 1993) showed that 68% of all nursing home residents had one or more psychiatric symptoms, including dullness, withdrawal, impatience, delusions, and hallucinations" (p. 46). Some 65% had at least one symptom of depression, and about 30% had psychotic symptoms. Women were likelier to have multiple psychiatric symptoms than men, but men exhibited more behavioral problems than women. The most common behavioral problems were "getting upset or yelling (31%), followed by wandering (11%) and physically hurting others (11%)" (p. 46).

Burgio, Jones, Butler, and Engel (1988) defined a behavior problem as a "diverse array of patient responses which are considered noxious to staff, other patients, or the patient himself" (p. 31). They also noted that "few data are available that delineate the prevalence of behavior problems in nursing homes." These authors studied the behavior problems of 160 residents in one nursing home. Although they primarily studied physical problems such as mobility, incontinence, and dressing, "an unexpected finding was the high number of aberrant and acting-out behaviors such as physical aggression" (p. 32). Of the residents in their study, 25% had aberrant and acting-out behaviors, 25% demonstrated verbal abuse, and 20% displayed physical aggression (p. 33).

When nursing home staff are not able to care effectively for residents with major disruptive or violent behavior, the residents are often sent by ambulance to a nearby hospital (Tierney, Cronin, & Scanlon, 1986), where their behavior may worsen because of the change in the environment (often in the middle of the night), and where even the hospital staff may lack the knowledge or experience to care for a geropsychiatric patient without further referral and/or consultation.

❖ *Categories of Mental Health and Behavioral Problems*

The most common types of mental and behavioral problems among nursing home residents are (1) depression; (2) confusion and disorientation; (3) disruptive behaviors including physical, verbal, and sexual aggression; and (4) paranoid behaviors. Depression is probably the most common. However, it is less obvious to the staff and less disruptive to the facility than wandering and aggression. Symptoms of depression should not be overlooked, because much depression can be treated or prevented with specific nursing interventions.

Depression

Depression is the most common functional mental disorder among older adults. Nursing home residents are more prone to depression than other older adults in the community. Chronic physical problems that require institutionalization cause increasing dependence on others as well as feelings of helplessness, hopelessness, loss of control, and decreased feelings of self-esteem and self-worth.

Eisdorfer (1988) has estimated that 70% to 80% of nursing home residents have some symptoms of depression. However, the specific prevalence and causes of depression among nursing home residents have not been extensively studied. Also, most depressed older people in nursing homes do not have the benefit of specific mental assessment, diagnosis, treatment, or support by mental health professionals.

In one study of 708 subjects living in nursing homes and congregate apartments for older adults, 12% were classified with major depression and an additional 30% had marked depressive symptoms (Parmelee, Katz, & Lawton, 1989). These researchers also found that newly admitted residents were more likely to have symptoms of major depression than long-term residents, who were more likely to have cognitive defects and minor depression (p. M27). An important implication of these findings is that major depression of newly admitted residents may be reversible if there are "both administrative and professional vigilance to opportunities for support, counseling, or psychiatric treatment early in the period of tenure" (p. M28).

Withdrawal

Withdrawal is most common in residents who are depressed or who have given up because of their physical condition or what they perceive as a depressing environment. One older resident would lie in bed all day with his face turned toward the wall. He would not eat, take medications, or talk to anyone. He was losing weight and becoming weaker every day. A nurse on the psychiatric evaluation team discovered that he was depressed because he had been moved from a nursing home in a small community where he knew everyone and participated in all home activities to a nursing home in a large city. There was a relative in the same home to which he moved, but after he moved, the relative had a stroke and was no longer able to communicate with him. The resident who was severely depressed was admitted to a psychiatric hospital for a short stay. During hospitalization his anger was reduced and his general condition improved enough for him to be discharged. He was transferred to a different nursing home in a smaller community near some relatives and adjusted well to the new environment.

Too often withdrawal or depression is not assessed early enough in the nursing home setting. Hospitalization may be prevented if the nurse can assess the cause early. Careful placement of residents (an active mobile resident should not be placed in the same room with a completely helpless, aphasic, immobile resident), group therapy or reminiscence therapy led by a professional staff member and effective communication skills used by all staff members can help prevent reactive (environmental) depression in the nursing home resident.

Confusion and Disorientation

Many older persons are admitted to a nursing home because they can no longer function independently because of severe cognitive decline, for example, dementia of the Alzheimer's type. They display various degrees of confusion and disorientation.

There are many physical and mental causes for confusion (see Chapter 7). If the resident was beginning to be confused at home before admission, confusion will be more severe soon after relocation. One of the concerns is wandering.

Wandering

Wandering in nursing homes is common in cognitively impaired older residents. Staff fear that they will fall, injure themselves, or leave the facility and get lost or be injured. Since the implementation of the Omnibus Budget Reconciliation Act (OBRA) of 1987, residents may not be physically or chemically restrained because of wandering. Recent studies by Algase (1992) and others have attempted to describe the pattern of wandering, describing cycles and patterns over time.

According to Algase (1992), possible causes of wandering among the cognitively impaired are as follows:

- ◆ "A substitute for social interaction" (p. 31)
- ◆ "An indicator of worsening cognitive impairment" (p. 31)
- ◆ "An expression of agitation" (p. 32)

Other causes are overstimulation or understimulation of the senses by the environment, communication, or activities (Davidhizar & Cosgray, 1990). Loneliness, agitation, depression, confusion, and disorientation are also common causes.

It is important to assess the individual's reason for wandering so that interventions can be initiated, especially if the wandering is unsafe. Most interventions so far have focused on preventing residents from leaving the facility by the use of such electronic monitoring devices as neck, wrist, and ankle guards (Wandering Devices, 1992). Door alarms, video cameras, and other electronic devices also can be used. Other structural methods distort the floor, door, or doorknob so that residents do not go near the door or try to open it. Safe outdoor areas, which also provide fresh air and sunshine, are excellent. All of these methods are better than using physical or chemical restraints. However, the best approach is to determine the individual's pattern and cause of wandering and plan interventions accordingly (e.g., increase social contact, focus on orienting strategies, or decrease agitation) (Algase, 1992).

Other environmental and personal nursing interventions should also be used if safe wandering is not possible (Box 11-1).

Box 11-1 **How to Stop Wandering**

- Let patients look out a window to keep track of the seasons and time of day.
- Frequently repeat the name of the resident, names of staff, and locations of places in the health care facility. Wear an extra-large name tag and introduce yourself every time you encounter the patient.
- Make sure the residents have eye-glasses and hearing aids if they need them.
- Decorate residents' rooms with their favorite pictures, books, or quilts to give a sense of comfort and familiarity.
- Encourage visits by family members and friends.
- Provide continuity with the same staff, the same room assignment, and the same furnishings in the room.
- Convey warmth and reassurance through your physical presence. Communicate with a confused patient by speaking in a low tone of voice, using simple short words and brief phrases. Touch is reassuring and communicates warmth when words are not understood. Repeating words of reassurance and directions will have a calming effect on the patient.
- Avoid physical restraint unless absolutely necessary.
- Don't expect the resident to be able to interact with a large group of people for a long period of time.
- Involve residents in a variety of short-term, structured activities to reduce their anxiety and help them feel they are spending their time in a meaningful way.
- Allow time and opportunity to explore new areas and do a variety of things.
- Encourage all verbal and nonverbal forms of expression.
- Organize exercises, such as taking a long, vigorous walk each day. Even circular walks can be useful. Rocking chairs can provide a form of exercise too, and group exercise can provide social benefits as well as a method to use up excess energy.
- Place clocks and calendars in various spots around the facility.
- Allow residents some control over aspects of their environment, such as selecting activities or items of food.

From Davidhizar, R., & Cosgray, R. (1990). Helping the wanderer. *Geriatric Nursing, 11*(6), 281; with permission.

Aggression and Disruption

Aggression by nursing home residents is underreported and poorly documented, possibly because it is expected by nursing staff or they do not believe anything can be done about it. Beck, Robinson, and Baldwin (1992) stressed that aggressive behavior of nursing home residents should be systematically observed, reported, and documented "to develop adequate preventive measures and interventions for aggressive residents" (p. 23).

Many behaviors are caused by maladaptation to the environment or the aging process. If certain basic physiological needs are not met (e.g., preferred foods or relief of pain), anger and hostility can occur. Loss of personal control, either because of the more restricted environment of the nursing home setting or because of decreasing mobility, can cause feelings of decreased self-worth. Infantilization (being fed, being incontinent, or called Honey) causes the resident to lose self-respect and dignity. Some residents strike out at the caregiver in anger and frustration, especially if the caregiver does not treat the resident with dignity or demonstrate a caring attitude and approach.

Aggressive and violent behaviors are common reasons for requesting a psychiatric evaluation of nursing home residents (Box 11-2). Some nurse aides have been hit and kicked, causing them to need time off work. Other aides terminate employment because of their inability to cope with such behaviors. One man in one nursing home would not let anyone bathe him, so he did not have a bath for 4 weeks, which became a problem when the state licensing team arrived. One 85-year-old woman would attempt to hit anyone who approached her. Another nursing home resident would hit out at her daughter when she visited.

Beck et al. (1992) reported on a study of aggressive behavior of residents age 65 and older in a long-term geriatric unit of a hospital. Most of the aggressive behavior occurred in the bathroom (49%) and in the morning (86%) and was reported primarily by licensed practical nurses (41%). It is interesting that "55.1% of the aggressive residents did not have any visitors" (p. 22). The types of aggressive behavior reported were physical (57%), verbal (47%), and sexual (2%).

Constant yelling, day and night, is another type of disruptive behavior in nursing homes. If pain and physical discomfort have been ruled out as the primary cause of the behavior (most likely), it is usually due to organic brain changes rather than a psychiatric problem. This behavior is very tiring for the resident and very trying for the staff because of its constancy. Kikuta (1991) described a case study of a cognitively impaired 74-year-old man who yelled night and day, sleeping only a few hours at night. He was restrained because of wandering and unsteady gait and given several psychotropic medications. However, the yelling continued. A 2-month stay in a psychiatric hospital for assessment and medications did not produce much improvement.

Behavioral analysis was used to determine specifically what conditions increased his yelling (for example, when restrained in a chair or bed). "[This type of] analysis assists caregivers in identifying, modifying, and developing practical means to alleviate and monitor a problem" (Kikuta, 1991, p. 7). A companion was made

---

Box 11-2 **Common Disruptive Behavioral Problems among Nursing Home Residents**

- Refusing to eat
- Refusing medications or treatments
- Attempting to eat objects other than food (pica)
- Pacing the halls day and night
- Entering other residents' rooms without reason
- Stealing
- Climbing over bed rails
- Leaving without the knowledge of staff
- Destroying property
- Crying loudly
- Screaming
- Swearing and using foul and abusive language
- Threatening to hit or kick others
- Attempting to hit or kick others
- Hitting or kicking others
- Throwing objects at another person
- Spitting on another person, on walls, drapes, floor, etc.
- Biting
- Removing clothes in an inappropriate place
- Urinating or defecating in an inappropriate place
- Fecal smearing
- Sexual advances to others (for example, fondling other residents or sexual advances to staff)

---

available to walk with him 6 hours a day, 6 days a week. He sat down when he was tired, seemed less restless, and slept 9 hours at night. Change in the environment, reduced dosages of selected medications, and individualized nursing care (for example, two persons gave the nursing care so that it could be completed more quickly and he could walk sooner) produced results. He became more relaxed, more alert, smiled more, and listened to music on occasion. The resident confined to bed who yells constantly can be similarly analyzed. There is usually a specific cause for yelling, although it may be difficult to determine at times.

Hoarding is sometimes considered disruptive by nursing home staff. A resident may have her bedside table, bed, and floor near her bed stacked with boxes of mementos or clothing and paper sacks full of odds and ends. This kind of behavior may be an adaptive and harmless means of control over a few personal possessions when there have been many recent losses, or it may be a symptom of a mental illness that needs complete assessment and possible treatment (Hogstel, 1993).

Paranoid Behavior

Paranoid behaviors are common, although not normal, with increasing age. See Chapter 8 for a discussion of paraphrenia. The nurse should recognize that the residents really believe that others are stealing from them or trying to poison them. It is difficult to convince them otherwise. Although nursing home residents are not likely to have lethal weapons (such as a gun), they can use a walking stick, walker, furniture, or their hands to harm another resident or staff member. One nursing home resident who suddenly began having delusions and hallucinations, most likely because of a new medication dosage, cut her restraints and threw her walker through the window on the other side of the room. The 90-year-old resident in the bed near the window was very frightened but not hurt.

Buckwalter (1992) has observed that "persons who have both impaired sight and hearing may experience both phantom sounds and vision" (p. 46). These experiences are often labeled as hallucinations or delusions by nursing home staff although the person is not mentally ill. This process was described by Melzack (1992), who noted that phantom seeing and hearing occur in the brain as a result of decreased sensory stimuli. He concluded that this phenomenon is similar to phantom limb sensations following a leg amputation. These experiences probably cause more concern to staff than resident, and the resident should not be treated with antipsychotic medications if there are no other indications of mental illness (Buckwalter, 1992).

❖ Nursing Process

Assessment

A thorough assessment on admission to the nursing home is essential. It should include not only a complete physical assessment but also a psychosocial, functional, and mental status assessment. The initial assessment should be performed by a registered professional nurse. Too often the admission data are very brief and are limited primarily to obvious physical findings (e.g., skin lesions and prostheses) or functional assessment (e.g., ability to communicate and walk). A specific mental assessment tool should be selected and used routinely for each newly admitted resident. Many of these tools are simple and easy to use (see Chapter 4 and the appendixes).

An initial mental status assessment is essential because it (1) helps the staff in the preparation of the written plan of care; (2) provides baseline data for comparison purposes if and when the resident begins to exhibit mental or behavioral changes; (3) assists the physician in diagnosis and treatment when cognitive changes occur, thus helping to determine if the changes are temporary, reversible and treatable, or irreversible; (4) provides data for legal purposes (e.g., ability of the resident to manage his or her own resources or demonstrate the possible need for a legal guardian); (5) provides ideas for topics for staff development; and (6) provides data for research on the mental health and behavioral problems of nursing home residents.

The same mental status assessment tool should be used routinely for each resident, every few weeks if possible or whenever a resident exhibits a sudden change in mental status or intellectual functioning. Sudden changes in cognitive function should be carefully evaluated, because the cause may be physiological, reversible, and easily treated (e.g., infection, fluid and electrolyte imbalance, cardiac changes). See Chapter 7 for a detailed discussion of physical factors that can affect mental status. Behavioral problems caused by maladaptation to the nursing home environment may occur for weeks or months after admission (Brooke, 1989). Regular assessment of mental status may help to detect problems before they become severe.

Problems

Unfortunately, too often some nursing home staff and family members consider memory loss and disorientation a normal part of the aging process. Therefore when these or similar problems occur, they are not likely to seek evaluation and assistance. It is important that staff and family members realize that, although people of all ages forget sometimes, major memory loss, forgetfulness, and wandering are not part of the normal aging process. Normal mental capacity and functioning should continue well into the late 80s, 90s, and 100s until terminal decline, which probably occurs a few years before death (Riegel & Riegel, 1972).

Another problem that occurs is the older person's hesitancy to seek or accept mental health assessment or treatment because of possible stigmas from the past about psychiatric care (Buckwalter, 1985). One 87-year-old woman was seeing a geriatric psychiatrist for depression, but she did not want her friends to know that she was seeing a psychiatrist. The nurse can counteract this fear by helping clients to understand that they can benefit from medication or other types of psychiatric therapy.

Most nursing home residents are cooperative and willing to participate in the assessment process. Those who are severely confused and disoriented, paranoid, or hostile and aggressive are more difficult to assess. The nurse should be prepared for combative, hostile, aggressive behavior while assessing some clients. The initial approach of the nurse is very important. Remaining calm, accepting the resident's anger and hostility, being realistic and patient, and simply listening attentively will often change a very hostile and angry person into one who begins to open up and talk about problems and real feelings. These skills are essential for the nurse who assesses and plans the care for such residents. Nurse aides and technical nurses often are afraid to care for aggressive, hostile, combative residents. The residents sense their fear and take advantage of it by continuing their aggressiveness and hostility.

Psychiatric Assessment

Most physicians in general and psychiatrists in particular have not spent much time seeing residents in nursing homes, probably because of the extra time it requires to travel to different homes, the limited financial remuneration provided by visits, or a lack of general interest in the field of geriatrics.

Some psychiatric hospitals and geropsychiatric programs in general hospitals provide free psychiatric screening and evaluation by registered nurses prepared in psychiatry and mental health and gerontological nursing to nursing home residents in the community. In most instances the need for evaluation is brought to the attention of the hospital geriatric social worker by the director of nurses after receiving (sometimes requesting) an order from the attending physician. In some situations the family requests the psychiatric evaluation, and the physician usually agrees. The geriatric social worker at the hospital may briefly screen the request and refer the information to the nurses who do the initial screening assessment. Arrangements are made with the director of nurses to visit the nursing home resident within the next few days. However, if the resident requires immediate evaluation and treatment, he or she is admitted to the hospital as soon as possible; the social worker arranges for a staff psychiatrist to evaluate and care for the resident. If the resident has an alcohol problem, a staff member of the chemical dependency program visits the resident as soon as possible.

The assessment in the nursing home should consist of the following: (1) obtaining detailed information about the resident's behavior from the director of nursing or charge nurse on the unit where the resident is a patient; (2) reviewing the medical record (chart) for pertinent information in the history and physical examination, information about current prescribed medications, and nurses' notes for details of recent behavior of the resident; and (3) observing, interviewing, and performing a mental status assessment of the resident. See Appendix C for a sample guide for the screening assessment. The interview basically is nonstructured and varies according to the resident's behavior, condition, and needs.

A report (see Appendix C) should be written after the evaluation. The staff psychiatrist will decide whether to see the resident personally (by going to the nursing home or requesting that the family bring the resident to his office if possible), to suggest that the attending physician make changes in medication or dosage of medication, or to admit the resident to the hospital for further evaluation and treatment.

In some instances the family does not want the resident hospitalized even though it is recommended by the psychiatrist. Sometimes this presents a problem because the nursing home can no longer care for a resident who is a threat to other residents. The family then has to decide whether to find another placement for the resident or agree to hospitalization. If the resident does not agree to hospitalization and the family agrees that further evaluation and treatment is necessary (e.g., physical threats to self or others), the local mental health and mental retardation services are notified to help the family obtain a warrant for involuntary admission to the hospital for further evaluation, treatment, and care.

Planning

Planning to care for nursing home residents with mental and behavior problems involves teaching the staff how to care for these residents and how to use community programs and resources.

Staff Development

Because of the numbers of residents with mental and behavioral problems in nursing homes, the nursing staff should learn to recognize their special mental health needs and implement specific nursing interventions. Too often in-service education for all staff and on-the-job training for ancillary staff have centered on observation and care of the physical needs of residents. Although meeting the basic physical needs of residents is essential, the specific psychosocial and mental aspects of nursing care often have been neglected.

Table 11-1 lists examples of topics for staff development that relate to the psychosocial and mental health needs of nursing home residents. As previously mentioned, the nurse should perform a thorough assessment of each resident on

Table 11-1   Suggested Topics for Staff Development Related to the Psychosocial and Mental Health Needs of Nursing Home Residents

Category of personnel	*Suggested topics*

Professional staff
Administrators
Nurses (directors and supervisors)
Social workers
	Assessment
	  Psychosocial
	  Mental status
	  Family
	Group therapy and support
	  Resident (e.g., reminiscence and life review)
	  Family
	Community resources
	  Mental health and mental retardation
	    services
	  Geriatric psychiatrists
	  Geriatric psychiatry units in local hospitals

Other staff Staff registered nurses Licensed practical nurses Activity directors	Psychotropic medications Use of chemical and physical restraints Short mental status assessment tests

All staff
(including nurse aides)
	Developmental tasks of aging
	Sociological theories of aging
	Communication skills
	Sexuality in older adults
	Cognitive disorders (e.g., Alzheimer's
	  disease)
	Nursing interventions (see Table 11-2)
	  Depression
	  Confusion and disorientation
	  Aggressive and disruptive behaviors
	  Paranoid behaviors
	Caregiver support (individual and group
	  sessions)

admission. Assistance may be needed to obtain and learn the use of various types of assessment tools, especially mental status assessment instruments.

Nurses and social workers may need assistance in starting small group therapy sessions such as reminiscence therapy. Group sessions also are helpful for older residents who are moderately depressed. Staff may need assistance in learning to be group leaders or facilitators in such groups. Professional staff may also need assistance in starting and leading family support sessions. Family members often become quite upset and distressed when they see their aging parent or grandparent exhibiting behavior that is highly unusual and unacceptable. A dear, gentle grandmother may suddenly start cursing or striking out at personnel or family members whom she no longer recognizes. The nursing home can provide group sessions for interested family members so that they can not only share their frustrations and feelings, but also gain objective information about the older family member's condition and prognosis. A professional staff member or geropsychiatric nurse consultant who has had preparation and experience leading such a support group is needed. The primary focus of such group sessions should be education and support (Drysdale, Nelson, & Wineman, 1993).

Families also often need assistance in knowing what to do about the possessions and financial affairs of a resident who is becoming increasingly confused or disoriented. A professional member of the staff should know how to answer the questions of families regarding power of attorney and legal guardianship. If the resident becomes severely violent and abusive, with the danger of causing harm to self or others, commitment to a psychiatric hospital for evaluation and treatment may be necessary. If such is the case, the family may need guidance to learn how to arrange for such assistance.

The professional staff should become aware of all available resources in the community for older adults, particularly resources that might be needed for residents with mental and behavioral problems. Directors of nursing should know the names and addresses of geriatric psychiatrists in the community or psychiatrists who have a special interest in geriatric clients. An aging specialist who works for the local mental health and mental retardation services or mental health association may be a good source of information about mental health resources for older clients in the community.

Community Programs

Professional staff in the nursing home should become aware of and use resources in the community, not only for staff development, but also for services and programs for their residents. If there is a medical school or university in the community, psychiatrists, mental health and gerontological nurses, and other gerontologists can be asked to provide education for staff or act as consultants to the home.

Often the local mental health association or area agency on aging will provide speakers or consultants at no or low cost as a service to the community because they are funded by the United Way. In one community, the mental health association provides a Friendly Visitor program in which they train volunteers to visit nursing home residents who are lonely, withdrawn, depressed, or have no family or visitors. The staff of the nursing home contacts the aging specialist at the mental health association, which makes the arrangements. See Chapter 13 for other community resources that can be used in a nursing home setting.

Some psychiatric hospitals and geropsychiatric programs in general hospitals have developed comprehensive geriatric services that provide initial assessment in the community, the services of geriatric social workers, physician referral, complete inpatient evaluation, treatment and care, follow-up care, family therapy for those with mentally ill older relatives, and in-service education on mental health issues for staff in retirement centers and nursing homes. Most residents and their families cannot afford this type of care in addition to the other expenses of long-term care. There is a need for a mobile outreach service composed of a team of geriatric psychiatrists, geropsychiatric nurses, geriatric social workers, and other geriatric mental health workers not only to assess but also to initiate and provide medical supervision, group, and individual psychotherapy to nursing home residents who would benefit from such a service. There is a great need for more mental health care in the nursing home setting.

Some nursing home residents with mental and behavior problems are not appropriate for placement in psychiatric hospitals because most of these hospitals do not have the number or type of staff to care for patients who also have major physical problems, such as partial immobility and incontinence. However, many general acute care hospitals have also instituted geropsychiatric units to meet the mental and physical needs of older persons with mental and behavior disorders (see Chapter 10). Nursing home residents with mental health problems may be referred to one of these facilities for specific diagnosis, treatment, and care.

Nursing Diagnoses and Nursing Interventions

The 1992 list of nursing diagnoses (NANDA) may be found in Appendix F. The NANDA nursing diagnoses most common to older nursing home residents with mental and behavioral problems, along with contributing factors, defining characteristics, and specific nursing interventions, are listed in Table 11-2. These diagnoses and interventions have been grouped according to the most common problems observed in nursing home residents:

1. Depression
2. Confusion and disorientation
3. Aggressive and disruptive behaviors
4. Paranoid behavior

Additional Nursing Interventions

Aggressive behavior of nursing home residents with severe confusion and disorientation used to be controlled "as much as possible with physical restraints or

Table 11-2 Most Common Nursing Diagnoses, Contributing factors, Defining characteristics, and Nursing interventions for Nursing Home Residents with Mental and Behavioral Problems

Nursing diagnoses (NANDA)	Contributing factors	Defining characteristics	Nursing interventions
Category A: Depression Social interaction, impaired Social isolation Powerlessness Hopelessness Self-care deficit Self-esteem disturbance Grieving, dysfunctional Coping, ineffective individual Activity intolerance Nutrition, altered: less than body requirements Sleep pattern disturbance Relocation stress syndrome Constipation Self-mutilation, high risk for	Major depressive disorder (DSM-IV) Loss of home, work, income, friends, family, possessions Cognitive impairment Social isolation Infection Pain Medications Increasing dependency Multiple chronic illnesses	**Subjective:** Quiet Crying Expresses feelings of loneliness, low self-esteem, hopelessness, helplessness, being unloved, unlovable, abandoned, sad, vulnerable, alienated Suicidal ideation **Objective:** Does not want to bathe, shave, eat, or dress Withdraws from social contacts, friends, daily routines Cannot sleep or sleeps too much Stays in bed 24 hours a day Constipation Headache	Offer presence quietly Use gentle touch if appropriate Initiate and expect verbal communication Do not be too talkative or too cheerful Give positive sincere responses Suggest to the activities director that a special friend from the community be assigned to the resident Observe closely and validate for suicidal tendencies (especially men in their 80s) Determine interests and encourage methods of individual stimulation Encourage participation in support and activity groups (for example, reminiscence groups and exercise) Encourage resident to focus on current activities rather than ruminate or socially withdraw Reduce tendency of staff to withdraw from the resident Allow ventilation of anger Provide a safe environment to discuss fears of rejection and retaliation

Category B: Confusion and disorientation

Nursing diagnoses	Related factors	Signs and symptoms	Interventions
Thought processes, altered	Delirium	**Subjective:**	Use reality orientation or validation techniques
Adjustment, impaired	Dementia	Express feelings of loneliness, fearfulness, hopelessness	Use resident's last name consistently
Sensory/perceptual alterations	Amnestic disorders	Bored	Have realistic expectations and conversation
Communication, impaired verbal	Other cognitive disorders (DSM-IV)	Confused	Provide adequate foods and fluids
Sleep pattern disturbance	Brain and nerve disorders	Misses family and home	Reduce number of medications, especially hypnotics and sedatives, if possible
Self-care deficit: feeding, bathing/hygiene, dressing/grooming, toileting	Medications	Wants to go home	Regulate lights, especially at dusk and dawn, and provide window to show diurnal variation
Unilateral neglect	Infection	Looking for something to do	Ask the family to provide a videotape of family members to show to resident when they cannot visit often
Anxiety	Malnutrition	**Objective:**	Provide for proper functioning of eyeglasses and hearing aids
Fear	Dehydration	Not oriented to person, place or time	Provide for personal familiar objects in room (for example, pictures of family and label with names)
Injury, high risk for	Sensory deprivation or overload	Wanders, especially at night	Assign same personnel as much as possble
		Short attention span	Keep consistent schedule of activities
		Recent memory loss	Convey reassurance, warmth, safety, security
		Seeking a lighted area	Encourage verbal expression of feelings and needs
		Attempts to leave the home	If wandering occurs: Observe closely at a distance; assign a buddy (if another resident is willing) to watch the resident who wanders; use I. D. bracelets around arm or neck; notify close neighbors, business, police, and the postal carrier of possible wanderers; use magnetic device on clothes that will set off an alarm when going out a door; have alarms on all doors not constantly visible; use a one-to-one approach, talk and walk back to room
		Cries out	

Continued.

Table 11-2 Most Common Nursing Diagnoses, Contributing factors, Defining characteristics, and Nursing interventions for Nursing Home Residents with Mental and Behavioral Problems—cont'd

Nursing diagnoses (NANDA)	Contributing factors	Defining characteristics	Nursing interventions
Category C: Aggressive and disruptive behaviors			
Injury, high risk for	Dementia	**Subjective:**	Intervene when hyperactivity starts, divert to other activities (for example, food, music, walking)
Protection, altered	Delirium (DSM-IV)	Expressing feelings of anger, frustration, anxiety, hostility, loneliness, fear, helplessness, powerlessness, loss of control	Listen and be supportive; do not threaten verbally or physically
Violence, high risk for: directed at self/others	Fear of being dependent, being hurt physically, pain, dying		Give space; do not crowd
Adjustment, impaired	Unintended verbal or physical action by caregivers (for example, loud voice or removing clothing for bath without explaining to the resident)		Accept hostility; build trust
Coping, defensive		**Objective:**	Speak with a low, soothing, slow, calm voice using simple, concise, clear terms; do not argue
Fear		Agitated, argumentive, swearing	Reflect resident's underlying feelings or covert messages; that is, "It must be very frustrating being dependent on people you do not know for everything you need."
Powerlessness	Pain	Hits or threatens to hit others	Lower lights, turn off TV, reduce stimuli
Anxiety	Lack of contact with reality	Throws objects at others	Be gentle
	Clothes too tight, too warm, skin irritations	Removes clothes and bed linens	Work slowly, do not humiliate
		Urinates or defecates in an inappropriate place	Do not show defensiveness, anger, or hostility in return; show that you are in control, be direct and frank, kind but firm
			Determine what causes hostility and aggressive action so that the situation can be altered
			Do not use restraints unless absolutely necessary; if so get help (other staff or family)

		Use pillow or blanket around your arm if needed for protection; use distance; do not raise arms (perceived as intending to strike out; use of force or threat to use force is criminal act unless needed to protect resident or others)
		Provide love and a sense of a secure, stable environment
		Be consistent with care (for example, bath same time each day)
		If resident removes clothes or bed linens: cover gently and without great fanfare; do not scold; be supportive through touch, talking, and presence; button clothes in back, use shirts without buttons, buckle belt in back; put resident's hands to his side gently and say no each time it happens; tie sheets to side rails or use cradle with sheet over it on bed; determine when and why clothes are removed
Category D: Paranoid behavior	**Subjective:**	
Thought processes, altered	Expresses feelings of fearfulness, anger, anxiety, agitation, guilt, lack of self-esteem, insecurity, loneliness, suspiciousness	Enter the resident's space or territory carefully, gently, slowly
Protection, altered	Schizophrenia, paranoid type (DSM-IV)	Respect the resident's personal belongings in sight or in reach (clothes, items on and in bedside stand, etc.); replace items if they must be moved
Violence, high risk for: directed at self/others	Sensory losses, especially sight and hearing	Take the resident to see the food prepared in the kitchen
Sleep pattern disturbance	Thinks possessions are being stolen or that someone is trying to poison him or her	Taste some of the food to show the resident it is not poisoned
Coping, defensive	Loss of trusted family and friends	Offer foods and medications in unopened containers when possible
Fear	Relocation to a new environment	
Personal identity disturbance	Thinks everyone hates him or her	
	Attempts to fill in gaps in memory (compensation)	

Continued.

Table 11-2 Most Common Nursing Diagnoses, Contributing factors, Defining characteristics, and Nursing interventions for Nursing Home Residents with Mental and Behavioral Problems—cont'd

Nursing diagnoses (NANDA)	Contributing factors	Defining characteristics	Nursing interventions
	Sensory isolation Medications	Oversensitive Sees or talks to imaginary people Believes voices on the TV are real people **Objective:** Withdrawn Aloof Secretive	Assure medication intake by crushing or giving in liquid form Reflect feelings of fear Avoid arguing with paranoid delusion Do not argue or joke with the resident Help resident to understand that he or she is seeing things that are not there. Say, "You see it, but I do not." Do not agree with the resident about seeing things (reality testing) Provide more sensory stimulation such as realistic conversation Encourage more visitors Replace the hallucinations with real interactions

Appreciation is expressed to Ann Kirkham, RN, MS, CS, ANP, psychiatric clinical nurse specialist, Fort Worth, TX, for some of the suggested nursing interventions. Adapted from Baldwin, B. A., Stevens, G. L., & Friedman, S. D. (1995). Geriatric psychiatric nursing. In G. W. Stuart & S. J. Sundeen (Eds.). *Principles and practice of psychiatric nursing* (5th ed.). St. Louis: Mosby. American Psychiatric Association (1994). *Diagnosis and statistical manual of mental disorders*, (4th ed., revised). Washington, DC: Author. See Appendix E for a list of psychiatric diagnoses commonly found in older adults. Love, C. C. (1992). Applying the nursing process with the elderly. In H. S. Wilson & C. R. Kneisel (Eds.). *Psychiatric nursing* (4th ed., pp. 867-899). Menlo Park, CA: Addison-Wesley. NANDA *Nursing Diagnoses: Definition and Classification 1992-1993*. Used with permission. Stuart, G., & Sundeen, S. J. (1994). *Principles and practice of psychiatric nursing* (5th ed.). St. Louis: Mosby. Wilson, H. S., & Kneisel, C. R. (Eds.). (1992). *Psychiatric nursing* (4th ed.). Menlo Park, CA: Addison-Wesley.

psychotropic medications" (Ryden & Feldt, 1992, p. 35). Ryden (1992) suggested five major goals for caring for cognitively impaired adults with aggressive behavior. These goals and suggested nursing interventions are presented in Table 11-3. The ultimate goal of care for these residents is to improve their well-being, prevent their aggressive behavior, and provide humane care (Ryden & Feldt, 1992, pp. 40-41).

Nurse aides need help from professional staff in learning how to care for residents with major behavioral problems, particularly those with aggressive behavior. Otherwise, the nursing assistants have problems (e.g., frustration, despair, and frequent turnover) and residents may suffer (e.g., physical or psychological abuse). Feldt and Ryden (1992) implemented an educational program for nursing assistants in an attempt to reduce aggressive behavior in nursing home residents. The program also included role modeling and problem solving by a gerontological clinical nurse specialist. Although the nurse aides had received the required amount of education for basic care, they had not had much focus on communication skills. The educational program focused "on specific activities of daily living when aggression was likely to occur, such as bathing, grooming, toileting, or dressing" (Feldt & Ryden, 1992, p. 8). Then they concentrated on strategies to prevent aggressive behavior during specific activities (e.g., bathing). Although they recognized that it is impossible to stop all aggressive behavior, they taught strategies to keep the aggressive behavior from increasing. Some of their strategies were "resident and [nursing assistant] safety; removal of the stimulant for aggression; use of diversion

Table 11-3   Goals and Interventions for the Care of Cognitively Impaired Nursing Home Residents with Aggressive Behavior

Goal	*Nursing interventions*
For the client to feel safe	Avoid threatening stimuli in the environment (e.g., loud voices, other noises, touch perceived to be harmful)
For the client to feel physically comfortable	Prevent unnecessary pain; assess and relieve pain; be gentle during daily physical care (e.g., bathing and positioning)
For the client to have a sense of control	Allow the person to have some freedom of choice whenever possible (e.g., time of bath or other activity; if the person refuses a treatment, try again later)
For the client to have minimal stress	Maintain a balance between too much stimulation (e.g., traffic, noise) and lack of stimulation (e.g., some activity helps to maintain cognitive and physical functions)
For the client to feel pleasure	Encourage caregivers to provide pleasurable experiences (e.g., smell, taste, touch); replace aggressive behavior with pleasurable activities

Adapted from Ryden, M. B. (1992). Alternatives to restraints and psychotrophics in the care of aggressive, cognitively impaired elderly persons. In K. C. Buckwalter (Ed.). *Geriatric mental health nursing: Current and future challenges* (pp. 84-93). Thorofare, NJ: Slack, Ryden, M. B., & Feldt, K. S. (1992). Goal-directed care: Caring for aggressive nursing home residents with dementia. *Journal of Gerontological Nursing, 18*(11), 35-42.

distraction, or time out; and momentarily leaving the situation" (Feldt & Ryden, 1992, p. 9). The nurse aides were taught "not to shout, confront, reason or argue with, or touch an already agitated resident" (p. 9). As a result of this program and role modeling by the clinical nurse specialist, the care of residents with aggressive behavior improved, and the nursing aides found caregiving more rewarding and less frustrating.

"Staff members forget that clients with dementia often do not understand the meaning of words, but they are sensitive to voice tone and body language (Rosenheimer & Francis, 1992, p. 25). Nurse aides especially must be taught that their tone of voice and approach to the resident can be helpful or can trigger aggressive behavior. A slow approach and a kind, low-pitched calm voice is much less likely to cause a negative response than a loud, high-pitched fast voice and a hurried approach. Young women tend to have a high-pitched voice, and if they talk fast, the older resident has difficulty hearing and interpreting what is being said and may react aggressively.

Restraints

Physical and chemical restraints (e.g., psychotrophic medications) have been commonly used to control residents with mental and behavioral problems for about 50 years (Eigsti & Vrooman, 1992). Restraints were frequently used, for example, on residents with Alzheimer's disease to prevent them from wandering into other patients' rooms or out of the building, supposedly for their own safety but often more for staff convenience.

Physical restraints are defined as *any* device that limits mobility of the resident. This includes vest and wrist restraints, bed rails, and wander bracelets. It is well known that physical restraints can cause major problems (e.g., pressure ulcers, skin tears, urinary and fecal problems, aspiration, fractures, chafing, and loss of muscle function and ability to walk (Eigsti & Vrooman, 1992; Weick, 1992). Restraints can also increase agitation, withdrawal, and depression. The use of physical restraints ultimately requires more nursing time because of the frequent observations necessary to prevent the possibility of these complications (Blakeslee, 1988).

Primary reasons for use of restraints in the past have been the belief that they were for protection of the resident from falls and that the staff would be legally liable if the resident did fall. Thus, staff believed that they were protecting themselves from "reprimand, loss of employment or legal suit" and "that no alternatives to restraints exists" (Evans & Strumpf, 1990, p. 124). These and other myths, for example, "It doesn't really bother old people to be restrained" (Evans & Strumpf, p. 126) have made the removal of restraints slow.

The Omnibus Budget Reconciliation Act (OBRA), which was passed in 1987 and implemented in 1990, put strict limitations on use of restraints. Based on the OBRA legislation, restraints may be used only according to the following guidelines:

- ◆ Restraints may be used only in the treatment of a specific medical condition.
- ◆ There must be a written order by the physician except in specific emergencies.

◆ The order must state the length of time and circumstances for the use of restraints.

In addition, the Food and Drug Administration (FDA) now requires that all physical restraints be labeled with instructions for their use (e.g., label top and bottom) so that persons who use them will know the specific use and dangers (Weick, 1992). The FDA has also prepared specific detailed guidelines for the use of physical restraints (Weick, 1992, p. 77).

With the OBRA guidelines as an initial incentive, many nursing homes have become restraint free, or at least have substantially reduced the use of restraints. In a demonstration project on a 75-bed floor in one long-term care facility, restraints were removed from all 22 residents who had previously been restrained (Eigsti & Vrooman, 1992). Although the process is different for each individual resident, some of the techniques that can be used may be seen in Box 11-3. Many of these techniques are best tried slowly over a period of weeks to evaluate their safety and

---

Box 11-3 **Techniques Used to Provide a Restraint-Free Environment**

◆ Eliminate the problem that causes the need for restraints (e.g., social isolation).
◆ Plan daily individual activities based on personal needs (e.g., time and type of bath).
◆ Sensitively identify the rooms of residents with dementia for closer monitoring and surveillance.
◆ Add personal pictures, handmade objects, and artificial flowers to the room.
◆ Eliminate or minimize extraneous noise and other distractions (e.g., housekeeping noises and television).
◆ Provide comfort and relief of pain.
◆ Reposition the resident frequently.
◆ Implement a toileting regimen.
◆ Provide a sense of security.
◆ Adapt physical and activity therapy, including exercise and walking.
◆ Use contoured chairs, low beds, and alarms that go off when the resident attempts to get out of bed.
◆ Try rocking wheelchairs or a chair with wheels on the back legs to provide movement and exercise.
◆ Be consistent with daily care and staff assignments.

Adapted from Eigsti, D. G., & Vrooman, N. (1992). Releasing restraints in the nursing home: It can be done. *Journal of Gerontological Nursing, 18*(1), 21-23. Strumpf, N, Evans, L. K., & Swartz, D. (1990). Restraint-free care: From dream to reality. *Geriatric Nursing, 11*(3), 122-124.

effectiveness. Success often takes time, but it is very rewarding because it provides a better quality of life for the resident, more satisfaction for the family, and a sense of pride for the staff. Overall, "the impact of restraint reduction programs has been positive based on the overall decline in restraint use, but the effects of specific interventions on targeted resident care problems needs much more study" (Mion & Mercurio, 1992, p. 8).

Summary of Nursing Interventions

Many mental and behavioral problems of nursing home residents can be managed with creative nursing interventions. Making structural changes in the environment such as increased lighting and staffing changes such as consistent assignments may be helpful in decreasing the behavioral problems of nursing home residents. The staff should continue to orient new residents to their environment for several weeks after admission. All rooms should have large-type labels, the building should be secure, and staff should consistently use effective communication skills and the technique of reality orientation or validation for those residents for whom they would be helpful.

As mentioned previously, chemical or physical restraints should be a last resort as nursing interventions. All nursing home staff, particularly nurse aides who are with the residents every day, should use some of the nursing interventions listed in Table 11-2. Perhaps nurse aides cannot use all of the communication skills suggested to help change the patients' behavior, but they can learn to protect themselves, the resident, and others from physical harm.

The most important overall approach to the aggressive, hostile, angry, combative resident is to remain calm, stay in control of the situation, accept the resident's feelings of anger without accepting the aggressive behavior, and divert the resident's thoughts and actions to other more appropriate activities if possible.

The nurse should recognize that minor paranoid beliefs may become major paranoid delusions if not treated. An older resident who threatens to harm someone who he believes is stealing from him should be taken seriously and observed carefully. Observing such residents closely, remaining calm and in control, and directing attention of the resident to other activities may decrease such behavior.

Many residents who have been independent all of their lives find it difficult to learn to be dependent on others. Although specific nursing interventions depend on the nursing diagnoses, nurses should recognize that adapting to some of the physical and mental changes of aging and a new environment can be very difficult. To whatever extent possible, nursing home residents should be able to maintain some sense of control and feeling of independence in their daily lives. Specific nursing interventions should be based on these primary goals (Table 11-2).

Evaluation

The evaluation phase of the nursing process is perhaps the most difficult, probably because behavioral change is often so slow. Some initial assessment will be necessary to determine whether the goals have been met and the nursing interventions have been effective. Nurse aides should be taught to report when behavioral problems cease as well as when they begin.

A reduction in aggressive, violent, hostile behavior probably will be quite obvious. If psychotropic medications are used, their specific effects should be consistently reported and well documented in the medical record so that the smallest dosage possible eventually can be used. Residents who are withdrawn or depressed should be carefully assessed for (1) percentage of food eaten at each meal, (2) body weight each week, (3) amount of sleep each 24 hours, (4) daily participation in home activities, and (5) amount and type of communication with other residents, staff, and visitors.

A short weekly mental status assessment test should be used for residents who have cognitive impairment and are confused. The effect of reality orientation can be evaluated by the use of such a test. Nurse aides should be taught to report a decrease in wandering. A reduction in paranoid behaviors may be less obvious because the resident often stops making paranoid statements while maintaining paranoid tendencies. There should be careful observation and evaluation of residents with increasing paranoid tendencies.

❖ Summary

Many nursing home residents have mental and behavioral problems at some time during their stay in the institution. Sometimes these problems are a continuation of mental illness that began early in their lives. Other problems occur because of maladaptation to the changes of aging and a new environment.

The nursing process can be used to assess these behaviors and determine appropriate nursing diagnoses, goals, and interventions. The most common mental and behavioral problems among nursing home residents are (1) depression, (2) confusion and disorientation, (3) aggressive and disruptive behaviors, and (4) paranoid behaviors. Nursing home staffs should plan to employ permanent or consultation staff who can provide assessment and care of residents and educate or supervise other staff members in the care of those residents with behavioral problems. Community programs also can help the nursing home staff provide better care for their mentally disturbed residents.

Sample nursing diagnoses and specific nursing interventions have been included for each of the major categories of behaviors identified. Examples of methods to evaluate the nursing interventions are also presented.

❖ References

Algase, D. L. (1992). A century of progress: Today's strategies for responding to wandering behavior. *Journal of Gerontological Nursing, 18*(11), 28-34.

American Psychiatric Association (1994). *Diagnostic and statistical manual of mental disorders* (4th ed.). Washington, DC: Author.

Beck, C. M., Robinson, C., & Baldwin, B. (1992). Improving documentation of aggressive behavior in nursing home residents. *Journal of Gerontological Nursing, 18*(2), 21-23.

Blakeslee, J. A. (1988). Untie the elderly. *American Journal of Nursing, 88*(6), 833-834.

Brooke, V. (1989). How elders adjust. *Geriatric Nursing, 10*(2), 66-68.

Buckwalter, K. C. (1985). Integration of social and mental health services for the elderly. *Family Community Health, 8*(4), 76-87.

Buckwalter, K. C. (1992). Phantom of the nursing home. *Journal of Gerontological Nursing, 18*(9), 46-47.

Burgio, L. D., Jones, L. T., Butler, F., & Engel, B. T. (1988). Behavior problems in an urban nursing home. *Journal of Gerontological Nursing, 14*(1), 31-34.

Davidhizar, R., & Cosgray, R. (1990). Helping the wanderer. *Geriatric Nursing, 11*(6), 280-281.

Drysdale, A. E., Nelson, C. F., & Wineman, N. M. (1993). Families need help too: Group treatment for families of nursing home residents. *Clinical Nurse Specialist, 7*(3), 130-134.

Eigsti, D. G., & Vrooman, N. (1992). Releasing restraints in the nursing home. *Journal of Gerontological Nursing, 18*(1), 21-23.

Eisdorfer, C. (1988, June 10). Mental illness in older adults. Conference on Aging, Texas College of Osteopathic Medicine and Psychiatric Institute of Fort Worth, Fort Worth, TX.

Evans, L. K., & Strumpf, N. E. (1990). Myths about elder restraint. *Image, 22*(2), 124-125.

Feldt, K. S., & Ryden, M. B. (1992). Aggressive behavior: Educating nursing assistants. *Journal of Gerontological Nursing, 18*(5), 3-12.

Hogstel, M. O. (1991). Assessing mental status. *Journal of Gerontological Nursing, 17*(5), 42-43.

Hogstel, M. O. (1993). Understanding hoarding behaviors in the elderly. *American Journal of Nursing, 93*(7), 42-45.

Kane, R. A. (1986). Mental health in nursing homes: Behavioral and social research. In M. S. Harper & B. D. Lebowitz (Eds.). *Mental illness in nursing homes: Agenda for research.* Rockville, MD: National Institute of Mental Health.

Kikuta, S. C. (1991). Clinically managing disruptive behavior on the ward. *Journal of Gerontological Nursing, 17*(8), 4-8.

Levenson, S. A. (1987). Innovations in nursing home care. *Generations, 12*(1), 74-79.

Lucas, M. J., Steele, C., & Bognanni, A. (1986). Recognition of psychiatric symptoms in dementia. *Journal of Gerontological Nursing, 12*(1), 11-15.

Melzack, R. (April 1992). *Scientific American,* 120-126.

Mental health status of nursing home residents. (1993). *Journal of Gerontological Nursing, 19*(2), 46.

Mion, L. C., & Mercurio, A. T. (1992). Methods to reduce restraints: Process, outcomes, and future directions. *Journal of Gerontological Nursing, 18*(11), 5-11.

Parmelee, P. A., Katz, I. R., & Lawton, M. P. (1989). Depression among institutionalized aged: Assessment and prevalence estimation. *Journal of Gerontology, 44*(11), M22-29.

Riegel, K. F., & Riegel, R. M. (1972). Development, drop, and death. *Developmental Psychology, 6*(2), 306-319.

Rosenheimer, L., & Francis, E. M. (1992). Feasible without subsidy? Overnight respite for Alzheimers'. *Journal of Gerontological Nursing, 18*(4), 21-29.

Ryden, M. B. (1992). Alternatives to restraints and psychotropics in the care of aggressive, cognitively impaired elderly persons. In K. C. Buckwalter (Ed.). *Geriatric mental health nursing: Current and future challenges* (pp. 84-93). Thorofare, NJ: Slack.

Ryden, M. B., & Feldt, K. S. (1992). Goal-directed care: Caring for aggressive nursing home residents with dementia. *Journal of Gerontological Nursing, 18*(11), 35-42.

Smith, M., Buckwalter, K. C., & Albanese, M. (1990). Psychiatric nursing consultation: A different choice for nursing homes. *Journal of Psychosocial Nursing, 28*(3), 23-28.

Strumpf, N. E., Evans, L. K., & Swartz, D. (1990). Restraint free care: From dream to reality. *Geriatric Nursing, 11*(3), 122-124.

Tierney, J. C., Cronin, A., & Scanlon, M. K. (1986). . . . and don't send her back! *American Journal of Nursing, 86*(9), 1011-1014.

Wandering devices. (1992). *Journal of Gerontological Nursing, 18*(12), 39-40.

Weick, M. D. (1992). Physical restraints: An FDA update. *American Journal of Nursing, 92*(11), 74-80.

## Chapter 12

❖ *Care of the Mentally Ill Older Person in the Home*

Mildred O. Hogstel*

One of the areas most lacking in mental health care of the older population is home care. Unless family, neighbors, or friends become aware of an older person's unusual behavior and seek assistance for that person, these individuals often become recluses in their own homes and deteriorate both mentally and physically. If a person is living alone and develops a mental illness, some of the problems that family or friends might observe are a lack of personal care and hygiene (e.g., not bathing or wearing clean clothes), an unkempt house that is cluttered with trash and newspapers, poor nutritional intake with old food or no food in the kitchen, an obvious loss of weight, and reports by neighbors of unusual behavior.

Other more specific signs of mental illness in older people that family members should look for are these (Buckwalter and Stolley, 1991, pp. 136-139):

- ◆ Suspiciousness
- ◆ Jealousy
- ◆ Hallucinations
- ◆ Delusions
- ◆ Sadness, crying, severe depression

---

*With appreciation to Mary S. Harper and Mira Kirk Nelson for their contributions to this chapter.

- Withdrawal, isolation, passiveness
- Talking about suicide
- Changes in speech
- Inappropriate dress
- Poor hygiene
- Pacing, rocking

Often family members are not aware of the severity of these problems, especially if they do not live close to the older person, and are surprised when neighbors or friends tell them about it. The older person may not be aware that assistance (e.g., diagnosis and treatment) would provide an increased quality and length of life. "Sometimes the elderly are reluctant to seek mental health services because of, for example, the stigma attached to mental illness, transportation and geographic problems, perceived inability to be helped or to pay for services, and fear of loss of freedom" (Buckwalter and Stolley, 1991, p. 139).

Connecting the person and family with a service provider in the community is often the primary need. See Chapter 13 for detailed information on community services available for older adults.

Failing health of the older family member presents difficulties in daily living for the whole family. The greatest risk occurs when both the older family member and the caregiver are in poor health. If the ill person has Alzheimer's disease or other related dementia, the associated behavioral problems tend to create greater difficulties than physical problems. For example, it is very frustrating for family members constantly to fear that the older person will wander out of the house during the night or to hear a person ask the same question many times during the day. Families are usually able to manage major physical disabilities much more easily than behavioral abnormalities. Substance abuse by either the caregiver or the older person increases the difficulties in managing daily living. If the caregiver abuses substances, the result may be neglect or abuse of the older person. If the ill older person abuses substances, the result may be an increased physical and mental debilitation (Copstead & Patterson, 1986).

Adult family caregivers often do not have the knowledge, resources, or skills necessary to provide continuing, optimum support for older family members, especially those who have been diagnosed as having severe depression, Alzheimer's disease, or a related disorder. As a consequence, family relationships and the ability of the adult caregivers to care for their older family members may be less than satisfactory. These mental disorders add to the difficulty of caring for an ill older adult in the home.

A persistent and pervasive myth in both the public and professional spheres is that families tend to abandon older relatives. This belief arises first from a very real fear of abandonment that often accompanies mental and physical disability at any age and second from the kinds of older persons often encountered by professionals. However, abandonment is not the norm. Health professionals frequently see older adults who are childless or who have minimal family contact. Many older people seek professional help because of the lack of accessible, responsible family members to care for them. Most older people live within a short distance of members of their family and have contact with them frequently. "Contrary to the myth, families do not abandon frail elders" (Baldwin, 1990, p. 172).

This chapter will discuss the prevalence and problems of caring for the mentally ill older person in the home and potential effects on the family and the older person. The manner in which the nursing process can be applied to these families will be discussed. An overview of family support therapy and care for the caregiver, with its accompanying support groups, will conclude the chapter.

❖ *Prevalence and Problems*

Psychopathology is a serious problem among older adults. Approximately 15% to 20% of individuals aged 65 and over demonstrate functional psychiatric disorders. If persons with dementia are included, up to 25% of the older population may need neuropsychiatric evaluation and treatment. Approximately 65% of older persons with psychiatric disorders have significant physical disease. Often the mental illness is considered an inevitable consequence of the primary medical disorder or the aging process itself. Depression or other psychiatric disorders should not be considered a normal response to other disease or to aging.

In the literature for home health, geropsychiatric nursing care, and a study of mental health needs of older adults in 200 home health care settings (Harper & Gilchrist, 1988) some commonly observed and reported mental health disorders of older adults in the home health care setting include the following:

- ◆ Confusion and delirium
- ◆ Wandering and restlessness, especially at night
- ◆ Cognitive impairment
- ◆ Depression, sadness, and self-depreciation
- ◆ Feelings of hopelessness
- ◆ Dementia
- ◆ Frequent crying spells
- ◆ Suicidal ideation or expression of the wish to die
- ◆ Hyperactivity
- ◆ Confusion following surgery, strokes, cancer, hip fractures, and falls
- ◆ Agitation
- ◆ Behavioral and/or emotional problems associated with physical illness and/or drug-drug interactions and side effects
- ◆ Hostility
- ◆ Abuse of alcohol
- ◆ Polypharmacy
- ◆ Frequent use of psychotropic drugs for clients without a psychiatric diagnosis

The increase in life expectancy and the increase in the number of frail older people have resulted in a demographic shift toward the multigenerational family.

There has been a significant increase in the number of four- and five-generation families.

Conservative estimates show that at least 5 million people in the United States are involved in parent care at any given time. Another 4 million to 5 million are engaged in some type of family responsibility for older adults, whether on a consistent or transitional basis. This responsibility extends to the management of chronic physical and psychological or emotional disorders, which increase in complexity and intensity as a person ages (Baldwin, 1987). Adult children in their 60s and 70s are increasingly caring for parents in their 80s, 90s, and 100s, who usually need more care and support than the young-old group.

The number of families providing long-term care to older relatives is expected to increase substantially in the future as a result of major demographic and social trends. Changes in mortality and fertility rates and patterns of migration have contributed to increases in the number and proportion of persons in the population. The fastest-growing segment of the older population is age 85 and over (Atchley, 1994). This age group is most likely to develop some form of chronic physical and/or mental disorder.

A major demographic trend is the decline in birthrate and family size in recent years, which has resulted in a smaller number of adult children as potential caregivers, especially daughters. Therefore, there will be fewer siblings available to care for the older frail people (Hooyman & Lustbader, 1986.) The second trend concerns the increase in the number of women in the labor market. Among women 45 to 54 years old, the age group most likely to become caregivers, 60% are in the labor force. While not abandoning their caregiving responsibilities, women's employment status may necessitate more shared responsibility among both brothers and sisters. These trends indicate that sons may be increasingly called on to become caregivers to their older parents.

The adult caregiver is usually a woman, most likely an adult daughter, wife, sister, or daughter-in-law. The wife may be older with health problems and often is not able to be the primary caregiver. Women tend to live closer to their families of origin than do men and generally interact more frequently with extended family members. Older women are more likely than older men to move in with their children when they find it difficult or impossible to live alone, and these children are usually daughters.

Despite these changing family patterns, most families attempt to maintain their older members at home as long as possible, generally at considerable personal sacrifice. Most older people with chronic mental or emotional problems are being cared for in their own homes or in the homes of family members.

❖ *Nursing Process*

The nurse in the home health care setting is in a unique position to use knowledge of gerontology and mental disorders of the older adult to improve the lives of mentally ill older persons and their families. Progressive chronic physical problems often cause mental problems. "Home health care nurses are frequently in the best position to detect and treat early imbalances" in mental or physical health (Buckwalter and Stolley, 1991, pp. 136-137). Although the nursing process is outlined in discrete steps for the purposes of discussion, the process is cyclical and carried out many times in each encounter with the ill older person and the family. An example of the interplay between steps in the nursing process is that while assessing a depressed older person, the nurse also spends time listening to the concerns that person expresses, which helps to improve the client's self-esteem. Because assessment is a form of intervention, it is important for the nurse to evaluate the impact of the assessment on the individual and the family.

Assessment

Most mentally ill adults who are cared for in the home are chronically mentally ill (e.g., they have Alzheimer's disease or a similar type of dementia). They previously have been referred for a complete evaluation and treatment (if appropriate) and returned to the home for long-term care. An accurate initial assessment of the family and the chronically mentally ill older person is necessary to maintain or restore effective management of daily living in the family. Copstead and Patterson (1986) suggest that the assessment should include the patterns of daily living, the demands placed on both the caregiver and the mentally ill older person, the available internal and external resources for managing the requirements of daily living, and the deficits that are present. A reliable family member who sees the mentally ill older person regularly is usually able to provide information about the client before and after the onset of the illness; these data are critical to an adequate assessment. The client's relatives, neighbors, or friends may also be able to provide pertinent information for the assessment.

Copstead and Patterson (1986) believe that the nurse should work at the family's pace in making a family assessment to allow them sufficient time to share their perceptions of the situation. Throughout the assessment, the nurse should maintain a neutral, objective attitude in the collection of data. Areas of assessment include the following:

- Perception of the primary problem areas and how they occurred
- Problem-solving strategies attempted and how they worked
- Goals for the older client and for the family
- Patterns of daily living of the caregiver and the older person relevant to the situation
- The nature of the home environment relevant to the older person's functional status
- Internal and external resources available to resolve problems
- Additional external assistance the family feels is needed and usable
- Assessment for abuse of the ill older family member
- Assessment for severe fatigue and stress in the caregiver

See Chapter 7 for additional information on assessment of the older adult with Alzheimer's disease and related disorders.

Nursing Diagnoses

When these areas have been assessed and organized, the nurse, in conjunction with the family and caregiver, formulates nursing diagnoses and plans for management. Some of the nursing diagnoses* commonly seen in older adults and families with a dependent mentally impaired older adult include the following:

Older Family Member
- Anxiety
- Coping, ineffective individual
- Hopelessness
- Self-esteem, chronic low
- Constipation
- Nutrition, altered: less than body requirements
- Self-care deficit: bathing/hygiene, dressing/grooming, toileting
- Thought processes, altered
- Violence, high risk for: directed at self/others
- Communication, impaired verbal

Family Members
- Fatigue
- Sleep pattern disturbance
- Adjustment, impaired
- Grieving, anticipatory
- Home maintenance management, impaired
- Caregiver role strain
- Family coping, compromised
- Family processes, altered
- Role performance, altered
- Social isolation
- Hopelessness

Planning

The nursing diagnoses should provide directions for planning care. The nurse assists the family in setting realistic goals and plans activities for each member. The most

---

* *NANDA Nursing Diagnoses: Definitions and Classification* 1992-1993. Philadelphia, PA.: North American Nursing Diagnosis Association; with permission.

important short-term goal is the provision of immediate support for the areas of unmet needs for both the family and the older adult. A long-range goal is establishment of a care system that will enable the family and the ill older adult to cope with life demands with minimum assistance. Making tentative plans for future placement of the mentally ill older adult in an alternative safe environment helps ensure that the decision will not have to be made hurriedly, possibly in a period of extreme stress. Specific goals will depend on the difficulties that the mentally ill older adult and the family encounter in daily living.

Interventions

Interventions are directed toward reducing or eliminating the causative or contributing factors related to the nursing diagnoses (Carpenito, 1993). The nurse should teach family members how to look for sudden changes of behavior in the older person, how to assess for suicidal ideation, if needed, how to supervise or administer the most effective drug regimen for the older person, and how to make environmental changes in the home that will help the older person who has cognitive deficits (e.g. labeling the bathroom and closet). The nurse can help family members to accept their feelings of helplessness, hopelessness, frustration, guilt, anger, or sadness as normal and expected. The family members may encounter difficulty with altered role relationships. The nurse can assist them by identifying specific changes that have occurred, noting the reactions that these changes have caused in each family member, and determining the reason for them. It may be helpful for the nurse to suggest some options for action to provide a sense of control over the situation. Options include discussion of altered role relationships and the need to establish expectations for these new roles among family members, and in situations in which this is not possible, identification of the areas of change, the reasons for the changes, and the acceptable options the caregiver has in adapting to the changes.

If the nurse notes that the emotional tone of a family member seems out of proportion to the situation, it may be that the individual is responding to some emotional backlog of feelings from earlier experiences and relationships. This history should be validated to assist the persons involved to understand and alter their behavior (Copstead & Patterson, 1986).

If there are insufficient financial resources, the nurse should assist the family in determining the availability of government programs to help in the care of the older family member. The family may not be aware of the full range of income-related benefits that are available. Applying to the various state and local agencies for assistance may be overwhelming for the family, especially if the family members have mobility or sensory deficits. Securing a trustworthy volunteer can assist greatly in the family's ability to benefit from government services (McConnell, 1988b).

Evaluation

Evaluation of the intervention may be made in terms of cessation or continuation of manifestations. Successful interventions will be reflected when caregivers and family members begin to report being happier with the living arrangement. The family members are better able to enjoy being in the presence of the older adult. There may be fewer complaints voiced by both the caregiver and the older person, reflecting a much happier atmosphere within the household. The caregiver and the older adult may report sleeping better, eating better, being less tired, and making fewer demands on each other. There may be improvements in the family financial situation and living environment, reflecting less crowding and greater comfort. Outside support services have been identified and used to improve the overall living arrangement of the family. It is important for the nurse to anticipate changes in the family situation and to offer support when needed (Copstead & Patterson, 1986).

❖ *Effects on the Family*

When the family brings a mentally ill older person to live with them, there will be many changes in their lives. Each family member will be affected in different ways by an older person's presence in the home. Changes in family roles occur when the adult child becomes the caregiver and supporter for the older person.

"Roles are different from responsibilities," and clarification is important for each member of the family. "Roles include who you are, how you are seen, and what is expected of you." A person's role is his place in the family, such as the father, who is probably the head of the household, and the mother, who is the probable caregiver of the ill members of the family. "Roles are established over many years and are not always easy to define." "Responsibilities are the jobs each person has in the family." New responsibilities can be learned by various family members, such as washing clothes, balancing the checkbook, or buying the groceries. Learning new responsibilities can be difficult, especially when family members are faced with the everyday needs of the mentally ill older person. Understanding that each person's roles and responsibilities can change will help family members to understand other personal feelings and problems that may arise in the family (Mace & Rabins, 1991, p. 183).

Changes may occur in the husband-wife relationship in which the wife's major role previously was to care for the husband and children. Conflict may develop with the addition of responsibilities of caring for an older adult. Changes in lifestyle and adjustments in relationships will be experienced by all family members as the ill older person becomes a member of the family.

Potential Family Problems and Conflicts

There are many decisions to be made before moving an older person into the family home. The family, including members who live elsewhere, should meet to discuss openly the potential problems and determine the best solutions for the whole family (see Fig. 12-1). The family must agree about where the older person will live and who will provide the needed everyday care. If possible, the desires of the ill older family member should be considered. If family members who live elsewhere must contribute financially to the older person's care expenses, an agreement should be

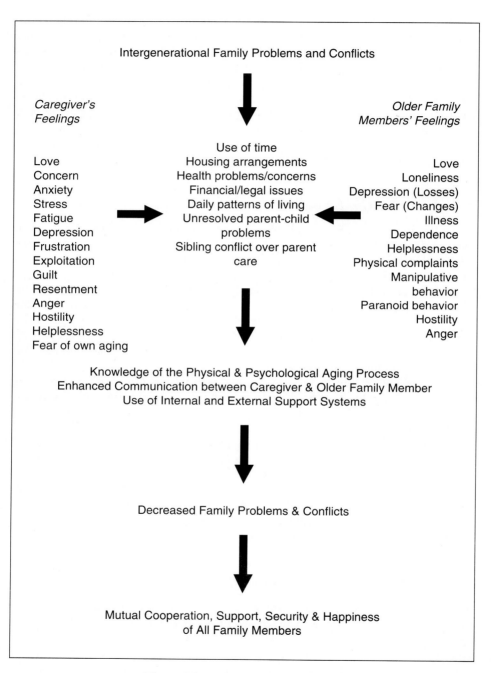

Figure 12-1 Intergenerational issues

made in advance for a fixed amount of money to be sent each month to the family who will provide care of the older person in their home. It is essential to have open and frank discussions of all problems, particularly finances, to prevent misunderstandings, anger, and hostility among family members.

Expenses

Caring for a mentally ill older person in the home can be an expensive undertaking. The expenses for many of the care needs are not reimbursed by insurance companies, Medicare, or Medicaid. One of the primary problems will be the added expense for food, home maintenance, and utilities. The purchase of additional or different kinds of food, especially if the older person is on a special diet, can be expensive for the caregiving family. The purchase of medications or medical supplies may be a major expense. Necessary modifications of the home could be expensive, especially if the older person uses a wheelchair. There will be additional expenses for utilities, since the thermostat would have to be set higher in the winter because older persons get cold easily (McConnell, 1988a; Williams, 1985).

Space

The older person needs a space to call his or her own, which could be a small apartment in or near the family home (called an *echo* home) or a private bedroom. A communication system is important to alert family members to problems or needs that arise. If a family member must give up a bedroom to be used by the older person, conflict can develop because this person will not have his or her private space. Privacy is very important to most family members so that they each have a personal retreat where they can unwind from stress-producing activities. Older persons should move some of their personal possessions into the family home to make the transition easier. Some family members may not like the possessions or have room for them; therefore the total family must decide which possessions will be moved into the home and what adjustments will have to be made.

A possible solution to the space problem may be to convert an attached double garage into a living area for the older family member. Adding a bathroom and carpeting the living area would provide comfortable space for the older person. A separate heating system with a thermostat in the room would allow the temperature to be adjusted as the older person desired. An electrical signal system installed in this area and connected to the family living area would serve as a safety precaution. Some of the living room and bedroom furniture and other belongings of the older person could be used to make the new surroundings feel more like home. Although this would require considerable expense, the arrangement would eliminate many of the potential problems of bringing an ill older person to live in the home.

Excessive Noise

Excessive noise can be very disturbing to the older person with a mental or behavioral problem, especially confusion. Loud stereo music that is enjoyed by teenagers and dishes banging in the kitchen sink can interfere with television viewing and can be particularly disturbing or frightening to many older adults. The older adult may be startled by or misinterpret normal sounds such as door chimes or telephone rings. Care must be taken to prevent as much loud extraneous noise as possible.

Environmental Factors

McConnell (1988b) states that the essential aspects of the physical environment include a room temperature between 65° and 80° F, freedom from disease-carrying pests, access to clean drinking water, toilet facilities, cooking and refrigeration facilities, and adequate space for sleeping.

It may be necessary to change the environment to avoid accidents and to ensure safety for the confused person. Adaptations may be required in stairs, rails, or bathrooms. The bathroom is one of the most dangerous places in the home for a confused older person. Bathrooms are a frequent site of falls, and the surrounding hard surfaces contribute to the severity of the injuries. A neat house is safer than a cluttered one, which necessitates removing things that cause problems. Clutter is always dangerous, especially when a person is confused or misinterprets what he or she sees. Medications, cleaning products, paint, knives, power tools, and other hazardous items must be removed or locked up so the confused older person does not have access to them. Many simple things can be done, such as removing the knobs from the stove to prevent its use without supervision. A rope could be installed to guide the confused person from the bedroom to the bathroom. Wandering is a potential problem, because the confused person may try to leave the premises during the night. Management of wandering depends on the cause (see Chapters 7 and 11). It is often helpful to install locks that are difficult to operate or are unfamiliar to the confused person. A lock installed at the bottom of the door may suffice to keep the confused person from leaving the house without supervision. Any of several electronic devices will alert the caregiver that the older person is getting out of bed or going out the door (Mace & Rabins 1991, pp. 92-95).

A simple but frustrating problem is maintaining a temperature comfortable for both young and middle-aged active adults while providing a safe and comfortable temperature for the older adult, who may have decreased metabolism and slowed circulation. In winter a higher room temperature is probably necessary for the older adult to prevent chilling and possible accidental hypothermia. A locked cover could be installed over the thermostat to prevent the older person from frequently changing the temperature in the home. The older adult should be encouraged to wear more clothes during the daytime and use an electric blanket or more covers at night. In the summer the older person may not be accustomed to air conditioning and should be encouraged to wear a light sweater or shawl to keep from getting too cold. Excessive heat in the house can be frustrating for the already overworked caregiver. If there are guns, razor blades, knives, or other dangerous objects in the home, they should be removed or kept locked, particularly if the older person is severely depressed and talks of suicide or has threatened other people. See Chapter 7 for other safety measures and environmental changes that are especially useful when caring for a demented older person in the home.

Responsibilities and Chores

With a mentally ill older person in the home, the caregiver will have more responsibilities and less time to accomplish the necessary everyday chores of maintaining a household. If physically and mentally able, the older person could assume some of the responsibilities around the home, such as folding laundry, working in the yard, taking out the trash, or cleaning his or her own bedroom. However, if the instructions or tasks are very complex, it will be too frustrating for the cognitively impaired older person.

Entertainment

There will be times when individual members of the family will want to entertain friends in the home without including each other in their plans. This can be achieved by asking the other family members in advance if they can have this night just for their friends. The other family members can remain in their rooms, or arrangements can be made to care for the older person elsewhere during this time (Williams, 1985). Many families hesitate to invite friends into the home because of potential embarrassment caused by the presence of an older person with mental or behavioral problems.

Stress

The potential problems previously discussed are a source of stress for an ill older person, a caregiver, and other members of the family. Stress is a problem for the family, especially when the older person has Alzheimer's disease or a similar dementing illness that requires both physical care and emotional support. It is also very stressful when an older depressed person continually talks about suicide, particularly if another family member has comitted suicide.

Baldwin (1987) states that the responsibilities of family caregiving are accompanied by stress, strain, and perhaps a sense of burden. Physical, emotional, and financial strain begins to take its toll. There may be unresolved family issues or conflicts that influence the roles of various family members. Adult children may resent assuming the role of caregiver. It may be especially difficult for middle-aged women who care for an aging parent in addition to their own spouse, children, and sometimes grandchildren.

The physiological and psychobiological symptoms of stress in family members include changes in sleeping patterns, especially if the older parent or spouse is a restless sleeper, altered eating habits or patterns, increased blood pressure, and, with some individuals, hypertension, gastrointestinal changes or upsets, diarrhea, bouts of depression, insomnia, headaches, extreme mood swings, and in all cases, fatigue. The onset of these symptoms varies in combination and degree, but they have been identified with the time when the caregiving responsibilities began (Baldwin, 1987).

Many psychosocial stressors are identified by caregiving families, including alienation from friends and other family members not involved in direct caregiving, feelings of being abandoned by other family members who lack the desire to assist in the caregiving responsibilities, feelings of being trapped in a situation from which there is little or no relief, feelings of isolation with no one to turn to for help or understanding, and feelings of resentment, anger, and frustration over their responsibilities. The caregivers also feel that there is a marked decrease in their own participation in social activities, such as eating out and visiting with friends, taking vacations, and having friends into their home for social events (Baldwin, 1987).

Copstead and Patterson (1986) outline stressful problems associated with continuous care:

- The planning required for a substitute caregiver who is acceptable to the client whenever it is necessary to leave home
- The tension of not knowing what is going to happen to the older client in a given day, such as falls, wandering, mood changes, not eating, setting fires, developing infections
- The tension created when the older person cannot tolerate any change in schedule or environment and becomes agitated if changes occur in any activities of daily living
- The concern of how long the situation will continue and whether changes in the client's status will require placement in a nursing home or hospitalization
- Serious deprivation of other family members if major portions of funds are required for the care of the ill older person

Interpersonal tensions between the primary caregiver and the mentally ill older person or between the primary caregiver and other family members can generate stresses in daily living. The nurse should be alert to anticipate these factors, which increase the risk of these problems.

Copstead and Patterson (1986) identify situations that arise from competing, continuing demands on a primary caregiver as follows:

- Differences in perceptions of what is needed, such as the client wanting more help or contact than is feasible or actually required, or the caregiver giving more help than the client wants
- Giving of time or resources to the client to the deprivation of younger family members or spouses
- Feeling of guilt when the caregiver is unable to meet his or her own expectations of what is needed
- Conflict between expectations or values of self and others, for example, institutionalization of the client versus care at home

Some primary caregivers face a combination of these problems, regardless of whether that person is an adult child caring for parents, a sibling, or spouse.

The nurse in the home health care setting can offer care and support to families with a mentally ill older adult in the home. Family members are at high risk for developing problems in daily living associated with trying to meet their own needs and those of the dependent older adult in their care. The nurse can identify risk factors and intervene so that primary caregivers receive the support they need to provide care for those who depend on them (Copstead & Patterson, 1986).

❖ *Elder Abuse*

Feelings of frustration over the responsibilities of caring for a mentally ill older person in the home can lead to mistreatment or abuse by the caregiver. Abuse of older people is a phenomenon with identifiable causes and consequences. Individuals and family groups are extremely complicated. Different types of treatment of older people are probably caused by various combinations of personal traits of the people involved, household finances, the interpersonal relationships that have developed over time, external events that affect the household, and similar factors. The presence or absence of motivation to cause harm to an older person is a principal consideration that distinguishes some forms of mistreatment from others (Douglass, 1987; Fulmer & O'Malley, 1987).

If there has been a positive relationship in the past, it is likely that the caregiver will provide adequate care for the ill older person. However, if the past relationship has been negative or if the older adult was a child or spouse abuser, the caregiver will probably be reluctant to expend the tremendous amounts of physical and emotional energy needed to provide adequate care for the ill older family member (Copstead & Patterson, 1986).

The prevalence of violence in our society is an influence on neglect and abuse of older people. Some people have been taught that violence is a means of solving problems or resolving conflicts. When the caregiver is confronted with a new problem, the reflex may be violent or abusive behavior. This response may be a result of the caregiver's inadequate understanding of the mentally ill older person's behavior (McConnell & Matteson, 1988). "An estimated 1.5 million elderly Americans are abused each year, often by their own children. . . " (*Exposing Statistics,* 1990, p. 4). However, it is difficult to determine the exact prevalence because "states, cities, and other units of government use different definitions and reporting methods" (Douglass, 1987, p. 4).

Under Title II mandate, virtually all states have enacted adult protective services legislation to assist adults who are unable to protect their own interests and are therefore in danger of abuse, neglect, or exploitation (State Policy and Practice, 1986, p. 12; United States Department of Health, Education and Welfare, 1978). Although this is useful, it is limited to some extent because a situation must reach crisis or near-crisis proportions before any protective action occurs. To benefit from protective services intervention, the older client must generally be legally incompetent; this situation leaves the majority of older people still unprotected (Kinderknecht, 1986).

A review of the literature revealed that the words *elder abuse, battered elderly, granny battering,* and *maltreatment* are used interchangeably to refer to physical abuse, neglect, exploitation, and violation of rights of older adults (O'Rourke, 1981; Block, 1983; Giordano & Gordano, 1984). Elder maltreatment is the nonaccidental situation in which an older person suffers physical trauma, deprivation of basic physical needs, or mental injury as a result of an act or omission by a caregiver or guardian. Curry and Stone (1994) have defined the following types of elder maltreatment: physical abuse, physical neglect, psychological abuse, psychological neglect, material abuse, material neglect, active maltreatment, passive maltreatment, violation of personal rights, self-abuse, self-neglect, domestic maltreatment, and institutional maltreatment.

All 50 states have laws or policies that govern elder abuse or suspected abuse, and 49 have reporting systems established by statutes. Fourteen states require anyone with a knowledge of or reasonable cause to believe that an abuse incident has occurred to report it. States differ in their definition of abuse and their requirements for reporting. It is imperative that nurses know the definition of abuse, neglect, and exploitation in their states and know where to report it. In some states the penalty for failing to report abuse is $1000 and 1 to 6 months' imprisonment (State Policy and Practice, 1986).

The most common forms of abuse are physical abuse, neglect, psychological abuse, violation of rights, and exploitation (Kimsey, Tarbox, & Bragg, 1981; Valentine & Cash, 1986; Goldstein, 1987). Examples of physical abuse are burns, beatings, and hittings that cause bruises and fractures. Neglect can be lack of food, medicines, and other essential necessities of living. Some older persons who live alone, especially those with mental illness, often suffer from self-neglect and need to be reported to a community agency such as Adult Protective Services if no family or friends are available to help them. Psychological abuse involves name calling, verbal assaults, threats, and social isolation. Examples of violation of rights include lack of privacy and lack of information or consent related to medical treatment and care. A common example of exploitation is using older persons' resources, such as selling their personal possessions or cashing their Social Security checks for one's own use without the older person's consent.

Prevention of Abuse

Abuse of older family members in the home is the result of many contributing factors that must be recognized in order to prevent it. Most caregivers are initially capable of meeting the needs of the dependent person, but they become overwhelmed by increasing frailty of the dependent person, additional disabilities, their own illness, or a combination of these problems. Neglect can be the first consequence of the caregiver's fatigue and frustration, which can lead to abuse or physical harm. Prevention requires making alternative plans in advance for providing care, not when the caregiver's ability begins to be inadequate (Douglass, 1987).

Primary Prevention
Primary prevention of abuse is possible only when the causes of a specific type of mistreatment are clearly understood and predictable. These cases may include the physical disability of the caregiver, a history of family violence, alcohol abuse by the caregiver or the dependent, exhaustion of the family's financial resources, or an emotional or psychiatric problem of the caregiver. A combination of causes increases the chances for mistreatment. Few sources can furnish information needed to anticipate situations in which mistreatment might occur. The extended family can be

instrumental in preventing neglect or abuse by recognizing the possibility of such mistreatment and taking action immediately. Much of the responsibility for primary prevention rests on individuals who act in their own best interests (Douglass, 1987).

Secondary Prevention

Nurses should observe family interactions closely and assess older clients carefully for possible abuse during home visits. Older people often do not report abuse because they fear abandonment or retaliation from the caregivers. If intervention becomes necessary, it can include a plan for preventing further abuse, which is called secondary prevention. Secondary prevention efforts include initial recognition of cases with low levels of damage and the introduction of training, counseling, personal assistance, respite for caregivers, or crisis intervention to protect the life or property of a victim. Preventive activities can be initiated to limit or eliminate the risk of someone becoming a victim of abuse or to limit or eliminate the risk of someone becoming neglectful of or abusive to another person (Douglass, 1987).

❖ *Family Support*

Many families feel alone in their care of a mentally ill person. The situation seems intolerable and the future appears bleak, empty, and meaningless. It is not unusual for family caregivers to feel sad, discouraged, alone, angry, guilty, tired, or depressed (Mace and Rabins, 1991). Mental health professionals agree that time spent with an older person's family as well as the identified client facilitates coping and positive outcomes. Psychologists, social workers, psychiatric nurses, clergy, and other professionals have excellent therapeutic and counseling skills. Talking about feelings and problems helps to clarify them. A good counselor can help to separate the problem into more manageable parts and help the family members to understand their feelings. Then the family will be able to continue their care of the ill older adult.

The Family Medical Leave Act passed by Congress in 1993 will allow some employed family caregivers to take an unpaid leave of absence of up to 12 weeks to care for an ill family member in the home. While 12 weeks is not very long when considering the care needed for a chronically mentally ill older person in the home, it may give the caregiver some time to help an older family member who is beginning to have mental problems get a diagnosis and beginning treatment or to provide the caregiver time to be with a family member in the last stages of Alzheimer's disease.

❖ *Care of the Caregivers*

The older person's well-being depends on the well-being of the caregiver. It is essential for the caregiver to find ways to care for himself or herself and not exhaust his or her own emotional and physical resources (Mace & Rabins, 1991). The emotional burdens of providing care tend to be greater than the physical or financial costs, since most caregivers sacrifice their own leisure time, vacations, and privacy. As a result of multiple responsibilities, stress and depression become major problems for caregivers. Caregivers need to be alert to signs of stress and depression that take their toll on those providing care. These are some of the warning signs for stress and depression:

- ◆ Loss of energy or fatigue
- ◆ Difficulties with concentration
- ◆ Neglect of vital physical needs
- ◆ Uncharacteristic crying or agitation
- ◆ Difficulty sleeping at night
- ◆ Increased use of sleeping medications, alcohol, or caffeine
- ◆ Decreased resistance to illness
- ◆ Marked changes in appetite
- ◆ Signs of impatience in giving care

These signs usually develop gradually and can remain unrecognized in caregivers for long periods. For example, a caregiver may wake up early in the morning, dreading to face the day. A short temper caused by fatigue may cause the caregiver to yell at the older person for trivial reasons. The caregiver maintains a frenetic pace to accomplish everything that needs to be done. The caregiver may refuse to allow anyone else to help with the care, feeling that the older person would be upset by anyone else's care. At night the caregiver falls into bed exhausted but is unable to sleep, thinking of the many problems in the family. Despite good intentions, the caregiver may eventually harm the older person and the family. Unrealistic expectations about handling multiple demands, the reluctance to accept help, and refusal to take time off are common causes of stress and depression among caregivers.

Support Groups

Support groups have become an increasingly important counseling resource. These groups are a vital link in the network for families caring for a mentally ill older person in the home. These groups meet on a regular basis to provide mutual support for persons with similar concerns. According to Ebersole and Hess (1994), support groups help the families (1) find a balance of responsibility between self, children, and parents, (2) make decisions about duties and obligations to parents and how these decisions can be facilitated, and (3) deal with parents in a mature way by letting go of residual conflicts, rebellions, and hurts.

Various national and local organizations help caregivers and their families understand the problems and assist them in caring for chronically mentally ill older persons. The Alzheimer's Association, founded in 1980, is a privately funded national not-for-profit health organization. The association has more than 1600 support groups and 215 chapters and affiliates nationwide. It promotes public awareness and serves as a clearinghouse for information pertaining to Alzheimer's disease. "The Alzheimer's Association is the oldest and largest national voluntary health organization dedicated to research for the causes, cure and prevention of Alzheimer's disease and to providing education and support services to Alzheimer patients, their families and caregivers" (Alzheimer's Disease and Related Disorders Association, 1993, p. 2). There are similar national and local support groups for families who care for a person with Parkinson's disease.

Education Groups

A number of educational programs help caregivers and their families learn how to cope with aging family members. These programs provide specific information about the aging process and facilitate communication among caregivers who can share their problems, concerns, and sources of support. One such group is Children of Aging Parents (CAPS) which provides lists of support groups for different states and caregiving booklets (see Appendix G). These groups meet routinely to assist adult caregivers in better understanding the behavior and problems of their aging parents.

Respite Care

Relief from the unrelenting responsibility of caring for a chronically mentally ill older person can be provided by planned periods of respite. "The single most important service we can give families . . . is respite" (Baldwin, 1990, p. 173). Respite care encompasses a wide range of services for both those who give care and those who receive it. These services may involve simply sitting with the older person for an hour or so or direct physical care over time if needed. Respite care provides support to the family member by providing some time to be away from the mentally ill older family member. Caregivers need to get away periodically to renew their energy. "The awareness that the caregiver is an 'invisible victim' has grown" (Baldwin, 1990, p. 173). An example of respite care is a program of the Visiting Nurse Association in Fort Worth, Texas, that provides home health aides to stay with a patient with Alzheimer's disease in the home for a few hours during the week to allow the caregiver some relief. Payment is on a sliding scale. The Visiting Nurse Association also provides care to clients with Alzheimer's disease while family members attend monthly program meetings of the local Alzheimer's Association. This type of care is free at the site of the meeting.

The type of respite care provided is based on the physical and psychological needs of the dependent person and on the convenience, availability, and cost of the service. Respite care can be delivered in the home or in institutional settings such as adult day care centers, nursing homes, and acute care hospitals. "All respite programs appear to have a common goal: delaying institutionalization" (Rosenheimer & Francis, 1992, p. 22).

Short-term respite care is available to persons who have qualified for the hospice care benefit under Medicare. For example, individuals in the later stages of Alzheimer's disease in a hospice program may be admitted to an inpatient facility for "no more than 5 days in a row," giving temporary relief to the person who regularly gives care in the home (The Medicare 1994 Handbook, 1994, p. 19).

One unique, innovative program of respite care for families of clients with

Alzheimer's disease was developed in California (Rosenheimer & Francis, 1992). This program provided short-term overnight respite for caregivers. Although the respite unit was in a county hospital, the care was to be essentially the same as that delivered at home. Care was provided by personal care attendants with nurse supervision and emergency care available if needed. A total program was available (for example, nutrition, medications, activities). They also developed an outreach program for referral of families to other resources in the community.

One of the major problems was attempting to provide homelike care in a hospital setting. For example, clients brought their medications from home, but they often did not match the physician's orders, so personnel were reluctant to give them. One of the reasons for the discrepancy was that "Alzheimer's clients see their personal physicians infrequently because families perceived little need for regular visits for a condition that was supposedly untreatable" (Rosenheimer & Francis, 1991, p. 25).

Also, staff found it difficult to allow clients to wander at night, sleep on the floor, or launder clothes soiled by incontinence (personal clothing could not be sent to the hospital laundry). However, those were exactly the reasons the clients were there, to give the caregiver a rest from these activities at home. Another problem was that the more affluent caregivers did not want to take their family member to a county hospital. Although an excellent program, use was lower than anticipated and there was lack of long-term funding, so the program closed after almost 3 years.

Volunteer Short-Term Programs

The family may want to find individuals who will volunteer to provide care in the home for the older person on a short-term basis. Inquiries could be made with friends, neighbors, church groups, or social organizations to find persons who will stay with the mentally ill older person on a volunteer basis for several hours. If the responsibilities for care are rotated among several neighbors and friends, no one individual is pressured.

It may become necessary to secure and pay for the services of a visiting nurse association or other home health care agency to provide homemaker, personal care, and adult-sitter services in the home. These services include physical care, chore services, food preparation, laundry, light housework, and grocery shopping (Copstead & Patterson, 1986; Mace & Rabins, 1991).

Adult Day Care

In some communities, adult day care centers offer several hours a day of structured recreation for older people with limited abilities. Adult day care centers provide a variety of health, social, and related support services in a protected setting; however, they vary with regard to type of staff, services offered, and clients accepted. Payment for care depends on the facility and its funding source. A client may pay privately, usually on a sliding scale. Services may be paid by a federal or state government agency according to eligibility regulations. Some day care centers may have a nurse or social worker on staff. Through the day care center program, confused people can receive a hot midday meal, some form of exercise program, and mental stimulation within their own capabilities. They frequently seem to enjoy life more, sleep better, and be more manageable at home once they are established in a day care program. It may be difficult to find adequate day care centers for people with severe mental impairment or who wander or cannot follow directions. However, a few adult day care centers specialize in the care of older adults with Alzheimer's disease. Some centers specialize in stroke patients, older alcoholics, or patients who can be rehabilitated (Copstead & Patterson, 1986; Eide, Steffl, & Burnside, 1988; Mace & Rabins, 1991).

Nursing Homes

Another method of obtaining respite care for the caregiver is to admit the older person to a 24-hour facility (usually a nursing home) for a time. Some nursing homes will consider a short-term stay for an older person when the family needs respite care. By using this program, a family would be able to attend a family reunion, go out of town on business or vacation, or accomplish other necessary tasks. Occasionally, the nursing home program could be used in an emergency, for example, when the caregiver becomes ill or hospitalized (Copstead & Patterson, 1986).

Regardless of the type of respite care selected, it is important for the caregiver to get out of the house or leave the client to get some benefit from this source of relief. The outcome of a break in the responsibilities through the respite care program may be an improvement in a relationship that is important to both the caregiver and the mentally ill older person (Copstead & Patterson, 1986).

Respite care programs are not used as much as they could be. "As a whole, respite care has not been embraced by the community" (Rosenheimer & Francis, 1992, 29), in terms of understanding, use by families, or funding. Caregivers are often reluctant to let go, even for a few hours or days. They may see it as a last resort, believe that they should give the care, feel guilty about meeting their own needs, not want a stranger in their home, or be unable to afford the cost (Rosenheimer & Francis, 1992, 28). However, respite care will most likely increase with a greater emphasis on community and home-based care in the changing health care delivery system. Home care is generally more satisfying to the older person and the family as well as less expensive if assistance is available on a part-time basis. More community groups such as social organizations and churches should be made aware of this great need for volunteer respite services that could be provided by their members.

❖ *Summary*

The increase in human life expectancy and thus the number of frail older adults will result in a substantial increase in the number of families who provide long-term care to chronically ill older family members. Psychopathology is a serious problem for persons aged 65 and older. Older persons with functional psychiatric disorders and those who have dementia comprise up to 25% of the older population. Some type of dementia, such as Alzheimer's disease, is the most common mental health problem of older clients in the home. The major responsibility for care of the older relative tends to be provided by middle-aged female family members.

A thorough assessment of the older person and the family, including the patterns of daily living, demands on the caregiver and needs of the client, and the available internal and external resources, provides the nurse in the home setting with data on which to base nursing care. The nurse, together with the family members, formulates the nursing diagnoses, goals, and interventions for which each member will be responsible. The overall goal is to restore or maintain effective management of daily living for the entire family.

The family as a whole is affected in different ways by an ill older person living in the home. Changes in relationships, roles, and responsibilities require adjustments in lifestyle by all family members. Potential problems include insufficient financial resources, insufficient space, and inadequate home environment, all of which are a source of psychosocial stress for the family members. Caregivers express feelings of alienation from friends and from other family members who are not involved in direct caregiving. Often caregivers feel abandoned by other family members who lack the desire to assist in the caregiving responsibilities. They also have feelings of isolation, resentment, anger, and frustration over the responsibilities.

Stress and the emotional responses of the caregiver can result in mistreatment or abuse of the chronically mentally ill older adult. The extended family can be instrumental in preventing neglect or abuse by recognizing the possibility of such mistreatment and taking immediate action. Prevention activities such as education and counseling for the caregiver can limit or eliminate the risk of the client becoming a victim of neglect or abuse.

Family support includes nurses, counselors, and other health-related professionals to assist the family in managing the depression and discouragement that result from caring for a mentally ill older person in the home. These people can assist the family in understanding their feelings and enable the family to continue the care. Caregivers must understand that they cannot do everything alone in caring for the older adult, but must care for themselves, having time away from the client for rest and renewal. Other family members or outside help should be sought to assume some of the responsibilities of everyday care of the client.

Support and educational groups are invaluable in assisting the caregiver to voice feelings and to obtain information about the disease and problems inherent in caring for an ill older adult. Respite care is a means of obtaining outside help in performing the caring responsibilities. This care can consist of finding volunteers to perform the care for short periods in the home, adult day care centers, or admitting the older person to a nursing home for a time to allow the caregiver and the family some relief from the responsibilities of caring for the chronically mentally ill older family member in the home.

❖ *References*

Alzheimer's Disease and Related Disorders Association, Inc. (1993). *Alzheimer's disease: Fact sheet*. Chicago: Author.

Atchley, R. C. (1994). *Social forces and aging* (7th ed.). Belmont, CA: Wadsworth.

Baldwin, B. A. (1987). The family caregiving role: Stresses and effective coping. In H. J. Altman (Ed.). *Alzheimer's disease: Problems, prospects and perspectives.* New York: Plenum Press.

Baldwin, B. A. (1990). Family caregiving: Trends and forecasts. *Geriatric Nursing, 11*(4), 172-174.

Block, M. D. (1983). Abuse of the elderly. In S. H. Kadish (Ed.). *Encyclopedia of crime and justice* (pp. 1635-1637). New York: Free Press.

Buckwalter, K. C., & Stolley, J. (1991). Managing mentally ill elders at home. *Geriatric Nursing, 12*(3), 136-139.

Carpenito, L. J. (1993). *Nursing diagnosis: Application to clinical practice* (5th ed.). Philadelphia: Lippincott.

Copstead, L. E., & Patterson, S. (1986). Families of the elderly. In D. L. Carnevali & M. Patrick (Eds.). *Nursing management for the elderly* (2nd ed., pp. 219-227). Philadelphia: Lippincott.

Curry, L. C., & Stone, J. G. (1994). Maltreatment of older adults. In M. O. Hogstel (Ed.). *Nursing care of the older adult* (3rd ed., pp. 468-518). Albany, N.Y.: Delmar

Douglass, R. L. (1987). *Domestic mistreatment of the elderly: Towards prevention.* Washington, DC: American Association of Retired Persons.

Ebersole, P., & Hess, P. (1994). *Toward healthy aging: Human needs and the nursing response* (4th ed.). St. Louis: Mosby.

Eide, I., Steffl, B., & Burnside, I. (1988). Community care. In I. Burnside (Ed.). *Nursing and the aged: A self-care approach* (3rd ed., pp. 950-983). New York: McGraw-Hill.

Exposing statistics on elders as victims. (1990, May 1). *Fort Worth Star Telegram,* Sec. 5, p. 4.

Fulmer, T. T., & O'Malley, T. A. (1987). *Inadequate care of the elderly: A health care perspective on abuse and neglect.* New York: Springer.

Giordano, J. A., & Gordano, N. H. (1984). Elder abuse: A review of literature. *Social Work, 29,* 232-236.

Goldstein, R. K. (1987). *Violence in the home: 2. Battered parents and the battered elderly.* Belle Mead, NJ: Carrier Foundation Letter #126.

Harper, M. S., & Gilchrist, A. (1988). A study of mental health needs of the elderly in home health care settings. Unpublished report. Rockville, MD.

Hooyman, N. R., & Lustbader, W. (1986). *Taking care of your aging family members.* New York: The Free Press.

Kimsey, L. R., Tarbox, A. R., & Bragg, D. F. (1981). Abuse of the elderly: The hidden agenda, the caretakers and the categories of abuse. *Journal of the American Geriatrics Society, 29*(10), 465-472.

Kinderknecht, C. H. (1986). In home social work with abused or neglected elderly: An experiential guide to assessment and treatment. *Journal of Gerontological Social Work, 9,* 29-42.

Mace, N. L., & Rabins, P. V. (1991). *The 36-hour day: A family guide to caring for persons with Alzheimer's disease, related dementing illnesses, and memory loss in later life* (revised ed.). Baltimore: Johns Hopkins University.

McConnell, E. S. (1988a). Nursing diagnoses related to psychosocial alterations. In M. A. Matteson & E. S. McConnell (Eds.). *Gerontological nursing concepts and practice* (pp. 528-586). Philadelphia: Saunders.

McConnell, E. S. (1988b). Nursing diagnoses influenced by setting of care. In M. A.

Matteson & E. S. McConnell (Eds.). *Gerontological nursing concepts and practice* (pp. 686-719). Philadelphia: Saunders.

McConnell, E. S., & Matteson, M. A. (1988). Psychosocial problems associated with aging. In M. A. Matteson & E. S. McConnell (Eds.). *Gerontological nursing concepts and practice* (pp. 480-527). Philadelphia: Saunders.

The Medicare 1994 handbook. (1994). Health Care Financing Administration (HCFA 10050). Baltimore: U.S. Department of Health and Human Services.

O'Rourke, M. (1981, March 23-25). *Elder abuse: The state of the art.* Paper presented at the National Conference on the Abuse of Older Persons, Boston.

Rathbone-McCuan, E., & Voyles, B. (1982). Case detection of abused elderly parents. *American Journal of Psychiatry, 139*(2), 189-192.

Rosenheimer, L., & Francis, E. M. (1992). Feasible without subsidy? Overnight respite for Alzheimer's. *Journal of Gerontological Nursing, 18*(4), 21-29.

State policy and practice related to elder abuse (elder abuse project). (1986). Washington, DC: American Public Welfare Association, p. 12.

U.S. Department of Health, Education and Welfare. (1978, December). *Public policy and the frail elderly.* Washington, DC: Author.

Valentine, D., & Cash, T. (1986). A definitional discussion of elder maltreatment. *Journal of Gerontological Social Work, 9*(3), 17-27.

Williams, S. D. (1985). The role of the family in home helath care. In M. O. Hogstel (Ed.), *Home nursing care for the elderly* (pp. 45-65). Bowie, MD: Brady Communications.

Chapter *13*

❖ *Community Programs*

Kathleen C. Buckwalter
Kay Weiler
Jacqueline Stolley

The changing demographics and economics of aging have forced a reconceptualization of care of geropsychiatric clients from that of exclusively institutional settings to the broader community perspective. The community approach to care mandates a system in which the needs of older psychiatric clients are articulated with an appropriate mix of services, many of which are examined in this chapter. The system of community programs should ensure that geropsychiatric clients receive the least restrictive care in an affordable manner. Thus, mentally ill older adults should be protected from premature and inappropriate placement in long-term care facilities if adequate home care, community programs, and other supportive services are available. It has been estimated that between 25% and 40% of the residents of long-term care facilities, many of whom have emotional or cognitive disabilities, do not need to be in such facilities. This unfortunate circumstance can be rectified only by the increasing availability of a range of alternative programs and care services in the community. This chapter presents an overview of the community services needed by geropsychiatric clients, identifies common barriers to the use of community-based mental health services by older adults, and examines a number of community programs that have overcome those barriers, including outreach programs, day care, case management services, peer counseling, prevention programs (bereavement groups), respite programs, projects for the homeless, self-help groups, supportive transportation and nutritional services such as home-delivered meals, phone-a-friend programs, friendly visitors, and programs sponsored by area agencies on aging and the Council on Aging. Area agencies on aging frequently supply information and referral services to assist older persons and their caregivers obtain appropriate services. These agencies may also coordinate services to prevent fragmentation and duplication of services as well as to improve continuity of care.

❖ *Overview of Service and Research Needs*

Ideally, community services for geropsychiatric clients and their families are comprehensive, including an array of residential and treatment settings that complement rather than impede the efforts of informal support networks such as family and neighbors (Bachrach, 1986). In most cases treatment for mentally ill older adults should be multidimensional, multidisciplinary, and long term (Bellack & Mueser, 1986) and should integrate client and family needs with those of treatment programs (Shern, Wilson, Ellis, Bartsch, & Coen, 1986). As noted in a report of the White House Conference on Aging (1981, pp. 112-121), there is widespread agreement that a long-term care system should promote the independence of the person in making decisions and in performing everyday activities. It should encourage support services in the least restrictive environment, preferably at home or in other community settings. It should try to make available appropriate, cost-effective, accessible, and humane care to all persons who need it while supporting the care provided by family and friends. For chronically impaired individuals who must receive care in nursing homes and institutional settings, it should ensure the quality of their care and seek to maximize their quality of life. Finally, public policy for long-term care should make maximum use of family, community, and other private sector initiatives to achieve these objectives.

Certainly this section of the White House Conference on Aging report sets the stage for discussion of the concept of a continuum of care for mentally ill older adults. The report clearly suggests that every older person who needs long-term care, mental, physical, or both, is entitled to receive it. The continuum may be viewed as having two complementary groups of services for older persons: first, supportive services not directly related to health but of great significance in the lives of most older persons, and second, more direct health-related services (Morris, 1987).

For effective continuity of care, geropsychiatric clients need access to a variety of community-based services—services that provide for both sustenance and growth. Examples of supportive services necessary to foster independent community living include information and referral, transportation, nutrition, telephone, friendly visitation, housing (low-rent public housing and group homes), legal and protective services, comprehensive senior centers and recreation, handyman and chore services, homemaking, and sheltered employment (Morris, 1987).

The continuum of health-related services for older adults includes outreach or case-finding services, comprehensive assessment services, primary medical, dental, and nursing services, home health care, adult day care centers, residential care facilities, intermediate care facilities, skilled nursing facilities, outpatient and inpatient rehabilitation (day hospital) units, respite care, and hospices.

The availability and accessibility of these services vary greatly from setting to setting, and some have eligibility requirements. Also, some mentally ill older clients may resist these services. Geropsychiatric nurses should conduct research on the use of these services where they are available, on alternative modes of service delivery, particularly in rural settings, and on reluctance and barriers to use of community-based services by impaired older persons. If resistance to service utilization is widespread, the problem must be addressed and innovative delivery mechanisms developed and tested.

Despite the recommendations of the White House Conference on Aging report, at present long-term home health care and other nonhospital, community-based services are not sufficiently available, nor are the funds to meet the needs of the Medicare population adequate (Kelly, Shea, & Ross, 1987). These inadequacies contribute to morbidity and recidivism among geropsychiatric clients discharged from acute care settings in particular. Nursing research efforts must also be directed toward determining whether older mentally ill clients and their families would use in-home care services if such services were more widely available and less costly. In addition, researchers should determine whether such home care services would help to delay or prevent institutionalization. The best method of assuring quality of care for home care services has yet to be decided. Also, the extent to which home care services support the informal caregiving network of family, friends, and neighbors is not yet clear. In terms of cost effectiveness, researchers must evaluate whether home care services substitute for informal caregiving and thus add to the financial burden of local, state, and federal governments (Haber, 1986).

❖ *Barriers to Utilization of Community Mental Health Services by Older Adults*

Mentally ill older adults are an underserved population. Historically they have always received the poorest and most restrictive types of care (Gatz, Smyer, & Lawton, 1980). Today aged persons receive mental health services at less than one fourth the rate of persons 25 to 44 years old despite their demonstrated need for such services.

Epidemiological studies suggest that between 15% and 25% of persons over the age of 65 need some form of mental health services (Kermis, 1986; Roybal, 1984). More than 25% of those who commit suicide in the United States are age 65 or older, and these statistics are probably an underestimate of the true incidence of suicide (Pfeiffer, 1977). Suicide rates for older adults rose from 17.1 per 100,000 in 1981 to 21.5 per 100,000 in 1986 (Brandt & Osgood, 1990). Furthermore, the risk of institutionalization for both mental and physical conditions increases with age; 25% of older people living in the community and 50% of those in institutions take some form of psychoactive medication (Peterson, 1983).

Community mental health services have been largely unresponsive to the needs of older people as reflected in the following statistics:

◆ Only about 6% of clients in outpatient community mental health centers (CMHCs) are older adults (Hagebak & Hagebak, 1983).

◆ Fewer than 7% of older people receive private psychiatric services (Kermis, 1986).

◆ The lowest rate of increase in the use of CMHC services has been among older people (Hagebak & Hagebak, 1983).

◆ Less than 1% of the total time given to psychiatric patients in CMHCs is provided to older clients (Mental Health and Aging, 1982).

◆ Fewer than 18% of CMHCs have created any kind of special geriatric program. Current caseloads are far below the known need.

These statistics, along with what is known about the incidence of mental disorders in older adults, suggest that community-based treatment of older people has not increased to keep pace with their needs (Buckwalter, 1986). Some of the barriers to use of mental health services by older people, including societal and professional biases, organizational and structural barriers, and the attitudes of older persons themselves, are examined in the following sections.

Societal Biases

Ageism, or negative and prejudicial attitudes about older adults (Butler, 1968), is an important factor contributing to poor mental health services for older people. Ageism implies that psychiatric illness is an inevitable part of aging, that mental illness in older adults is irreversible, and that opportunities for therapeutic success are extremely limited (therapeutic nihilism). This attitude is perhaps best reflected in the large quantities of medications prescribed for older adults, often merely as a stopgap measure.

It is important that psychiatric nurses and other health professionals become sensitized to aging issues and recognize their personal biases. Gerontophobia, or fear of aging, is still prevalent in the United States, especially in our youth-glorifying Pepsi generation culture. Furthermore, the media reflect our culture and reinforce many of the myths and ageist biases pervasive in our society. Older persons continue to be featured in negative or stereotypical ways, particularly in advertisements for prunes, laxatives, pain formulas, vitamins, denture adhesives, and life insurance.

Biases of the Mental Health Profession

The mental health establishment has traditionally concerned itself primarily with the needs of the young. Until recently few concepts, goals, or evaluation criteria had been developed regarding the mental health needs of the aged. A conceptual base for mental health and aging was lacking, and until the 1970s there were few attempts to define mental health with respect to aging.

The societal attitude toward aging (that it is dismal to grow old) has been largely shared by mental health professionals (Pfeiffer, 1977). Health care professionals must recognize the heterogeneity of the older adult population and avoid stereotypical images of elders (Ory, 1989). Often there is little motivation or incentive for psychiatric nurses and other professionals to work with the aged, many of whom they consider unpleasant crocks to be avoided. Working with older people is still unprestigious, and many health professionals believe that the aged are the least deserving when it comes to the distribution of resources and services (Kermis, 1987; Pfeiffer, 1977).

Traditionally, psychiatric thinking in the United States has been influenced by Freud, who had little interest in older adults because he believed that their emotional disturbances were not subject to modification. Kaufman (1940, p. 74) quotes Freud as follows:

Near and above the 50's, the elasticity of the mental processes on which treatment depends is, as a rule, lacking. Old people are no longer educable, and on the other hand, the mass of material to be dealt with would prolong the duration of treatment indefinitely.

Furthermore, there are insufficient numbers of mental health professionals, including psychiatric nurses, trained to work with older adults. However, some important changes have occurred in gerontological nursing in the past decade, especially in North America. These changes include a new focus on maximizing the older persons' capacity throughout the aging process. The Council on Gerontological Nursing, a division of the American Nurses' Association, has published its own standards of practice (American Nurses' Association, 1987). The need for nurses prepared in geropsychiatric nursing continues, however. If only 10% of the population age 65 and older (an underestimate) require the services of a geriatric mental health nurse, the number of such persons in need of services is 3,230,000. If the more reasonable 20% need estimate is applied, the estimated number of such persons in need of mental health services is 6,460,000. Clearly, when these figures are compared with the actual number of psychiatric nurses who work with older patients, the picture is bleak. Geriatric mental health nurses must be recruited, educated, and have their services reorganized if even present demands are to be met.

Similar shortages and lack of appropriate education and training are evident among other geriatric team members, including geropsychiatrists; psychologists; social workers; dentists; speech, occupational, and physical therapists; and pharmacists.

Organizational and Structural Barriers

Mental health professionals are not solely responsible for the failure to provide adequate community mental health services to the older population. The entire mental health system requires scrutiny and reassessment. Many barriers are organizational or structural in nature and are rooted in our laws and reimbursement regulations. For example, Medicare coverage is noticeably skewed against reimbursement for outpatient mental health care and has shortcomings in other reimbursement and support programs that relate to older clients. The system also lacks enough alternative living arrangements for older people, which often results in inappropriate nursing home placement and other forms of institutionalization.

The United States needs a federal policy commitment to build mental health programs for older adults, combined with a transfer of money from custodial care programs to home care and rehabilitation programs for older persons (Walz & Elliot, 1983). Currently 85% of mental health care for the aged is provided in inpatient settings (Kermis, 1987). Prospective payment systems such as diagnostic related groups (DRGs) and resource utilization groups (RUGs) will probably further reduce services provided to older Americans. The average length of stay in an acute care hospital has decreased 5.6 days since 1968 and an additional 2.1 days since 1980 (Fowles, 1993). Harlow and Wilson (1985) noted that after the institution of DRGs, area agencies on aging encountered increased demands for services from older clients discharged from acute care settings, including a 365% increase in case management services, a 196% increase in skilled in-home nursing services, and a 63% increase in personal care services. Under the RUG system, low reimbursement rates for the mentally impaired and physically frail, especially those with behavioral problems, confusion, and diminished ability to perform activities of daily living, may restrict their access to health care as they become economically less desirable clients (Kermis, 1987). As a result mentally compromised older adults are inappropriately shunted to adult homes, emergency rooms, and programs for the homeless.

DRGs in particular are based on an acute care model of disease and care. It is not appropriate for chronically mentally ill older persons, who often need prolonged treatment in a variety of settings including family-based and protective care settings. At present inpatient psychiatric services are exempt from DRGs. However, for the psychiatric patient admitted to a medical service, DRGs may prevent appropriate medical and nursing intervention unless otherwise documented by a psychiatrist. Medicare will cover psychiatric services in the home for older persons if they are homebound, have the appropriate diagnosis, and have orders for in-home services written by a psychiatrist. In summary, these prospective payment systems are potentially very damaging to mental health services for older clients (Kermis, 1987).

Medicaid and Medicare (which consumes 90% of the federal health care budget) reimbursement guidelines also require revision so that they no longer discriminate against mental health treatment. Coverage should be extended to include CMHC services, unlimited reimbursement for outpatient services, reductions in copayment percentages, and extension of mental health inpatient coverage comparable to that allocated for physical problems (Walz & Elliot, 1983). At present, Medicare is woefully inadequate in its coverage of psychiatric care for older patients; furthermore, unless waivers are obtained, mental health services can only be provided by psychiatrists or psychologists working under their authorization. Psychiatric nurses practicing autonomously are ineligible for Medicare reimbursement (Kermis, 1987). Basically federal reimbursement policies have "limited the development and use of community-based alternatives" and have encouraged "institutional placement outside the mental health system (or family) for older persons" (Kermis, 1987, p. 273). Further, the narrow physician-oriented view of professional autonomy seriously limits access to services for many older people, especially those in rural environments, and encouraged "the use of inappropriate and costly health care services" (Kermis, 1987, p. 273). Walz and Elliot (1983) note that "Federal policy should recognize the interplay of medical, social, and psychiatric problems and provide the elderly with aid in paying for medical and mental treatment" (p. 103). Psychiatric nurses can no longer afford only to react to enacted legislation. Instead they must actively apply clinical and research findings to the formation of health care policy. Without the support of policymakers, even the most innovative and effective mental health programs cannot fulfill their potential.

It is hoped that health care reform under development will help to alleviate problems associated with inadequate community services. Medicare part B helps to pay for covered services received from clinical nurse specialists and nurse practitioners in certain facilities or in certain locations in collaboration with a physician (The Medicare Handbook, 1994, p. 23), and state boards of nursing are further defining the role of the advanced practice nurse.

Attitudes of Older Adults

Older adults must also take some responsibility for their situation because they have traditionally done little to promote their needs with respect to mental health. Some of the attitudes and factors that contribute to their underutilization of services include the following (Hagebak & Hagebak, 1983):

- ◆ Accessibility problems, especially limited transportation
- ◆ Decreased financial resources
- ◆ Lack of awareness of services available within the community
- ◆ Feeling stigmatized, including the notion that emotional problems indicate personal weakness or just punishment
- ◆ Belief that confusion and mental illness are natural by-products of aging
- ◆ Feelings of hopelessness and worthlessness that no type of services can overcome problems

The older adult cohort in general is not accustomed to talking therapies or discussing their feelings with others. In fact, older persons tend to somaticize their emotional problems, and more than 80% go to a primary care physician rather than a mental health professional when they have difficulties. As a result, many underlying psychiatric disorders are masked by physical complaints and are treated with sedatives or hypnotics by uninformed practitioners. However, research has shown that older adults can be just as responsive to cognitive and behavioral interventions, and even psychodynamic approaches, as other clients.

❖ *Implications for Geropsychiatric Nursing Services*

Care of older adults and their families must be evaluated against the overall criterion of continuity of care, a concept that mandates access to a variety of medical, psychiatric, and supportive services over an unknown, unpredictable, and changing clinical course. If possible, the older client and the family should be treated together, because a change in status of one family member affects all family members. Continuity of care is currently more an ideal than a reality. Most mental health service delivery systems are fragmented and characterized by unrelated agencies variously involved in the care of older clients and their families. As Bachrach notes, continuity of care can be achieved "only when there exists true access to needed services" (1986, p. 171). She sets forth four dimensions essential to continuity of care and relevant to psychiatric services: (1) longitudinal access—because of the long-term nature of many psychiatric illnesses, services must be available over long periods; (2) psychological access—systems of care must be easily accessible and helpful and leave older clients and their families with positive feelings about their use; (3) financial access—older clients and their families must be able to pay for needed services; and (4) geographical access—older clients and their families must be able to get where care is provided or the services must be taken to them (Bachrach, 1986, p. 171). Achievement of these access dimensions is one yardstick against which psychiatric nurses can measure current and proposed mental health delivery systems.

In summary, overcoming these societal, professional, organizational, and structural barriers to use of mental health services by older adults is a difficult task, one compounded by the temptation (in light of reduced funding for many CMHCs) to reduce specialized services rather than to expand them. The next section of this chapter addresses solutions to some of the problems and examines strategies and community programs designed to improve the delivery of mental health services to older adults.

❖ *Community-Based Strategies and Programs for Geropsychiatric Clients*

Outreach Programs

Outreach programs provide an effective approach for delivery of services to geropsychiatric clients, particularly mentally ill older adults in rural environments, because those most at risk do not come to mental health and social service agencies (Toseland, Decker, & Bliesner, 1979). Outreach programs can diagnose and treat homebound clients with physical limitations or major psychiatric illnesses who are socially isolated or who have a combination of problems. Outreach has proved helpful in treating geropsychiatric clients who might not otherwise enter mental health programs until a crisis necessitates hospitalization (Wasson et al., 1984).

Evaluations of outreach programs in the literature suggest that they provide rapid and effective mental health assessment and treatment and minimize disruptions caused by premature institutionalization of older clients (Reifler et al., 1982).

One effective outreach program, the Mental Health of the Rural Elderly Outreach Project (EOP), was implemented at the Abbe Center for Community Mental Health in Linn County, Iowa, and is briefly described as a model for such community-based outreach programs.

EOP was designed to identify older persons in need of mental health care, to deliver services, and to initiate and coordinate referrals to appropriate medical and social service agencies. EOP addresses the problem of inadequate mental health services and inappropriate hospitalization by taking services to the people most in need of them, mentally ill older adults. It also addresses another service delivery problem that is especially common in rural areas, the sparse concentration of mental health professionals. In EOP, persons in need of mental health, medical, and social services are identified through a combination of five approaches (Fig. 13-1): (1) psychosocial screening at local sites, such as congregate meals; (2) referrals through the county case management team and its associated agencies (see description of case management later in this section); (3) training of nontraditional referral sources, known as gatekeepers, such as mail carriers and meter readers, to locate and refer high-risk persons; (4) mental health outreach specialists who serve as liaisons between EOP and service agencies in the community; and (5) contact with discharge planning departments of mental health and health care institutions in the community. After referral to EOP, a multidisciplinary outreach team conducts comprehen-

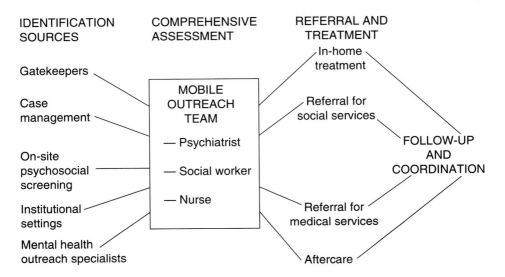

Figure 13-1 Rural outreach model.

sive in-home mental health evaluations, and implements and coordinates an appropriate treatment plan, including referrals to medical and social service agencies. Services are provided to geropsychiatric clients through existing service delivery mechanisms or home-based care.

Peer Counseling and Peer Helpers

Peer counselors or helpers are senior volunteers trained to provide support and assistance to older adults who have difficulties coping with their life situation. Peer counseling can overcome many of the barriers to use of mental health services by older adults. This relatively new strategy for alleviating the emotional distress of older clients began in the mid-1970s and uses the life experiences and skills of older adults in a self-help approach (Bratter, 1986). Peer counselors and helpers are empathic and respectful and do not share the negative view of many mental health professionals toward working with older people (Cohen, 1976). Moreover, emotionally disturbed older adults are more likely to seek counseling from a peer. This approach destigmatizes help seeking, promotes rapport, allays fears of negative consequences such as institutionalization, and costs less. An important by-product of the counseling approach is the positive role modeling that peer counselors and helpers provide for their older clients. For a program of this type to be successful, peer counselors and helpers must be carefully selected and trained and provided with ongoing supervision (Hoffman, 1983). They should receive training in the following areas: (1) the processes and issues of aging, (2) special emotional difficulties, (3) the range of emotional responses to loss, (4) the listening skills necessary to help older adults identify and work through their problems, and (5) identification of resources in the community to provide further assistance. Geropsychiatric nurses in both inpatient and community settings are in an excellent position to provide leadership in the recruitment, training, and supervision of peer counselors for older adults. Those interested in starting such programs should consult the works of Becker and Zarit (1978), Byers-Lang (1984), France and McDowell (1982), Poser and Engels (1983), and Walters, Fink, and White (1976).

Self-Help Groups

Peer counseling programs have been extended to include older people who serve as role models and helpers to others with similar needs (Storandt, 1983). With their emphasis on activity and responsibility for clients, these self-help groups can promote better understanding of emotional disorders in later life as well as increased compliance with therapeutic regimens among less impaired community-based persons. Self-help groups provide a "reference group of persons with the same condition, provide emotional support and a program of activities encouraging members to assume greater responsibility for the future course of their lives" (Cole, O'Connor, & Bennett, 1979, p. 328). Thus geropsychiatric clients who participate in self-help groups may undergo a transformation from a perception of themselves as passive victims of their mental illness to assumption of a more active role in preventing future mental health problems. Self-help groups can be categorized according to four major concerns: (1) rehabilitation and adjustment to new life situations, (2) behavioral change among persons with addictions, (3) primary care groups, and (4) those which forestall acute episodes of chronic illness by encouraging adherence to prescribed diet, medication, and exercise regimens (Gartner & Riessman, 1977). Self-help groups can provide mentally ill clients and their families with an emotional and social support system and group identification. Change in attitude and values often follows change in behavior rather than understanding, as support group members collectively seek strategies to enable them to cope more effectively with the stresses imposed by their mental illness and aging process (Cole et al., 1979).

Prevention Programs

Specific problems that occur in later life should be addressed by the mental health system to help prevent the onset of psychiatric disorders or deterioration of those already afflicted. Widows and widowers comprise one such target group, and bereavement groups are thus an important community program. The literature has documented that older widows and widowers are at higher risk for morbidity and mortality than their married peers (Maddison & Viola, 1968; Parkes, 1972). Many fine community programs specifically for widows are based on the Boston widow-to-widow program, in which widows are trained as outreach workers for the more recently bereaved. Thus the loneliness and isolation of widowhood are addressed by an empathic peer, who can provide support through the initial phases of grieving.

Some communities have staffed congregate apartments for deinstitutionalized chronically mentally ill adults (Matzo & Bernsee, 1990). For example, the Massachusetts Department of Mental Health established such apartments when it became apparent that they would be more beneficial and less restrictive to mental hospital patients than nursing home placement. Heritage House is one such project. It is based on milieu therapy—varied group activities geared to assisting tenants to gain control of their environment (Matzo & Bernsee, 1990). Together with staff, residents plan group activities, solve problems, and foster a sense of responsibility for the community. Residents attend day care, and the local mental health center coordinates a team to provide resources for residents (Matzo & Bernsee, 1990). Low-income chronically mentally ill persons are resocialized into the community, often with excellent results. However, some patients are unable to adjust to this type of setting and are eventually placed in a more restrictive environment.

The last (1981) White House Conference on Aging focused on education, public information, and prevention of illness. Over the past decade, many voluntary and lay organizations have become more active in educating older people and their family members on topics related to mental health and aging. For example, the National Institute on Aging produces *Age Page;* fact sheets on several issues have been published by the National Institute of Mental Health; and a variety of reports on topics that include the use of psychotropic medication, suicide in late life, and alcoholism have been distributed by the American Association of Retired Persons (AARP). Further, the National Council on the Aging has offered many programs intended to enhance the quality of life of elders (Finkel, 1993).

Council on Aging

Most councils on aging, which are funded with Older Americans Act monies governed by area agencies on aging, encompass a variety of resources available to the older population. Some of the services commonly provided include the following.

Business Assistance and Financial Counseling Programs

These programs assist older adults with the completion of business and financial forms such as food stamp applications, water affidavits, property tax credit forms (both federal and state), assistance in understanding health insurance policies, Medicare and Medicaid, investigation of possible overcharges and fraud to the older consumer, and assistance with managing daily financial affairs such as checkbook balancing and ensuring that bills are paid on time. Many councils also promote discounts for senior citizens by local businesses and provide eligible persons with discount cards.

Chore Services

These organizations provide basic lawn mowing and snow clearing services, in addition to small home repairs, for older people who meet income guidelines. Referral-for-hire lists of service persons are also available.

Escort Services

Such services provide volunteers to accompany older persons on trips to the doctor or shopping.

Social Support Programs

Social support programs include the friendly visitor program, in which volunteers visit older persons to decrease loneliness and social isolation, and Phone-a-Friend, whose volunteers call older persons for similar purposes. Telecare programs that provide a daily health check call with emergency procedures that go into effect if the telephone is not answered may also be available.

Housing

Rent-supplemented and federally subsidized low-cost housing is available for qualified older renters. Many councils also sponsor shared housing programs that match individuals interested in sharing a home with others, or co-op housing plans in which homes owned by the council on aging are shared by three unrelated older persons who share household responsibilities. Some households share expenses, and some exchange services for rent. For example, a homebound homeowner may prefer having someone do housework, shopping, yard work, or other errands in exchange for free lodging (AARP, 1988). Community action programs can also provide eligible low-income people with home winterization and insulation. Most councils on aging provide assistance with housing relocation, home repair, and limited maintenance.

Retired Senior Volunteer Program (RSVP)
RSVP is a program for persons age 60 and older who are retired and want to be involved in their community through worthwhile and meaningful activities. For example, a retired clerical worker might assist a community organization with the preparation and mailing of a promotional brochure, or a retired nurse might take weight, blood pressure, and temperature readings at the well adult clinic.

Nutrition Programs
Congregate meals provide a nutritious noon meal and socialization opportunities for persons age 60 and older. Transportation is available to various community sites. Hot meals can also be delivered (Mobile Meals Program) at noon to persons who have difficulty preparing meals. Special diets are prepared as needed, and a donation is suggested for both meal programs. Many homemaker services also have trained homemakers who provide meal preparation and shopping for food. The council on aging also sponsors the delivery of government commodities to homebound people by volunteers. Many community action programs have a food bank where grocery items are available on an emergency or short-term basis.

Transportation
Door-to-door bus service for mobility-impaired persons age 60 and older within the city limits is available in most communities. Modest fares and reservation 2 days in advance are required. Many transit authorities also provide reduced rates for older residents using the city bus system. An application and identification card are usually required.

Respite Programs
Respite is a service that provides family caregivers with periods of relief from the burden of caregiving and social and recreational opportunities for geropsychiatric clients. Adult day care programs provide an important form of community respite. Other forms of respite, such as in-home programs with trained volunteers or paid caregivers and respite provided by community-based agencies such as churches and synagogues, also offer services to the older mentally ill and their families.

Telephone Counseling
Innovative social service programs are increasingly using telecommunication technology to provide safety for frail older persons, live training conferences for health

care professionals, suicide prevention hotlines, and conference call groups for the disabled older adults and/or their caregivers (Evans & Jaureguy, 1982; Evans, Smith, Werkhoven, Fox, & Pritzl, 1986). Recent research has documented that telephone networks can successfully provide support for family caregivers of patients with Alzheimer's disease. Reported benefits of the teleconferencing strategy include (1) a sense of shared struggle, (2) satisfaction from helping, (3) open exchange, (4) increased confidence, and (5) increased self-awareness (Goodman & Pynoos, 1988). Given the large number of older persons and their caregivers who are homebound because of lack of transportation and physical or mental disabilities, alternative means of providing social support, such as telephone networks, must be considered.

Research on cognitive behavioral group therapy by telephone with visually impaired older people suggests that telephone group participants experienced phenomena (e.g., affiliation, confrontation, acceptance, and termination) similar to those of more traditional modes of group therapy. Furthermore, telephone contacts were particularly useful in "reassurance, intimacy, impulse, expression . . . and periodic efforts to break out of depression and isolation" (Evans & Jaureguy, 1982, p. 83), which provided the older clients with a sense of control and a feeling of anonymity.

Day Programs

There are three basic models of day programs: (1) social day care, (2) active treatment, or day hospital model (also called partial hospitalization), and (3) maintenance (Steingart, 1991). Social day care provides supervised and structured group recreational activities; active treatment emphasizes the medical and restorative model; and maintenance provides a combination of social and treatment models. Day care is oriented primarily to socialization, counseling, and recreational activities.

Social Day Care

Because this type of day care is the most widely available and affordable service, it is the most popular form of respite service. Impaired older adults are typically placed in supervised day care one or more days a week (excluding weekends). This allows the caregiver to run errands, enjoy social activities, or continue employment. The cost for adult day care, which can be as high as $40 a day, is not covered by Medicare (AARP, 1988). However, sliding fee scales are widely available.

The clients in day care centers are primarily persons with dementia, physically frail older persons, and older adults who need socialization or continued physical activities. Some day care centers specialize in persons with specific needs, such as those associated with dementia.

Physicians are not a part of this model, as clients are expected to get medical care from their private physicians. Clients are not formally admitted or discharged, but attrition occurs for a variety of reasons: the person is dangerous to self or others, cannot toilet or is incontinent, wanders, is institutionalized, or moves away.

A new program sponsored by the Robert Wood Johnson Foundation provides day care assistance for persons with dementia and their caregivers. Partners in Caregiving offers technical assistance and some grant support to adult day centers that serve people with chronic cognitive disorders and their families (Partners in Caregiving, 1993). The first program focused primarily on persons with dementia and their caregivers. More recent efforts expand the focus to include adults with other chronic cognitive disorders such as developmental disabilities, AIDS, and chronic mental illnesses.

Active Treatment Model

Adult day care centers in hospitals or community mental health programs often are called day hospitals, geriatric day programs, or partial hospitalization programs. They provide intensive medical, psychiatric nursing and rehabilitative services to individuals who do not require 24-hour nursing care but would need inpatient care if the day program were not available (Persily & Albury, 1991; Steingart, 1991). These services can best be provided in a hospital. This service may be reimbursed by Medicare and/or Medicaid, and rehabilitation-oriented therapies such as physical therapy and occupational therapy are usually covered. Receiving therapy in a day hospital keeps clients within the hospital or CMHC's circle of care without continued hospitalization. For clients who do not require 24-hour care, day treatment programs can provide services such as speech, physical, and occupational training in the activities of daily living as well as recreational outings and social activities (Persily, 1991). Somatic treatments such as pharmacotherapy and electroconvulsive therapy may be provided (Steingart, 1991). A psychiatrist usually heads a treatment team consisting of occupational therapists, social workers, and nursing staff. Discharge is expected when the client shows sufficient improvement.

Day treatment programs have been available for alcoholics and polydrug abusers, but most of these programs are targeted to those who have health insurance. Some outpatient programs are several months long, and clients are expected to participate up to 8 hours each day during the week (Vourakis & Bennett, 1990).

Day hospital or partial hospitalization is one of the services expected of the CMHC. Programs are not necessarily geared to the geropsychiatric client but include mentally ill persons over age 18. One such program in Davenport, Iowa, is at the Vera French Community Mental Health Center (personal communication from Annabel Flaherty, MA, RN, June 14, 1993.) The program admits chronically mentally ill clients over 18 years old, including elders. Groups consist of persons with similar concerns, and an interdisciplinary team meets daily to plan care and evaluate progress. Clients either retain a personal psychiatrist or are treated by the medical director of the center. A physician's orders are required for admission and discharge, but referrals can be made by a variety of sources including family and community agencies. Medicare covers partial hospitalization, and in some cases Medicaid will pay for this treatment. The Davenport program reports successful outcomes and is expected to continue.

Maintenance Model

Persons at high risk for institutionalization may benefit from maintenance care, long-term day care that delays or prevents permanent institutionalization (Steingart, 1991). Client mix includes frail persons who suffer from chronic psychiatric disorders such as schizophrenia, treatment-resistant affective disorders, personality disorders, and dementia. Services are generally available 5 days a week to provide respite for family members. A physician referral usually initiates placement and a multidisciplinary team including a psychiatrist plans care. Some active treatment may be implemented, but for most clients no improvement is expected. Discharge is most often to a more intensive level of care such as an inpatient hospital or nursing home (Steingart, 1991).

Geriatric Assessment

Comprehensive geriatric assessment includes use of a multidisciplinary team to evaluate an older person's medical, psychological, socioeconomic and environmental needs. This procedure is most often performed by a physician, nurse, and social worker, with other specialists consulted as necessary. The team determines the client's full set of health and social service needs, evaluates resources and support services, and produces a comprehensive plan of treatment and management. In 1987 the National Institute of Health's Consensus Conference on Geriatric Assessment concluded that geriatric assessment is a valuable tool in the treatment of certain subgroups of frail older adults. In addition, geriatric assessment has been demonstrated to improve diagnostic accuracy, functional status, and cognition. It is also associated with decreased nursing home placement and medication usage. Geriatric assessment programs can be conducted on either an inpatient or outpatient basis, and many include an assessment of the home. To date there is no universally accepted model for geriatric assessment programs (Statewide Geriatric Healthcare Issues, 1992).

The assessment effort is costly because of the heavy use of professionals and the amount of time the comprehensive assessment takes. Under the Medicare coding system there is no means to account for the additional time, previsit and postvisit work, and ancillary staff required for comprehensive assessment. Inadequate reimbursement for these services will continue to deter the establishment of geriatric assessment programs. Assessment clinics often lose money, and many have been shut down. These financial disincentives must be addressed. Organizations such as the American Geriatrics Society are pursuing this issue at the national level through the Physician Payment Review Commission (Statewide Geriatric Healthcare Issues, 1992).

Projects for the Homeless

At least 30% of homeless persons suffer from some type of mental disorder. The unique problems and characteristics of older homeless mentally ill clients require adjustments in the delivery of services.

The homeless mentally ill generally are unable or unwilling to participate in traditional mental health treatment (i.e., outpatient, evaluation, or partial hospitalization services). Even in outreach work, contact over long periods may be necessary to establish trust. Flexibility with regard to the timing and location of the interventions is essential to successful treatment. Fragmentation and lack of cooperation and coordination among various needed services (mental, social, medical, public assistance, shelters) can cause additional problems for this population. The disabling qualities of the mental illness may cause the older person to be less tolerant of administrative red tape (for example, waiting for services, filling out forms), which can interfere with their ability to get along in the system. Because of these barriers, often the geropsychiatric client does not receive needed services.

Aggressive outreach approaches have proved successful in identifying and helping older chronically mentally ill homeless people. Outreach and screening occurs wherever the homeless mentally ill are located, that is, river banks, shelters, lobbies of public buildings, and parks.

❖ Case Management (Care Coordination)

Continuity of services is achieved through active coordination to ensure that older clients and their families do not "fall between the cracks of the service delivery system" (Bellack & Mueser, 1986, p. 178); yet to date the smorgasbord of program supports has lacked coordinating and integrating centers. Thus, while community-based services for older people do exist, a true system of long-term care services often does not. A major barrier is the lack of tradition among service provider agencies in terms of functioning as a system (Walz, 1983).

Case management is a method of assessing a person's total care needs, arranging for necessary services, and coordinating their delivery. Since care problems rarely occur one at a time and services may be fragmented, this service can be used by caregivers to coordinate a care plan (AARP, 1988). The term *case management* can mean many things but in this chapter is the monitoring and coordination of services for the client, and in some cases for the family. It begins on hospital admission and continues post discharge. A team of professionals, which may include the attending physician, nurses, social workers, and mental health therapists, works together to develop a plan of care for the client (DeVito, Persily, Zubkoff, & Albury, 1991). Seven fundamental functions are key components of the process: (1) intake and screening, (2) geriatric assessment, (3) care planning, (4) arranging for services, (5) ongoing monitoring, (6) reassessment, and (7) discharge (DeVito et al., 1991).

Key features of case management include (1) assumption of responsibility for mobilizing medical, social, and health services to ensure continuity of care; (2) comprehensive and systematic assessment and planning with involvement of multidisciplinary personnel; and (3) assumption of responsibility to provide or coordinate the multiple services needed by the client and family over time (Brody, 1984). The National Council on Aging uses the term *care management* in its standards because it conveys that the process is the management of care rather than the case or the person (National Council on Aging, 1988). Terms such as *care coordination, service coordination,* and *service management* are used interchangeably with *case management.*

Case management models and methods vary widely according to setting. Case management has been defined by Kane (1989) as "the coordination of a specified group of resources and services for a specified group of people" (p. 5). Most often, case management provides community-based services to frail and vulnerable older people who are unable to meet their multiple and complex needs without assistance, in an effort to help them avoid inappropriate institutionalization. Case management, whether provided by a solo practitioner, agency, or the family, should facilitate the development and implementation of individualized case plans to improve the quality of care provided to older persons. Kane (1989) has identified the essential tasks of any case management model as (1) case finding/screening, (2) comprehensive multidimensional assessment, (3) care planning, (4) implementation of the plan, (5) monitoring of progress, and (6) formal reassessment at periodic intervals (p. 5).

The assessment is designed to improve the quality of the in-home care received by the older person and to ensure that the appropriate mix and level of services are made available to them (Walz, 1983). The assessment data must be translated into specific types and amounts of services required by the older client through the development of a case plan. In an agency-based model, clients who meet the criteria for case management in terms of age, functional limitations, and needed services are asked to sign a release of information to allow their case to be reviewed by all the member agencies of the case management network, which generally meet on a regular basis to develop the case plan in cooperation with the older client and the family. The case management team reviews each case for its priority needs and makes a staffing decision based on those needs. The contact agency usually acts as an advocate for the individual case being discussed but may not automatically assume the role of case manager because of specific actions recommended by the team. Case managers can request or suggest referrals to other members of the network, and a coordinator maintains records of the case as it is served by various agencies. Case managers report regularly on progress of their older clients during staff meetings. Periodic reassessment of the older client's problems, follow-up or termination, and periodic review of the cost-benefits ratio of community-based care are also part of the best case management systems. Clients may be charged for the services provided by individual agencies, although there are usually no additional costs for case management. The major benefits of this approach to community-based, long-term care services for older adults are as follows: (1) the older clients can remain in their own homes, (2) the coordination of services reduces confusion, (3) the case plans address current and future needs before emergencies arise, (4) duplication of services is eliminated, and (5) clients receive appropriate care to meet their needs. Thus case management services increase the availability of services and enhance joint resource management.

Information Exchange

A final component of continuity of care is the need to aggregate and exchange client information bases with all service agencies concerned with care of clients. Today's world is one of data-based planning and policy making. Continuity of care has grown increasingly dependent on the ability of data information systems to span the network of all service contributors (Walz, 1983). An effective data information system requires standardization of service definitions, measures of service activity, record-keeping procedures, and computer entry protocols.

❖ *Legal Options in Case of Decision-Making Incapacity*

Options of the Mentally Capable Adult

As a result of mental illness or dementia, many geropsychiatric clients temporarily or permanently lose decision-making capacity. Several legal options are available for the mentally ill older client who retains periods of decision-making capacity to plan for personal, health care, and financial decisions. There are also processes available to the family or friends of a client who is no longer able to make the necessary decisions.

Two major classifications of substitute decision making are available to the individual who is planning for incapacity: private and public documents (Table 13-1). Private documents include the power of attorney for health care and financial decisions and the living will for health care decisions. The geropsychiatric client may work with a private attorney to explore and draft the power of attorney, a private document that will transfer limited and designated decision-making authority to another person, the agent. All states recognize an adult's authority to transfer financial decision making to another person by the execution of a power of attorney (Hunzeker, 1990). The power of attorney sets forth the type and scope of authority subject to transfer and the person who has been designated to exercise the authority. The power of attorney was originally applied to the delegation of financial authority; however, 32 states have now expanded the power of attorney to include health care treatment decisions (Alexander, 1991).

A living will is a personal document that sets forth the health care treatment decisions individuals want carried out in the event that they are unable to decide for

Table 13-1   Ways for a Competent Adult to Plan for Decision-Making Incapacity

	Private agreements	*Court-appointed makers*
Health care treatment decisions	Durable power of attorney for health care Living will	Standby guardianship
Financial decisions	Durable power of attorney Power of attorney	Standby conservatorship

themselves. Forty-five states now have living will legislation (Alexander, 1991). Each state statute is different. Many statutes specify conditions that must be met before a living will is invoked (for example, need for life-sustaining procedures, terminal illness, likelihood of impending death).

Both the durable power of attorney for health care and the living will may express personal preferences about specific health care treatments such as artificial nutrition and hydration, artificial respiration, dialysis, and cardioversion. The private documents are maintained in confidence between the client who has signed the document, the agent, the attorney and the physician's records and hospital medical records.

Some states also allow all adults to file public documents, such as a standby guardianship or conservatorship, that name an individual to assume certain health care or financial authority if the client becomes mentally incapacitated. These public documents must be filed by a mentally competent adult and indicate a substitute decision maker. The documents are a matter of public record and are usually available for review at the local courthouse. Guardianships and conservatorships are established by the court according to information that the potential ward is no longer mentally competent and needs such service.

The major advantages of using public documents is that the court monitors the guardian's or conservator's actions. Generally, the guardian or conservator must file an annual report with the court that outlines the decisions and actions taken in the previous year. The guardian or conservator must also seek prior court approval for decisions detailed by state statute, for example, moving the ward to a more restrictive living environment.

Options of the Family of a Mentally Incapacitated Adult

Not all geropsychiatric adults are capable or choose to plan for incapacity to make decisions. This lack of planning leaves many family members and friends with limited ability to make essential decisions for the geropsychiatric client. Concerned family members and friends may encounter situations in which the mentally ill older adult is unable to make essential health care treatment decisions, for example, essential surgery and adherence to dietary or medication regimens. The client, as a result of lack of planning and cognitive incapacity, may have placed his or her own life or physical health in serious jeopardy.

Family members may try to work with health care professionals to identify the best health care treatment options. However, health care professionals may be reluctant to implement care that requires informed consent if the client is not capable of giving that consent and no other adult has the legal authority to do so. This hesitancy by health care professionals may stem from uncertainty regarding the validity of the consent or fear of a lawsuit if the treatment outcome is unfavorable.

One legal mechanism that family members may pursue is the establishment of a court-appointed guardianship. With a guardianship, family members or friends must file a petition with the court stating that the geropsychiatric adult is no longer able to make personal or health care decisions and that some decisions are required. In addition to filing the petition, some states require that the petition name the guardian (Iowa Code, 1992). After reviewing the petition and hearing evidence from various sources, the court grants or denies the petition. If the guardianship is granted, the incapacitated adult becomes a ward of the court and the named guardian must pledge to make decisions that reflect the best interests of the ward.

The main advantage of the standby guardianship is that the court maintains judicial overview of the guardian-ward relationship. As compared with private legal documents, this judicial oversight provides a forum in which other concerned family members, friends, or health care professionals may challenge decisions of the named guardian. The primary disadvantage of the guardian-ward relationship is the fact that it is a public record.

All states have statutory language that allows for the naming of a substitute decision maker for financial concerns (Hunzeker, 1990). Some states refer to this relationship as a conservatorship, and others use a very broad definition of guardianship to encompass these financial concerns. Still other states refer to this relationship as a committee. Regardless of the statutory label, all states recognize the need for this conservator-ward relationship that allows the designated individual to act for the ward in fulfilling essential financial obligations such as depositing income checks and paying debts.

The conservator, like the guardian, is appointed by the court and has a corresponding obligation to base decisions upon the ward's best interests. This obligation prohibits the conservator from using the ward's financial assets for personal gain. The conservator is also responsible to the court for an annual accounting of the ward's financial assets, and the relationship is open for public inspection.

Adult Protective Services

The incidence of violence in American society is increasing, and older adults are not immune. Elder abuse, neglect, and mistreatment are recognized forms of societal violence that affect 700,000 to 1.5 million elders each year (Fulmer, 1992). Abuse consists of a variety of violent and nonviolent acts ranging from brutal physical treatment to subtle acts such as withholding money or affection or repeatedly threatening the older adult with isolation or nursing home placement. Elder abuse may occur in the home, community, or institutional setting. Therefore, the nurse in the community must be alert to potential abuse in all settings.

All 50 states have legislation designed to protect vulnerable adults. Some states categorize the legislation as elder abuse legislation, and other states have adult protective services legislation (Hunzeker, 1990). Even though all states have legislation concerning elder abuse, the substance of the legislation varies. All states recognize physical harm or injury as abuse (Hunzeker, 1990). However, the nurse must know whether the more subtle forms of abuse such as psychological abuse, abandonment, and financial exploitation are included in the state's definition of mistreatment.

States vary in the definition of who specifically is covered by the statutory language, for example, aged, vulnerable, or dependent adults. The statutes also vary regarding who is expected or required to report suspected abuse and whether the reporting is voluntary or mandatory for selected groups of professionals.

In states that have mandatory reporting, not all states penalize a mandatory reporter who fails to report the suspected abuse. However, states do typically protect from civil liability those who provide a good faith report of suspected abuse. This immunity provides protection from a civil or criminal suit that may arise from the reporting of the suspected abuse. The state laws also specify which agency has the responsibility for receiving and investigating the suspected abuse report.

From the perspective of determining whether an elder client needs adult protective services, the nurse in the community should determine (1) whether the person exhibits signs or symptoms of elder abuse, neglect, or mistreatment; (2) whether the person meets the state's definition of an adult who is protected under the statute; (3) whether the nurse is a mandatory reporter; and (4) which agency should receive the report of suspected abuse.

❖ *Summary*

Clearly the community-based approach to care of mentally ill older adults is long overdue and is a welcome addition to the continuum of services that health care professionals must use to ensure appropriate services at the least restrictive level. Although this chapter has focused on noninstitutionalized aspects of the continuum of care for the geropsychiatric client, the community care system clearly should include protocols for effective coordination with hospital and extended care facilities as well.

Geropsychiatric clients challenge nurses and other health care professionals committed to continuity of care. Many clients become acutely ill and chronically disabled and require both temporary and permanent health care assistance. An equally large number eventually return home but require a full range of community-based health, mental health, social, and supportive services to function at an optimal level according to the principle of least restrictive care. The continuum of community resources from the least restrictive (e.g., in-home services) to the most restrictive (e.g., day programs) must be used according to the needs of the client. Geropsychiatric clients and their families must be made aware of their rights, including legal considerations. It is important that these concerns be given full attention, particularly while the client remains capable of decision making.

Health care professionals and social service providers must overcome traditional communication and turf barriers if continuity of care for this population is to be achieved. Health care professionals must view the client holistically and value each modality of care. In this way, optimum mental and physical functioning is most likely to be achieved.

❖ *References*

AARP, American Association of Retired Persons. (1988). *Tomorrow's choices*. Washington, DC: Author.

Alexander, G. (1991). Time for a new law on health care advance directives. *The Hastings Law Journal, 42,* 555-778.

American Nurses' Association. (1987). *Standards and scope of gerontological nursing practice*. Kansas City, MO: Author.

Bachrach, L. (1986). The challenge of service planning in chronic mental patients. *Community Mental Health Journal, 22*(3), 170-174.

Becker, F., & Zarit, S. H. (1978). Training older adults as peer counselors. *Educational Gerontology, 3,* 241-250.

Bellack, A. S., & Mueser, K. T. (1986). A comprehensive treatment program for schizophrenia and chronic mental illness. *Community Mental Health Journal, 22*(30), 175-189.

Brandt, B. A., & Osgood, N. J. (1990). The suicidal patient and long-term care institutions. *Journal of Gerontological Nursing, 16*(2), 15-18.

Bratter, B. (1986). Peer counseling for older adults. *Generations, 10*(3), 49-50, Spring.

Brody, S. J. (1984). DRGs: The second revolution in health care for the elderly. *Journal of the American Geriatrics Society, 32*(9), 676-79.

Buckwalter, K. C. (1986). Integration of social and mental health care services for the elderly. *Family and Community Health, 8*(4), 1-9.

Butler, R. N. (1968). Toward a psychiatry of the life cycle: Implications of sociopsychologic studies of the aging process for the psychotherapeutic situation. *Psychiatric Research Report, 23,* 233-248.

Byers-Lang, R. E. (1984). Peer counselors, network builders for elderly persons. *Journal of Visual Impairment and Blindness, 78,* 193-197.

Cohen, G. D. (1976). Mental health services and the elderly: Needs and options. *American Journal of Psychiatry, 133*(1), 65-68.

Cole, S. A., O'Connor, S., & Bennett, L. (1979). Self-help groups for clinic patients with chronic illness. *Primary Care, 6*(2), June, 325-340.

DeVito, C. A., Persily, N. A., Zubkoff, W., & Albury, S. R. (1991). Case management initiatives in eldercare. In N. A. Persily (Ed.). *Eldercare: Positioning your hospital for the future* (Chapter 6). Chicago: American Hospital Association.

Evans, R. L., & Jaureguy, B. M. (1982). Phone therapy outreach for blind elderly. *The Gerontologist, 22*(1), 32-35.

Evans, R. L., Smith, K. M., Werkhoven, W. S., Fox, H. R., & Pritzl, D. O. (1986). Cognitive telephone group therapy with physically disabled elderly persons. *The Gerontologist, 26*(1), 8-11.

Finkel, S. I. (1993). Mental health and aging: A decade of progress. *Generations, 17*(1), 25-30.

Fowles, D. (Ed.). (1993). *A profile of older Americans*. Washington, DC: American Association of Retired Persons.

France, M. H., & McDowell, C. (1982). Seniors helping seniors: A model of peer counseling for the aged. *Canada's Mental Health 30,* 13-15.

Fulmer, T. (1992). Clinical outlook: Elder mistreatment assessment as a part of everyday practice. *Journal of Gerontological Nursing, 18*(3), 42-43.

Gartner, A., & Riessman, F. (1977). *Self-help in the human services* (pp. 69-96). San Francisco: Jossey-Bass.

Gatz, M., Smyer, M. A., & Lawton, M. P. (1980). The mental health system and the older adult. In L. W. Poon (Ed.), *Aging in the 1980s: Psychological issues.* Washington, DC: American Psychological Association.

Goodman, C., & Pynoos, J. (1988). Telephone networks connect caregiving families of Alzheimer's victims. *The Gerontologist, 28*(5), 602-604.

Haber, D. (1986). In-home and community-based long-term care services: A review of recent AoA projects involving self-determination. *Journal of Applied Gerontology, 5*(1), 37-50.

Hagebak, J. E., & Hagebak, B. R. (1983, January-February). Meeting the mental health needs of the elderly: Issues and action steps. *Aging,* 26-31.

Harlow, K. S., & Wilson, L. B. (1985). DRGs and the community-based long term care. Paper presented to the Committee on Education and Labor, Subcommittee on Human Resources of the U.S. House of Representatives.

Hoffman, S. B. (1983). Peer counselor training with the elderly. *The Gerontologist, 23*(4), 358-360.

Hunzeker, D. (1990). *State legislative response to crimes against the elderly.* Denver: National Conference of State Legislatures.

Iowa Code 235. (1992).

Kane, R. (1989). Introduction: Case management. *Generations, 12*(5), 5.

Kaufman, M. R. (1940). Old age and aging: The psychoanalytic point of view. *American Journal of Orthopsychiatry, 10,* 73-84.

Kelly, J. T., Shea, M. A., & Ross, J. E. (1987). Implications of Medicare hospital utilization trends for long term health care. *Pride Institute Journal, 6*(2), 14-18.

Kermis, M. D. (1986). The epidemiology of mental disorder in the elderly: A response to the Senate/AARP Report. *The Gerontologist, 26*(5), 482-487.

Kermis, M. D. (1987). Equity and policy issues in mental health care of the elderly: Dilemmas, deinstitutionalization and DRGs. *Journal of Applied Gerontology, 6*(3), 268-283.

Maddison, D. C., & Viola, A. (1968). The health of widows in the year following bereavement. *Journal of Psychosomatic Research, 12*(4), 297-306.

Matzo, M., & Bernsee, M. L. (1990). Independent after all these years! *Geriatric Nursing, 11*(6), 268-270.

The Medicare 1994 Handbook. (1994). Baltimore, MD: U.S. Department of Health and Human Services.

Mental health and aging: Approaches to curriculum development. (1983). (Publication No. 114, vol. 14). New York: Committee on Aging, Group for the Advancement of Psychiatry.

Morris, W. W. (1987, June 10). Handout for "Continuum of Care" Lecture. Iowa Geriatric Education Center, Summer Workshop, Iowa City, IA.

National Council on Aging. (1988). *Care management standards, guidelines for practice.* Washington, DC: Author.

Ory, M. G. (1989). Considerations in the development of age-sensitive indicators for assessing health promotion. *Health Promotion: An International Journal, 3*(2), 139-150.

Parkes, C. M. (1972). *Studies of grief in adult life.* Madison, CT: International Universities Press.

Partners in Caregiving selects 50 sites. (1993). *Respite Report, Winter.* Winston-Salem, NC: Bowman Gray School of Medicine, Wake Forest University.

Persily, N. A. (1991). Service options in eldercare. In N. A. Persily (Ed.). *Eldercare: Positioning your hospital for the future* (Chapter 5). Chicago: American Hospital Association.

Persily, N. A., & Albury, S. R. (1991). Health care service delivery. In N. A. Persily (Ed.). *Eldercare: Positioning your hospital for the future* (Chapter 3). Chicago: American Hospital Association.

Peterson, D. M. (1983). Epidemiology of drug use. In M. D. Glantz, D. M. Peterson, & F. J. Whittington (Eds.). *Drugs and the elderly adult.* Washington, DC: U.S. Department of Health and Human Services.

Pfeiffer, E. (1977). Psychopathology and social pathology. In J. E. Birren & K. W. Schaie (Eds.). *Handbook of the psychology of aging.* New York: Van Nostrand Reinhold.

Poser, E. G., & Engels, M. I. (1983). Self-efficacy assessment and peer group assistance in a preretirement intervention. *Educational Gerontology, 9* 159-169.

Reifler, B. V., Kethley, A., O'Neill, P., Hanley, R., Lewis, S., & Stenchever, D. (1982). Five year experience of a community outreach program for the elderly. *American Journal of Psychiatry, 139*(2), 220-223.

Roybal, E. R. (1984). Federal involvement in mental health care for the aged. *American Psychologist, 39*(2), 163-166.

Shern, D. L., Wilson, N. Z., Ellis, R. H., Bartsch, D. A., & Coen, A. S. (1986). Planning a continuum of residential/service settings for the chronically mentally ill: The Colorado experience. *Community Mental Health Journal, 22*(3), 190-202.

Statewide geriatric healthcare issues: A growing challenge for Iowa. (1992). Iowa City: University of Iowa Hospitals and Clinics.

Steingart, A. (1991). Day programs. In J. Sadavoy, L. Lazarus, & L. F. Jarvik (Eds.). *Comprehensive review of psychiatry* (Chapter 30). Washington, DC: American Psychiatric Press.

Storandt, M. (1983). *Counseling and therapy with older adults* (Series on Gerontology). Boston: Little Brown.

Toseland, R. W., Decker, J., & Bliesner, J. (1979). A community outreach program for socially isolated older persons. *Journal of Gerontological Social Work, 1,* 211-224.

Vourakis, C., & Bennett, G. (1990). Treating the drug abuser. In A. W. Burgess (Ed.). *Psychiatric nursing in the hospital and community* (5th ed., Chapter 34). Norwalk, CT: Appleton & Lange.

Walters, E., Fink, S., & White, B. (1976). Peer group counseling for older people. *Educational Gerontology, 1,* 157-170.

Walz, T. (1983). Social policies reader: An overview of long term care for, 42:185, Social Work Policy and the Elderly, Iowa City: University of Iowa.

Walz, T., & Elliott, M. (1983). The mental health of the rural elderly. In G. M. Jacobsen & P. K. Kelly (Eds.), Issues in rural mental health practice (Monograph, pp. 97-105). Iowa City: University of Iowa.

Wasson, W., Ripeckyj, A., Lazarus, L. W., Kupferer, S., Barry, S., & Force, F. (1984). *The Gerontologist, 24*(3), 238-242.

White House Conference on Aging. (1981). Final Report on Long Term Care (vol. 3). Washington, DC: Government Printing Office.

❖ *Bibliography*

Abrams, W. B., & Berkow, R. (Eds.). (1990). *The Merck manual of geriatrics*. Rahway, NJ: Merck Sharp & Dohme Research Laboratories.

American Nurses' Association Council on Gerontological Nursing Practice. (1987). *Standards and scope of gerontological nursing practice*. Washington, DC: Author.

American Nurses' Association (1994). *A statement on psychiatric-mental health clinical nursing practice and standards of psychiatric-mental health clinical nursing practice*. Washington, DC: Author.

American Psychiatric Association. *Diagnostic and statistical manual of mental disorders* (4th ed.). (1994). Washington, DC: Author.

Atchley, R. C. (1994). *Social forces and aging* (7th ed.). Belmont California: Wadsworth.

Baldwin, B., Stevens, G. & Friedman, S. (1995). Geriatric psychiatric nursing. In G. Stuart & S. Sundeen (Eds.). *Principles and practices of psychiatric nursing* (5th ed.). St. Louis: Mosby.

Brown, P., et al. (1987). Linking psychiatric nursing care to patient classification codes. *Nursing and Health Care, 8*(3), 156-163.

Burnside, I. M. (1988). *Nursing and the aged* (3rd ed.). New York: McGraw-Hill.

Busse, E. W., & Blazer, D. G. (Eds.). (1980). *Handbook of geriatric psychiatry*. New York: Van Nostrand Reinhold.

Butler, R. N., Lewis, M., & Sunderland, T. (1991). *Aging and mental health* (4th ed.) New York: Macmillan.

Carstensen, L., & Edelstein, B. A. (1987). *Handbook of clinical gerontology*. Elmsford, NY: Paragon Press.

Chaisson-Stewart, M. G. (1985). *Depression in the elderly: An interdisciplinary approach*. New York: Wiley.

Crook, T., Bartus, R., Ferris, S., & Gershon, S. (Eds.). (1986). *Treatment development strategies for Alzheimer's disease*. Madison, CT: Mark Peinley Associates.

Dye, C. A. (1986). *Assessment and intervention in geropsychiatric nursing*. Orlando, FL: Grune & Stratton.

Feil, N. (1982). *Validation*. Cleveland: Edward Feil Productions.

Ham, R. J. (1987). *Geriatric medicine annual*. Oradell, NJ: Medical Economics Books.

Harper, M. S., & Lebowitz, B. D. (Eds.). (1986). *Mental illness in nursing homes: Agenda for research*. Rockville, MD: National Institute of Mental Health.

Healthy People 2000. (1992). U.S. Department of Health and Human Services. Boston: Jones and Bartlett.

Hogstel, M. O. (Ed.). (1992). *Clinical manual of gerontological nursing*. St. Louis: Mosby.

Hogstel, M. O. (Ed.). (1994). *Nursing care of the older adult* (3rd ed.). Albany, NY: Delmar.

Hyman, S. E., & Arana, G. W. (1987). *Handbook of psychiatric drug therapy.* Boston: Little, Brown.

Jenike, M. A. (1985). *Handbook of psychiatric psychopharmacology.* Littleton, MA: PSG Publishing.

Jeste, D. V., & Zisook, S. (Eds.). (1988). Psychosis and depression in the elderly. *Psychiatric Clinics of North America, 11*(1).

Lidoff, L. (1990). *Caregiver support groups in America.* Washington, DC: The National Council on the Aging.

Mace, N. L., & Robins, P. V. (1991). *The 36-hour day* (revised ed.). Baltimore: Johns Hopkins University Press.

NANDA nursing diagnoses: Definitions and classification 1992-1993. (1992). Philadelphia: North American Nursing Diagnosis Association.

Resource directory for older people (1993). Bethesda, MD: National Institute on Aging.

Salzman, C. (Ed.). (1992). *Clinical geriatric psychopharmacology* (2nd ed.). Baltimore: Williams & Wilkins.

Stanley, M. & Beare, P. G. (Eds.) (1995). *Gerontological nursing.* Philadelphia: F. A. Davis.

Stuart, G. W., & Sundeen, S. J. (Eds.). (1995). *Principles and practice of psychiatric nursing* (5th ed.). St. Louis: Mosby–Year Book.

Talbott, J. A., Hales, R. E., & Yudofsky, S. E. (1988). *The textbook of psychiatry.* Washington, DC: American Press.

Verwoerdt, A. (1982). *Clinical geropsychiatry.* Baltimore: Williams & Wilkins.

Weiner, M. (Ed.). (1991). *The dementias: Diagnosis and management.* Washington, DC: American Psychiatric Press.

Wilson, H. S., & Kneisl, C. R. (Eds.). (1992). *Psychiatric nursing* (4th ed.). Menlo Park, CA: Addison-Wesley.

Wise, M. G., & Rundell, J. R. (1988). *Consultation psychiatry.* Washington, DC: American Psychiatric Press.

Wolfe, S. M., & Hope, R. E. (1993). *Worst pills, best pills II.* Washington, DC: Public Citizen Health Research Group.

❖ *Appendixes*

❖ *Health History Sample*

DATABASE

CLIENT PROFILE:

   I. Demographic data
     A. Name   Date
     B. Date of birth
     C. Address   Living arrangements
     D. Marital status
     E. Religion
     F. Level of education
     G. Family composition

  II. Health history
     A. Present
       1. Problems identified by client
       2. Chronic problems
       3. Mobility
       4. Allergies
     B. Past
       1. Medical
       2. Surgical
       3. Mental and emotional
       4. Trauma and injuries
       5. Childhood illnesses

 III. Family genogram (back two generations from client)

 IV. Medications
     A. Prescription
     B. Over-the-counter

V. Communication patterns during interview
  A. Interpretation of questions
  B. Affect
  C. Ability to communicate
  D. Attention span
  E. Behavior patterns
  F. Memory
  G. Orientation
  H. Abstract thoughts

VI. Review of systems
  A. Integument, hair, nails
  B. Head and neck
  C. Nose, mouth, teeth, and throat
  D. Eyes and ears
  E. Hematopoietic
  F. Lungs and respiratory
  G. Cardiovascular
  H. Gastrointestinal
  I. Renal
  J. Reproductive
  K. Musculoskeletal
  L. Neurological

VII. General health perceptions
  A. General health
    1. Appearance
    2. Speech
    3. Dress
  B. Chronic conditions
  C. Habits
    1. Smoking
    2. Alcohol intake
    3. Eating
    4. Coping patterns
    5. Medical regimen
  D. Self-concept
    1. Description of self
    2. Changes in body
    3. Changes in memory
    4. Changes in coping
    5. Changes in feelings
    6. Major life stresses
    7. Major life changes in past 2 years

E. Communications
   1. Interaction patterns
   2. Support persons
   3. Communication of needs
   4. Intelligence
F. Sexuality
   1. Feelings about gender relationships
   2. Feelings about self
G. Cognitive patterns
   1. Memory deficits
   2. Emotional responses to change
   3. Level of comprehension
   4. Mood
   5. Affect
   6. Insight
   7. Mental status
H. Interaction patterns
   1. Genogram
   2. Social relationships
   3. Living arrangements
I. Nutritional assessment
   1. Diet, 24-hour recall
   2. Weight gain or loss
   3. Exercise
   4. Appetite
   5. Socialization during mealtime
J. Sleep and rest patterns
   1. Number of hours sleep
     a. Night
     b. Day
   2. Restfulness after sleep
   3. Changes in sleep patterns
   4. Energy level

Appendix *B*

❖ *Short Portable Mental Status Questionnaire (SPMSQ)*

Eric Pfeiffer, M.D.

Instructions: Ask questions 1-10 in this list and record all answers. Ask question 4A only if patient does not have a telephone. Record total number of errors based on ten questions.

+	−

1. What is the date today? _____
   Month   Day   Year
2. What day of the week is it? _____
3. What is the name of this place? _____
4. What is your telephone number? _____
4A. What is your street address? _____
    (Ask only if patient does not have a telephone)
5. How old are you? _____
6. When were you born? _____
7. Who is the President of the U.S. now? _____
8. Who was President just before him? _____
9. What was your mother's maiden name? _____
10. Subtract 3 from 20 and keep subtracting 3 from each new number, all the way down.

_____ Total Number of Errors

SPMSQ reprinted with permission of E. Pfeiffer, M.D.

To Be Completed by Interviewer

Patient's name _____   Date _____

    Sex: 1. Male   Race: 1. White
          2. Female   2. Black
                                       3. Other

    Years of Education: _____   1. Grade School
                                      2. High School
                                      3. Beyond High School

    Interviewer's Name: _____

Pfeiffer, E. (1975). A short portable mental status questionnaire for the assessment of organic brain deficit in elderly patients. *Journal of the American Geriatrics Society, 23*(10), 433-441.

❖ *Scoring of the Short Portable Mental Status Questionnaire (SPMSQ)*

The data suggest that both education and race influence performance on the SPMSQ, and they must accordingly be taken into account in evaluating the score.

For scoring purposes, three educational levels have been established: (1) persons who have had only a grade school education, (2) persons who have had any high school education or who have completed high school, (3) persons who have had any education beyond the high school level, including college, graduate school, and business school.

For white subjects with at least some high school education but not more than high school education, the following criteria have been established:

0-2 errors	Intact intellectual functioning
3-4 errors	Mild intellectual impairment
5-7 errors	Moderate intellectual impairment
8-10 errors	Severe intellectual impairment

Allow one more error if subject has had only a grade school education.

Allow one less error if subject has had education beyond high school.

Allow one more error for black subjects, using identical education criteria.

❖ *Instructions for Completion of the Short Portable Mental Status Questionnaire (SPMSQ)*

Ask the subject questions 1 through 10 in this list and record all answers. All responses to be scored correct must be given by subject without reference to calendar, newspaper, birth certificate, or other aid to memory.

Question 1 is to be scored correctly only when the exact month, exact date, and the exact year are given correctly.

Question 2 is self-explanatory.

Question 3 should be scored correctly if any correct description of the location is given. "My home," correct name of the town or city of residence, or the name of hospital or institution if subject is institutionalized, are all acceptable.

Question 4 should be scored correctly when the correct telephone number can be verified, or when the subject can repeat the same number at another point in the questioning.

Question 5 is scored correct when stated age corresponds to date of birth.

Question 6 is to be scored correctly only when the month, exact date, and year are all given.

Question 7 requires only the last name of the president.

Question 8 requires only the last name of the previous president.

Question 9 does not need to be verified. It is scored correct if a female first name plus a last name other than subject's last name is given.

Question 10 requires that the entire series must be performed correctly in order to be scored as correct. Any error in the series or unwillingness to attempt the series is scored as incorrect.

❖ *Community Geropsychiatric Screening Assessment Guide*

Date _____

Patient name _____

Date of birth _____ Age _____ Social Security number _____

Marital status: M   W   S   D   Date of admission* _____

Family/Relative _____   Phone _____

_____   Phone _____

Address or name of facility* _____

_____   Phone _____

Primary physician _____   Phone _____

Medical diagnoses _____

_____

Behavior requiring consult

_____

*If an inpatient setting.

ASSESSMENT DATA

Pertinent data from medical record (if available)

Obvious physical data (e.g., use of wheelchair)

Medications

Pertinent data from staff/family   *Name of staff/family*

Mental status assessment* and other behavior/observations

Appearance

Orientation

Speech

---

* See p. 372

Affect

Mood

Memory

Intelligence

Abstract thinking

Attention span

Thought content

Thought process

Insight

Attitude

Other

Summary/impressions

Reported to   *Date*

Follow-up

Category	Approach	Record	Samples
Appearance	Observation	Sex	Male, female
		Size	Obese, thin
		Apparent age	Older than stated age
		Manner of dress	Casual, robe, conservative, inappropriate
		Personal hygiene	Clean, soiled shirt
		Hair	Gray, not combed
		Use of cosmetics	None used
		Mannerisms	Facial tic
		Personal habits	Smoking
		Position	Fetal in bed
		Posture	Slumped in chair
		Gait	Staggering, shuffling
		Gestures	Hand tremors
		Motor activity	Hyperactive
		Mobility	Ambulatory
		Eye contact	Good
Orientation	Ask about 1. *Time* (year, month, day of month, day of week, season, time of day, duration of hospitalization (e.g., "Tell me what day it is.") 2. *Place* (name of nursing home, hospital, city, state) 3. *Person* (first and last names, names of close relatives)	Degree of orientation	Oriented to person and place but not time Oriented to person, place, and time
	Or use one of the following 1. VIRO Orientation Scale	Exact score ____ Perfect score = 24	
	2. Mental Status Questionnaire	Exact score ____ 0-2 errors 3–8 errors 9–10 errors	None or minimal ⎫ ⎬ Brain syndrome Moderate ⎪ Severe ⎭
Speech	Listen	Volume	Loud, soft
		Clarity	Distinct, clear, garbled, slurred
		Speed	Rapid, slow, blocking

Category	Approach	Record	Samples
		Quantity	Dysarthria, monosyl-labic, mute, aphasic
		Tone	High, low
		Other	Monotonous
Affect	Immediately observable episodic feeling tone experienced through	Voice Facial expressions Demeanor	Crying, angry Alert, calm, dreamy, ecstatic, happy, adjusted, broad, constricted, tense, nervous, sad, depressed, worried, irritable, suspicious, flat (no fluctuations), blunted
Mood	Sustained emotion relatively enduring over time	Describe	Euthymic, calm, elated, euphoric, anxious, silly, appropriate for content of discussion, labile (wide swings in emotions), angry, agitated, suspicious, constricted, sad, depressed, crying
Memory	Evaluate 1. *Immediate* (name three objects, e.g., table, book, chair, and ask the patient to name these objects after several minutes *or* ask the interviewer's name at the end of the interview). 2. *Intermediate or recent* (ask about events in the past 24 hours such as what was eaten for breakfast) 3. *Remote or distant* (ask about historical events such as presidents, wars, previous occupation, or year of marriage)	Record for each one	Intact Impaired Severely impaired

Category	Approach	Record	Samples
Intelligence	1. Ask general question, such as "what is this?" pointing to a pencil, bed, chair. 2. Ask to repeat four numbers forward (3821) and backward (6857). 3. Note use of vocabulary and terminology. 4. Determine ability to perform simple calculations such as "What is 9 + 6 or 4 × 15?" 5. Ask to count serial 7s or forward or backward from 20 by 3s.	Degree of impairment	No mental impairment Average Impaired Severely impaired
	6. Use the Short Portable Mental Status Questionnaire	Exact score _____	See Appendix B
Abstract thinking	1. Capacity to conceptualize and to reason abstractly. 2. Ask about the meaning of simple proverbs, such as "A stitch in time saves nine," or "When it rains, it pours." 3. Ask how two things are similar, such as an apple and an orange. 4. Judgment—ask a simple question and compare to mature adult standards.	Degree	Acute (function response) Adequate Concrete (structure response) Limited Absent
Attention span	Determine ability to follow the discussion and to answer question asked.	Degree	No deficit Deficit Easily distracted Poor Absent

Category	Approach	Record	Samples
Thought content	Listen for 1. *Obsessions* (persistent thoughts or behaviors) 2. *Delusions* (recurring false beliefs) 3. *Hallucinations* (hears noises or sees things that are not there) 4. *Phobias* (fears) 5. *Ideas of reference* (belief that conversation or actions of others have reference to oneself), (e.g., TV talking about him)	Types of content	No disorder Cognitive impairment Paranoid beliefs Depressive thoughts Fear of enclosed places Suicidal ideation
Thought process	Observe manner of speech	Manner of thoughts expressed Flow of speech	No evidence of formal thought disorder Logical Able to complete sentences Spontaneous Jumps from topic to topic Loose associations Illogical Meaningless repetition of words Neologism (new words) Flight of ideas Word salad (no relationship) Tangential Perseveration (repetition of same words, phrases, answers) Bizarre
Insight	Determine awareness of and meaning of present illness, impairment, treatment	Degree	Good Fair Poor Absent

Category	Approach	Record	Samples
Attitude	Determine attitude toward interviewer	Describe	Cooperative Sociable Friendly Evasive Indifferent Passive Sarcastic Resistive Hostile Combative

Barry, P. D. (1984). *Psychosocial nursing: Assessment and intervention*. Philadelphia: Lippincott.

Bates, B. (1987). *A guide to physical examination and history taking* (4th ed). Philadelphia: Lippincott.

Interviewing the manic patient. (1988, May 12). University of Washington Instructional Media Services, TDK Electronics.

Kane, R. A., & Kane, R. L. (1981). *Assessing the elderly*. Lexington, MA: Lexington Books.

Kermis, M. D. (1986). *Mental health in late life*. Boston: Jones & Bartlett.

Mental status examination (revised). (1986, July). Missouri Division of Mental Diseases.

Nursing 3364 mental status exam. (1987, February). Fort Worth, Texas: Texas Christian University, Harris College of Nursing.

Wilson, H. S., & Kneisl, C. R. (1992). *Psychiatric nursing* (4th ed.). Redwood City, CA: Addison-Wesley.

Appendix **D**

❖ *Behavioral Assessment for Low Stimulus Care Plan*

Nurses sometimes are at a loss knowing when to institute a low-stimulus care plan. Cognitive decline may not be diagnosed initially on admission. This form will assist nursing staff in evaluating clients for potential cognitive decline or need for a low-stimulus environment. The following behaviors are associated with progressive dementing illnesses and are indicative of general cognitive decline. Assessments used for acute confusion may not be valid for a dementia assessment, such as the mini mental status examination or simply asking the patient's orientation to person, place, or time.

Check off the following losses that you have observed in your client or have been reported by staff or family members. Award 1 point for each reported behavior and 2 additional points for anything observed. Examples of behavior are listed.

Scoring:

Place the total sum obtained in each symptom cluster where indicated. If the patient demonstrates losses scoring a 6 or greater in the Cognitive, Conative, and Affective clusters and a score of 2 or greater in the first category, the person should be considered for a dementia evaluation and the lowered stimulus care plan should be implemented. All positive scores should be recorded on the patient's medical record.

From "Behavioral Assessment for Low Stimulus Care Plan" by G. R. Hall, 1988. Unpublished manuscript, University of Iowa Hospitals and Clinics, Department of Nursing, Iowa City. Reprinted by permission.

I. Progressively lowered stress threshold   Cluster Total _____

  1 Catastrophic behaviors .... _____

    a. Becomes confused

    b. Becomes agitated

    c. Wakes up confused at night

    d. Has panic attacks

    e. Becomes violent or combative

    f. Has sudden psychotic symptoms (see above)

    g. "Sundown behaviors" such as late-day confusion

    h. Fearful behavior

    i. Purposeful wandering to get away from environment

    j. Packing to leave

  2. Purposeless behavior .... _____

    a. Purposeless wandering, touching everything

    b. Continuous sorting through objects

    c. Daytime sleeping other than naptime

    d. Staring into space

    e. Fantasy behavior such as carrying briefcase,
       carrying dolls, stuffed animals, or clients stating
       they are at place other than where they really are

    f. Purposeless conversation to others or no one in
       particular

  3. Avoidance of stimuli .... _____

    a. Refusal to participate

    b. Avoidance of potentially misleading stimuli, such as
       TV, radio, social gatherings

  4. Compulsive repetitive behaviors .... _____

II. Conative (planning) and functional losses   Cluster Total _____

  1. Starts activity, wanders easily .... _____

  2. Starts activity, becomes mixed up .... _____

  3. Starts activity, becomes frustrated .... _____

  4. Refuses to start activity .... _____

  5. Unable to initiate activities but can perform once
    started .... _____

  6. Is confused or loses function if daily routine is
    changed .... _____

  7. Incontinent .... _____

  8. Motor apraxia .... _____

    a. Gait disturbances

    b. Problems with sitting or standing

    c. Becoming "frozen to spot" while walking

    d. Rigidity

  9. Unable to plan day .... _____

 10. Unable to plan events .... _____

11. Any sign of decline in function .... _____
    a. Money management
    b. Legal affairs
    c. Shopping
    d. Transportation
    e. Housecleaning
    f. Home maintenance
    g. Bathing
    h. Choosing clothing or dressing
    i. Cooking
III. Cognitive losses   Cluster Total _____
    1. Loss of memory .... _____
       a. Difficulty remembering recent events
       b. Distorts past events
       c. Difficulty remembering past events
       d. Asks same question repeatedly
       e. Missed appointments
    2. Loss of time sense .... _____
       a. Repeatedly asks what time or day it is
       b. Preoccupied with a coming event as to when it will
          occur
       c. Dresses or prepares for appointments or events
          early
       d. Confuses day with night, or time of day
       e. Obvious confusion over time of past events; did
          something occur one week or year ago
    3. Inability to abstract .... _____
       a. Calculate checkbook
       b. Respond to reasoning or explanations
       c. Lack of concern for safety
       d. Inability to problem solve
    4. Inability to make choices or decisions .... _____
       a. Cooks same food for dinner repeatedly
       b. Wears same clothing for days
       c. Asks others what to order when in restaurant
       d. Defers most choices to others
       e. Defers answers to direct questions to family members
    5. Poor judgment .... _____
       a. Has problems with financial matters
       b. Has legal problems
       c. Has made unusually large or inappropriate purchases
       d. Dresses inappropriately for weather
       e. Drives unsafely, refuses to stop
       f. Refuses to pay bills

      g. Eats spoiled food

      h. Sweeps, rakes leaves, mows grass or performs similar task for hours and despite completion, inclement weather, or other cues to stop

      i. Unrealistic about limitations and abilities

  6. Loss of language ability .... _____

      a. Unable to read or comprehend writing

      b. Has word-finding difficulties or substitutes inappropriate word

      c. Does not initiate conversation in social situations

  7. Attempts to compensate for losses .... _____

      a. Defers judgments, decisions, questions to others

      b. Keeps lists, calendars

      c. Becomes increasingly secretive

      d. Makes statements such as "I think I'm going crazy," "I think I'm losing my mind," "I keep forgetting," "something is wrong with my (head, memory, mind)"

IV. Affective losses   Cluster Total _____

  1. Loss of affect .... _____

      a. Loss of "sparkle" (loss of affect)

      b. Loss of sense of humor

      c. Loss of spontaneity

      d. Loss of personality, increasingly dull affect

      e. Loss of quickness, slow to respond to environment or in social situations

  2. Inability to inhibit .... _____

      a. Emotionally labile, quick to anger or cry

      b. Makes spontaneous or inappropriate remarks

      c. Displays disinhibited behavior, such as public undressing, making socially inappropriate comments, or being unable to wait for what is wanted

      d. Lack of patience

      e. Negative personality traits intensify or become dominant, person is "more of who they have always been"

      f. Increase in temper over increasingly trivial things

  3. Social withdrawal .... _____

      a. Withdraws from past social groups

      b. Prefers to stay at home

      c. Leaves or requests to leave social gatherings early

      d. Leaves dinner table early or abruptly

      e. Quits clubs or social organizations

      f. Avoids large groups, such as day room activities

  g. Intolerant or becomes upset after multiple or
      high-stimulus activities
4. Self-preoccupation .... _____
  a. Apparent selfishness
  b. Apparent lack of concern or ability to understand
      needs of others, including spouse
  c. Need for immediate gratification (food, activity,
      toileting)
  d. Withdrawal from family group
  e. Appears to withdraw into self or become seclusive or
      even reclusive
  f. Develops preoccupation with bodily needs, such as
      bowels, toileting, or food consumption, fear of
      gaining weight or constant eating
5. Psychotic manifestations .... _____
  a. Paranoia, making accusations or fearing persons are
      stealing or plotting against
  b. Hallucinations, delusions, illusions
  c. Distorted perceptions of environmental stimuli,
      such as thinking TV pictures or situations are
      real, misinterpreting pictures, or mirror images
6. Loss of recognition of people .... _____
  a. Friends
  b. Family
  c. Self in mirror
7. Antisocial behavior .... _____
  a. Loss of social graces
  b. Family complains of being embarrassed
  c. Inappropriate use of everyday objects, such as stuffing
      objects into toilet, taking down drapes, or ingesting
      cleaning fluids
  d. Smearing food or body wastes
  e. Yelling, screaming

❖ *Psychiatric Diagnoses Commonly Found in Older Adults Based on DSM-IV Classification*

Delirium, Dementia, and Amnestic and Other Cognitive Disorders

293.0	Delirium Due to . . . (General Medical Condition)
780.09	Delirium NOS
290.xx	Dementia of the Alzheimer's Type, With Early Onset
.10	Uncomplicated
.11	With Delirium

Adapted and reprinted with permission from the *Diagnostic and Statistical Manual of Mental Disorders, Fourth Edition.* Copyright 1994, pp. 13-24, American Psychiatric Association.

.12	With Delusions
.13	With Depressed Mood
290.xx	Dementia of the Alzheimer's Type, With Late Onset
.0	Uncomplicated
.3	With Delirium
.20	With Delusions
.21	With Depressed Mood
290.xx	Vascular Dementia
.40	Uncomplicated
.41	With Delirium
.42	With Delusions
.43	With Depressed Mood
294.1	Dementia Due to Parkinson's Disease
294.1	Dementia Due to Huntington's Disease
290.10	Dementia Due to Pick's Disease
290.10	Dementia Due to Creutzfeldt-Jakob Disease
294.1	Dementia Due to . . . (General Medical Condition)
294.8	Dementia NOS

Substance-Related Disorders

303.90	Alcohol Dependence
305.00	Alcohol Abuse
303.00	Alcohol Intoxication
291.8	Alcohol Withdrawal
291.9	Alcohol-Related Disorder NOS
305.90	Caffeine Intoxication
292.89	Caffeine-Induced Anxiety Disorder
292.89	Caffeine-Induced Sleep Disorder
292.9	Caffeine-Related Disorder NOS
305.10	Nicotine Dependence
292.0	Nicotine Withdrawal
292.9	Nicotine-Related Disorder NOS
304.10	Sedative, Hypnotic, or Anxiolytic Dependence
292.9	Sedative-, Hypnotic-, or Anxiolytic-Related Disorder NOS
304.90	Other (or Unknown) Substance Dependence
305.90	Other (or Unknown) Substance Abuse

Schizophrenia and Other Psychotic Disorders

295.xx	Schizophrenia
.30	Paranoid Type
.10	Disorganized Type
.20	Catatonic Type

.90	Undifferentiated Type
.60	Residual Type
297.1	Delusional Disorder
293.xx	Psychotic Disorder Due to . . . (General Medical Condition)
.81	With Delusions
.82	With Hallucinations
298.9	Psychotic Disorder NOS

Mood Disorders

296.xx	Major Depressive Disorder
.2x	Single Episode
.3x	Recurrent
300.4	Dysthymic Disorder
311.	Depressive Disorder NOS
296.xx	Bipolar I Disorder
.0x	Single Manic Episode
.40	Most Recent Episode Hypomanic
.4x	Most Recent Episode Manic
.6x	Most Recent Episode Mixed
.5x	Most Recent Episode Depressed
.7	Most Recent Episode Unspecified
296.89	Bipolar II Disorder
301.13	Cyclothymic Disorder
296.80	Bipolar Disorder NOS
293.83	Mood Disorder Due to . . . (General Medical Condition)
296.90	Mood Disorder NOS

Anxiety Disorders

300.3	Obsessive-Compulsive Disorder
300.02	Generalized Anxiety Disorder
293.89	Anxiety Disorder Due to . . . (General Medical Condition)
300.0	Anxiety Disorder NOS

Somatoform Disorders

307.xx	Pain Disorder
.80	Associated with Psychological Factors
.89	Associated with Both Psychological Factors and a General Medical Condition
300.7	Hypochondriasis
300.81	Somatoform Disorder NOS

Sexual and Gender Identity Disorders

607.84	Male Erectile Disorder Due to . . . (General Medical Condition)
625.0	Female Dyspareunia Due to . . . (General Medical Condition)
625.8	Other Female Sexual Dysfunction Due to . . . (General Medical Condition)
608.89	Other Male Sexual Dysfunction Due to . . . (General Medical Condition)
302.70	Sexual Dysfunction NOS

Sleep Disorders

307.42	Primary Insomnia
307.44	Primary Hypersomnia
780.59	Breathing-Related Sleep Disorder
780.xx	Sleep Disorder Due to . . . (General Medical Condition)
.52	Insomnia Type
.54	Hypersomnia Type
.59	Parasomnia Type
.59	Mixed Type

Adjustment Disorders

309.xx	Adjustment Disorder
.0	With Depressed Mood
.24	With Anxiety
.28	With Mixed Anxiety and Depressed Mood
.3	With Disturbance of Conduct
.4	With Mixed Disturbance of Emotions and Conduct
.9	Unspecified

Other Conditions that May Be a Focus of Clinical Attention

333.82	Neuroleptic-Induced Tardive Dyskinesia
995.2	Adverse Effects of Medication NOS
V61.1	Physical Abuse of Adult
V61.1	Sexual Abuse of Adult
V15.81	Noncompliance With Treatment
780.9	Age-Related Cognitive Decline
V62.82	Bereavement
V62.89	Phase of Life Problem

Appendix *F*

❖ *Nursing Diagnoses— North American Nursing Diagnosis Association*

❖ *NANDA Approved Nursing Diagnoses*

This list is the NANDA approved nursing diagnoses for clinical use and testing (1992).

Pattern 1: Exchanging

1.1.2.1	Altered Nutrition: More than body requirements
1.1.2.2	Altered Nutrition: Less than body requirements
1.1.2.3	Altered Nutrition: Potential for more than body requirements
1.2.1.1	High Risk for Infection
1.2.2.1	High Risk for Altered Body Temperature
1.2.2.2	Hypothermia
1.2.2.3	Hyperthermia
1.2.2.4	Ineffective Thermoregulation
1.2.3.1	Dysreflexia

*	1.3.1.1	Constipation
	1.3.1.1.1	Perceived Constipation
	1.3.1.1.2	Colonic Constipation
*	1.3.1.2	Diarrhea
*	1.3.1.3	Bowel Incontinence
	1.3.2	Altered Urinary Elimination
	1.3.2.1.1	Stress Incontinence
	1.3.2.1.2	Reflex Incontinence
	1.3.2.1.3	Urge Incontinence
	1.3.2.1.4	Functional Incontinence
	1.3.2.1.5	Total Incontinence
	1.3.2.2	Urinary Retention
*	1.4.1.1	Altered (Specify Type) Tissue Perfusion (Renal, cerebral, cardio-pulmonary, gastrointestinal, peripheral)
	1.4.1.2.1	Fluid Volume Excess
	1.4.1.2.2.1	Fluid Volume Deficit
	1.4.1.2.2.2	High Risk for Fluid Volume Deficit
*	1.4.2.1	Decreased Cardiac Output
	1.5.1.1	Impaired Gas Exchange
	1.5.1.2	Ineffective Airway Clearance
	1.5.1.3	Ineffective Breathing Pattern
#	1.5.1.3.1	Inability to Sustain Spontaneous Ventilation
#	1.5.1.3.2	Dysfunctional Ventilatory Weaning Response (DVWR)
	1.6.1	High Risk for Injury
	1.6.1.1	High Risk for Suffocation
	1.6.1.2	High Risk for Poisoning
	1.6.1.3	High Risk for Trauma
	1.6.1.4	High Risk for Aspiration
	1.6.1.5	High Risk for Disuse Syndrome
	1.6.2	Altered Protection
	1.6.2.1	Impaired Tissue Integrity
*	1.6.2.1.1	Altered Oral Mucous Membrane
	1.6.2.1.2.1	Impaired Skin Integrity
	1.6.2.1.2.2	High Risk for Impaired Skin Integrity

Pattern 2: Communicating

2.1.1.1	Impaired Verbal Communication

Pattern 3: Relating

3.1.1	Impaired Social Interaction
3.1.2	Social Isolation
* 3.2.1	Altered Role Performance

3.2.1.1.1	Altered Parenting
3.2.1.1.2	High Risk for Altered Parenting
3.2.1.2.1	Sexual Dysfunction
3.2.2	Altered Family Processes
# 3.2.2.1	Caregiver Role Strain
# 3.2.2.2	High Risk for Caregiver Role Strain
3.2.3.1	Parental Role Conflict
3.3	Altered Sexuality Patterns

Pattern 4: Valuing

4.1.1	Spiritual Distress (distress of the human spirit)

Pattern 5: Choosing

5.1.1.1	Ineffective Individual Coping
5.1.1.1.1	Impaired Adjustment
5.1.1.1.2	Defensive Coping
5.1.1.1.3	Ineffective Denial
5.1.2.1.1	Ineffective Family Coping: Disabling
5.1.2.1.2	Ineffective Family Coping: Compromised
5.1.2.2	Family Coping: Potential for Growth
# 5.2.1	Ineffective Management of Therapeutic Regimen (Individuals)
5.2.1.1	Noncompliance (Specify)
5.3.1.1	Decisional Conflict (Specify)
5.4	Health Seeking Behaviors (Specify)

Pattern 6: Moving

6.1.1.1	Impaired Physical Mobility
# 6.1.1.1.1	High Risk for Peripheral Neurovascular Dysfunction
6.1.1.2	Activity Intolerance
6.1.1.2.1	Fatigue
6.1.1.3	High Risk for Activity Intolerance
6.2.1	Sleep Pattern Disturbance
6.3.1.1	Diversional Activity Deficit
6.4.1.1	Impaired Home Maintenance Management
6.4.2	Altered Health Maintenance
* 6.5.1	Feeding Self Care Deficit
6.5.1.1	Impaired Swallowing
6.5.1.2	Ineffective Breastfeeding
# 6.5.1.2.1	Interrupted Breastfeeding
6.5.1.3	Effective Breastfeeding
# 6.5.1.4	Ineffective Infant Feeding Pattern

*	6.5.2	Bathing/Hygiene Self Care Deficit
*	6.5.3	Dressing/Grooming Self Care Deficit
*	6.5.4	Toileting Self Care Deficit
	6.6	Altered Growth and Development
#	6.7	Relocation Stress Syndrome

Pattern 7: Perceiving

*	7.1.1	Body Image Disturbance
*	7.1.2	Self Esteem Disturbance
	7.1.2.1	Chronic Low Self Esteem
	7.1.2.2	Situational Low Self Esteem
*	7.1.3	Personal Identity Disturbance
	7.2	Sensory/Perceptual Alterations (Specify) (Visual, auditory, kinesthetic, gustatory, tactile, olfactory)
	7.2.1.1	Unilateral Neglect
	7.3.1	Hopelessness
	7.3.2	Powerlessness

Pattern 8: Knowing

8.1.1	Knowledge Deficit (Specify)
8.3	Altered Thought Processes

Pattern 9: Feeling

*	9.1.1	Pain
	9.1.1.1	Chronic Pain
	9.2.1.1	Dysfunctional Grieving
	9.2.1.2	Anticipatory Grieving
	9.2.2	High Risk for Violence: Self-directed or directed at others
#	9.2.2.1	High Risk for Self-Mutilation
	9.2.3	Post-Trauma Response
	9.2.3.1	Rape-Trauma Syndrome
	9.2.3.1.1	Rape-Trauma Syndrome: Compound Reaction
	9.2.3.1.2	Rape-Trauma Syndrome: Silent Reaction
	9.3.1	Anxiety
	9.3.2	Fear

New diagnostic categories approved 1992

* Categories with modified label terminology

From *NANDA Nursing Diagnoses: Definitions and Classification 1992-1993*. Philadelphia PA: North American Nursing Diagnosis Association. Reprinted with permission.

All of the nursing diagnoses are listed because older adults often have physical as well as mental or emotional problems.

❖ *Agencies and Organizations*

Administration on Aging
330 Independence Avenue S.W.
Washington, DC 20201

Alzheimer's Association
919 North Michigan Avenue, Suite 1000
Chicago, IL 60611

American Association for Geriatric Psychiatry
P.O. Box 376-A
Greenbelt, MD 20768

American Association of Homes and Services for the Aging
901 E Street, N.W. Suite 500
Washington, DC 20004-2037

American Association of Retired Persons
601 E Street N.W.
Washington, DC 20049

American Association of Retired Persons Andrus Foundation
601 E Street N.W.
Washington, DC 20049

American College of Nursing Home Administrators
4650 East-West Freeway
Washington, DC 20014

American Geriatrics Society
770 Lexington Avenue, Suite 300
New York, NY 10021

American Health Care Association
1201 L Street N.W.
Washington, DC 20005

American Nurses' Association
Council on Gerontological Nursing Practice and Division on Psychiatric and Mental
Health Nursing Practice
600 Maryland Avenue S.W., Suite 100W
Washington, DC 20024-2571

American Parkinson's Disease Association
60 Bay Street, Suite 401
Staten Island, NY 10301

American Psychiatric Association
1400 K Street N.W.
Washington, DC 20005

American Psychiatric Nurses' Association
6900 Grove Road
Thorofare, NJ 08086

American Psychological Association
750 First Street N.E.
Washington, DC 20002

American Society on Aging
833 Market Street, Suite 512
San Francisco, CA 94103

Association for Gerontology in Higher Education
1001 Connecticut Avenue N.W.
Washington, DC 20036-5504

Children of Aging Parents
1609 Woodbourne Road, Suite 302-A
Levittown, PA 19057

Family Caregiver Alliance
425 Bush Street, Suite 500
San Francisco, CA 94108

Federal Council on the Aging
330 Independence Avenue S.W., Room 4280 HHS-N
Washington, DC 20201

Gerontological Society of America
1275 K Street N.W., Suite 350
Washington, DC 20005-4006

Gray Panthers
1424 16th Street N.W., Suite 602
Washington, DC 20036

National Association for Home Care
519 C Street N.W.
Washington, DC 20002

National Association of Area Agencies on Aging
1112 16th Street N.W., Suite 100
Washington, DC 20036

National Caucus and Center on the Black Aged, Inc.
1424 K Street N.W., Suite 500
Washington, DC 20005

National Council on the Aging
409 Third Street S.W., Suite 200
Washington, DC 20024

National Council of Senior Citizens, Inc.
1331 F Street N.W.
Washington, DC 20004

National Institute on Aging
Federal Building
Room 5C27, Building 31
9000 Rockville Pike
Bethesda, MD 20892

National Institute of Mental Health Public Inquiries Office
Room 15C-05
5600 Fishers Lane
Rockville, MD 20857

National League for Nursing
350 Hudson Street
New York, NY 10014

National Mental Health Association
1021 Prince Street
Alexandria, VA 22314-2971

Older Women's League
666 11th Street N.W., Suite 700
Washington, DC 20001

Social Security Administration
6401 Security Blvd.
Baltimore, MD 21235

❖ *Journals and Other Publications*

Write to the addresses listed for subscription prices and frequency of publication.

AARP News Bulletin
AARP Fulfillment
AARP Publications
3200 East Carson Street
Lakewood, CA 90712

Age Page
National Institute on Aging
U.S. Department of Health & Human Services
U.S. Government Printing Office
Washington, DC 20402

Aging
Office of Human Development Services
Department of Health & Human Services
200 Independence Avenue S.W.
Washington, DC 20201

Archives of Psychiatric Nursing
W.B. Saunders Company
The Curtis Center
Independence Square West
Philadelphia, PA 19106-3399

Capsules and Comments in Psychiatric Nursing
Mosby–Year Book Inc.
200 N. LaSalle Street
Chicago, IL 60601

Changes—Research on Aging and the Aged
Superintendent of Documents
U.S. Government Printing Office
Washington, DC 20402

Generations
833 Market Street, Suite 512
San Francisco, CA 94103

Geriatric Nursing
Mosby–Year Book
11830 Westline Industrial Drive
St. Louis, MO 63146-3318

Geriatrics
For the Primary Care Physician
Harcourt Brace Jovanovich Publications
1 East First Street
Duluth, MN 55802

Gerontology Newsletter
Institute of Human Development and Family Studies
Main Building 2300
University of Texas at Austin
Austin, TX 78712

Hospital and Community Psychiatry
1400 K Street N.W.
Washington, DC 20005

International Journal of Psychiatry in Medicine
Baywood Publishing Co., Inc.
26 Austin Avenue
P.O. Box 337
Amityville, NY 11701

Journal of the American Geriatrics Society
Williams & Wilkins Company
428 East Preston Street
Baltimore, MD 21202-3993

Journal of Geriatric Psychiatry
International Universities Press, Inc.
59 Boston Post Road
P. O. Box 1524
Madison, CT 06443-1524

Journal of Gerontological Nursing
Slack Incorporated
6900 Grove Road
Thorofare, NJ 08086

Journal of Gerontological Social Work
The Haworth Press, Inc.
10 Alice Street
Binghamton, NY 13904-1580

Journal of Psychosocial Nursing and Mental Health Services
Slack Incorporated
6900 Grove Road
Thorofare, NJ 08086

Journal of Religious Gerontology
P.O. Box 248264
Coral Gables, FL 33124-4672

Long-Term Care Currents
Ross Laboratories
625 Cleveland Avenue
Columbus, OH 43216

Modern Maturity
Publication of the American Association of Retired Persons
3200 East Carson Street
Lakewood, CA 90712

Perspectives in Psychiatric Care
Nursecom, Inc.
1211 Locus Street
Philadelphia, PA 19107

Psychiatric Clinics of North America
W.B. Saunders Company
The Curtis Center
Independence Square West
Philadelphia, PA 19106-3399

Psychiatry
J.B. Lippincott Company
c/o Kevin Fenton
Washington Square East
Philadelphia, PA 19106

Research on Aging
A Quarterly of Social Gerontology & Adult Development
Sage Publications, Inc.
2111 West Hillcrest Drive
Newbury Park, CA 91320

The Gerontologist
Gerontological Society of America
1275 K Street N.W., Suite 350
Washington, DC 20005-4006

The International Journal of Aging and Human Development
Baywood Publishing Company, Inc.
26 Austin Avenue
P.O. Box 337
Amityville, NY 11701

❖ *Index*

A

Abandonment, 319-320

Abnormal protein model of Alzheimer's disease, 182-183

Abstract thinking as sign of dementia, 173

Acetophenazine (Tindal), 108*t*

Acetylcholine, 179

Acetylcholine model of Alzheimer's disease, 179

Acquired immunodeficiency syndrome (AIDS), effect on the central nervous system, 177

Acquired immunodeficiency syndrome (AIDS) dementia complex, 177

ACTH, 4-9, 113

ACTION, 32

Active treatment model, 355

Activities of daily living (ADL), assessment of, 86, 129, 143

Activity theory of aging, 23-24

Acute dystonic reaction, 109

Addictions nursing, 236, 237-238
  assessment in, 236, 238-241, 244-245
  health problems in, 241-243
  nursing care plan, 248-252, 255-258
  nursing diagnoses, expected outcomes, interventions, and evaluations in, 245-246
  psychosocial problems in, 243-244

Adjustment disorder with depressed mood, 127

Administration on Aging, 46

Admission to geropsychiatric unit
  criteria for, 268-270
  routes in, 270

Adult caregiver, 319
  characteristics of, 321

Adult day care, 336-337, 353

Adult protective services, 361-362

African-Americans
  as caregivers, 8
  leisure activities of women, 33

Ageism, 26
  as barrier to mental health care, 264-265, 344

Agencies and organizations, 397-399. *See also specific name*

Age Page, 351-352

Aggression
  in nursing home residents, 298-299
  managing in hospital, 282-283

Aging
  effects on central nervous system, 82
  social theories of, 22-25
  subjective indicators of successful, 22
  understanding in assessment of older adults, 74-75

Agitated wanderers, 198

Akathisia, 109

Akinesia, 109

Alcohol abuse, 225-226, 227-229
  in suicide assessment, 157
  treatment of, 230-233

Alcoholics
  early-onset, 229-230